D0713926

Practical Ethics in Occupational Health

Edited by

Peter Westerholm

Professor Emeritus in Occupational Epidemiology
National Institute for Working Life, Sweden

Tore Nilstun

Professor of Medical Ethics
University of Lund, Sweden

John Øvretveit

Director of Research
The Karolinska Institute Medical Management Centre, Stockholm
Professor of Health Policy and Management
The Nordic School of Public Health, Gothenberg
Bergen University Faculty of Medicine, Norway

WA
400
P8948
2004

RADCLIFFE MEDICAL PRESS
OXFORD • SAN FRANCISCO

Radcliffe Medical Press Ltd
18 Marcham Road
Abingdon
Oxon OX14 1AA
United Kingdom

www.radcliffe-oxford.com
The Radcliffe Medical Press electronic catalogue and online ordering facility.
Direct sales to anywhere in the world.

© 2004 Peter Westerholm, Tore Nilstun and John Øvretveit

All rights reserved. No part of this publication may be reproduced, stored in a retrieval system or transmitted, in any form or by any means, electronic, mechanical, photocopying, recording or otherwise, without the prior permission of the copyright owner.

British Library Cataloguing in Publication Data

A catalogue record for this book is available from the British Library.

ISBN 1 85775 617 7

Typeset by Anne Joshua & Associates, Oxford
Printed and bound by TJ International Ltd, Padstow, Cornwall

Contents

55989013

Foreword

This book addresses an area of fundamental importance for occupational health professionals. It is a core component of our professionalism. Competent professionals are expected to make decisions which are perceived as fair and equitable by both employees and employers. Other stakeholders influenced by our judgements include the work team and those affected by the impact of the enterprise on the wider biopsychosocial environment. Although the patients of general healthcare professionals increasingly have autonomy and real choice about their health treatments, healthcare workers have much less control over their work and socio-economic conditions, and may have no ability to choose their occupational health advisers, who have been appointed by their employers.

Into this picture in the past 20 or 30 years has come the growth of information technology and access to information for all, and much new legislation on equal opportunities, disability discrimination and employment conditions. Although evidence-based guidelines have been developed in occupational health, these have lagged behind some other areas of medical, nursing and safety practice. Scientific uncertainty creates ethical challenges and occupational health professionals regularly have to make judgements on extremely complex situations.

Thus it is no surprise that national and international ethical standards for occupational health practice have been produced, perhaps proportionately more than for any other area of healthcare. These are necessary reading for both occupational health professionals and their customers.

In the training of occupational health professionals competence in law and ethics is one of the more important aims. For occupational health physicians in Europe this was confirmed within the World Health Organization (WHO) publication on occupational medicine in Europe, *Scope and Competencies*,[1] and endorsed by the Occupational Medicine Section of the Union of European Medical Specialists in their Annex describing the common core competencies required in training occupational physicians. Similar emphases have developed in the training of occupational health nursing, safety, hygiene, ergonomic and other professions.

Across the European Union there is increasing universality of moral norms and shared values. The principles of free exchange of labour and capital have been established.

Implicit in good occupational health practice is the principle of respect for individuals, taking into account the needs of both society and enterprise.

This multi-author European text explores practical scenarios by use of a structured and analytical approach, and in so doing shows the reader how to apply and implement existing codes and guidelines in this increasingly complex professional area.

Dr Ewan B Macdonald
University of Glasgow
President, Section of Occupational Medicine
Union of European Medical Specialists
February 2004

Reference

1   WHO European Centre for Environment and Health (2000) *Occupational Medicine in Europe: Scope and Competencies*. Series: Health, Environment and Safety in Enterprises No. 3. WHO Regional Office for Europe, Copenhagen.

Preface

All censorships exist to prevent anyone from challenging current conceptions and existing institutions. All progress is initiated by challenging current conceptions and executed by supplanting institutions. Consequently, the first condition of progress is the removal of censorships. There is the whole case against censorship in a nutshell.

George Bernard Shaw (1856–1950)

This book deals with the ethical challenges confronting occupational health professionals in today's changing world of work. It is written, as the title of the book implies, with a view to the issues and problems occupational health professionals deal with in everyday practice. Commonly, occupational health professionals are commissioned for advisory and consulting tasks in the realm of occupational safety and health management by enterprises and organisations. They may be in the employment of companies using their services, or act as experts external to client firms or organisations.

Accordingly, the primary target group (the 'bull's eye', so to speak) of this book consists of occupational health professionals. This broad category includes occupational health physicians and nurses, physiotherapists and ergonomists, occupational hygienists and safety engineers, occupational psychologists, and social workers (to mention the most common groups), and also the managers of occupational health service units or organisations. As well as this primary target group, the book is designed to meet the needs of all those who purchase and use occupational health services – the services' customers and clients. They have legitimate interests in seeking services of good quality whilst seeking certainty that the ethical standards of the services on offer are reliable and trustworthy.

It is a daunting task to write a book on practical ethics, and possibly particularly with regard to occupational health services. The point of departure with regard to problems and observations has to be in the settings and organisations where occupational health professional care is practised. So, the context is thereby defined. This implies that readers seeking philosophical innovation are likely to be disappointed. The book emphasises the ethical issues inherent in the practical problems encountered by occupational health professionals. These may, however, illustrate and bring up more profound issues – questions and arguments that are, by analogy, similar to but not dependent on the context of the case material presented here.

Our starting point lay simply in a feeling that a book with a focus on the ethics of occupational health specialists was needed. The issues of professional ethics have been examined, and rules for the behaviour of occupational health professionals presented earlier, in the *International Code of Ethics for Occupational Health Professionals 1992*.[1] This was published as a set of norms in 1992 (revised in 2002) by the International Commission of Occupational Health (ICOH). Earlier, in 1980, the Faculty of Occupational Medicine (FOM) of the Royal College of Physicians in the UK published the document *Guidance on Ethics for Occupational Physicians*.[2] Now available in its fifth edition, this document takes the reader one step closer to the issues emerging in real life in different fields of occupational health practice. It also provides principled recommendations on ethical conduct. This book seeks to supplement both the ICOH *Code of Ethics* and FOM *Guidance on Ethics* by adding a dimension of reflection. There are problems in identifying pertinent facts and the ethical values involved, and using these as bases for arriving at considered decisions.

The book is structured according to the following logic. We start with three chapters of an introductory nature, providing an initial conceptual framework for the subject, which are then followed by a series of case-based chapters describing a problem or an issue in occupational health professional ethics from real life. Though the approach is somewhat different in these case chapters, they are similarly structured to include analysis of the specific problem or ethical dilemma at hand. The book concludes with a chapter designed to synthesise the editors' views in light of the preceding chapters.

We have no ambition to be exhaustive in dealing with the substance of professional ethics in occupational health and safety. The problems in the case chapters should be seen as examples that serve to demonstrate the use of three value criteria – namely autonomy (or the right to self-determination), beneficence (including non-maleficence) and justice (including equity). There are, of course, many other types of situations besides the ones described in the case chapters. They all give rise to ethical dilemmas for health professionals not covered by the book. It is our sincere belief, however, that its case material will be pertinent and give food for thought and reflection with regard to the challenges often met by occupational health professionals in their life at work.

It is important to remind readers that most of the chapter authors are, or have been, professional occupational health practitioners – from Belgium, Denmark, Finland, the Netherlands, Norway, Sweden and the UK. These are all countries from a relatively affluent region of the world, namely northern Europe. They have many common factors in their general functioning, structure and culture, and they are also characterised by relatively efficient public infrastructures and collaboration between private capital, the organs of the state and trade unions. These commonalities are likely to have enabled the various authors to converge in their views on the ethical values of beneficence, autonomy and justice. Indeed, they can be expected to have found much common ground in interpreting and using these value concepts. But it also implies that we do not claim universality in our descriptions of ethical problems, or in the mental processes we undergo in arriving at reflected opinions. We are convinced that a book written by people recruited on a more global basis would accept these values, but they would probably specify them differently, and also advocate a different balance between them.

Any introductory book on occupational health does not spring from any one single scientific discipline. In fact, the area is the common subject matter of a range of disciplines, in both the theoretical and applied sciences. It is concerned with the health, technical, psychological, organisational, social and political aspects of working life, and draws on scientific knowledge from many fields. This is a truly multidisciplinary arena, which carries the issues of ethics – with all their ramifications – into the realms of business, environment and politics.

Biomedical ethics has, at least until recently, focused primarily on individuals – in health services commonly referred to as the 'patient'. Patients' autonomy and integrity, and also their rights, are largely dependent on the judgements of health professionals and the complex workings of healthcare organisations, dominated as they are by hospital-based medicine. In issues of environmental ethics, however, issues of benefit or harm to the general public and society make up a significantly larger portion of our concerns. In the latter domain, individual autonomy is to be seen from a different perspective. It is often a source of harm to others – leading to a need not to expand, but rather to set limits to individual freedom. For example, biotechnological considerations commonly lead to state regulations on the emissions of pollutants or discharges of toxic waste and requirements for high safety standards. They may also lead to demands for international standards or regulations on environmental matters, which then become subject to enforcement by state authorities acting in concert across national borders.

Occupational health ethics occupy an intermediate position. They are clearly oriented towards individuals and their health concerns, but simultaneously focus on context and living conditions in the workplace. In this domain, the workplace – embedded as it is in the social organisation of an enterprise – constitutes a dominant component of the environmental setting of people at work. The workplace is not only the place where we earn our livelihood. It forms, in reality, the centre stage of key social processes and interactions between people. Many different interests and stakeholders meet in the workplace, and the outcomes of interactions between them affect people's lives in many ways. There are also health implications of such processes. The workplace is a setting where we acquire knowledge, learn skills, and develop. People emerge on this stage in the roles of manager or staff, as expert or consultant, as owner or trades unionists, or as representative of the state in one of its many guises. Thus, the physical and cultural settings of the real-life issues of professional ethics in the workplace are of considerable complexity. Our idea is that an awareness of this complexity and the multitude of interests involved in occupational health service will equip professionals better for the difficult tasks with which they are confronted.

This book has no normative intent. We do not approve or recommend any one or other of the solutions offered in the conclusions of our case chapter authors. But, if they provide incentives for fact-finding and for identifying and using relevant value criteria in structured ethical analyses, we will be content with what we have achieved. All along, our aim has been to provide occupational health professionals with tools for the ethical analysis of challenging and complex cases and situations, all of which impose the demand of arriving at a well-reflected professional decision.

Please note that in some of the reference lists throughout the book English translations have been given for titles of documents published in languages other than English. This is for the reader's benefit only and does not necessarily indicate that the publication is available in the English language.

Peter Westerholm, Tore Nilstun and John Øvretveit
February 2004

References

1 International Commission on Occupational Health (2002) *International Code of Ethics for Health Professionals 1992*. Updated version of the Code (2002) available (English and French languages) on ICOH website (www.icoh.org.sg).

2 Faculty of Occupational Medicine of the Royal Society of Medicine (1999) *Guidance on Ethics for Occupational Physicians* (5e). Royal Society of Medicine, London.

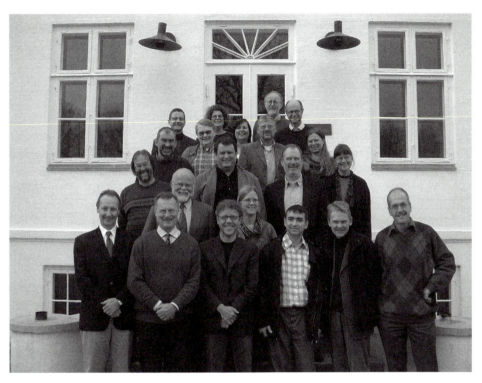

The editors and contributors

About the editors

Peter Westerholm MD, FFOM
Following his retirement in 2000, Peter Westerholm is now Professor
Emeritus in Occupational Epidemiology at the National Institute for
Working Life (NIWL), Sweden. He was born in Finland in 1935. After
clinical postgraduate training in general surgery he served as a surgeon in
the Royal Swedish Navy, as Deputy Medical Director of Sweden's National
Board of Occupational Safety and Health, a consultant epidemiologist at the
National Board of Health and Welfare, and a medical adviser to the Swedish
Confederation of Trade Unions. He was appointed Professor of Occupa-
tional Epidemiology to the NIWL in 1990. During the years 1993–2000 he
was Chairman of the ICOH Scientific Committee for Health Services
Research and Evaluation in Occupational Health.

Contact information
Office address: National Institute for Working Life, SE-113 91 Stockholm,
Sweden
Tel: +46 861 96972
E-mail: peter.westerholm@niwl.se

Tore Nilstun
Tore Nilstun has been Professor in Medical Ethics at Lund University in
Sweden since 2002. He was born in Norway in 1944.

Contact information
Office address: Department of Medical Ethics, St Gråbrödersgatan 16,
SE-222 22 Lund, Sweden
Tel: +46 46 22 21282
E-mail: tore.nilstun@medetik.lu.se

John Øvretveit PhD
Professor John Øvretveit, born in England in 1954, is currently Director of
Research at the Karolinska Institute Medical Management Centre (MMC),
Stockholm, Sweden. He is also Professor of Health Policy and Management
at the Nordic School of Public Health, Gothenburg, Sweden, and at Bergen
University Medical School, Norway. A theme underlying his work is
how practical research can contribute to healthy work organisation and
better patient care. He has undertaken health evaluation and development

projects in African countries, Yemen, Indonesia, Thailand, New Zealand, Australia, Japan, Sweden, Norway, Estonia and the USA. He was awarded the 2002 European Health Management Association Award and the Baxter Health Publication of the Year prize for 'Action Evaluation', and the 1992 award for 'Health Service Quality'. He also received the 1999 British Association of Medical Managers' publication award for 'Evaluating Health Interventions'.

Contact information
Office address: The Nordic School of Public Health, Box 12133, S-40242 Gothenburg, Sweden
Tel: +46 31 693900
E-mail: jovret@aol.com

About the contributors

Tommy Alklint MD

Tommy Alklint is an occupational health physician, currently working at Sweden's National Insurance Board, providing information and training for physicians concerning sickness certification and rehabilitation. He is also an occupational health adviser to Previa South, Sweden – an organisation providing occupational health services to the labour market. He is a former board member of the Association of Swedish Occupational Physicians. He was born in 1945 and has been a member of the board of the Union for Occupational Health Physicians of Sweden.

Contact information
Office address: FK Lund, Box 104, S-22100 Lund, Sweden
Tel: +46 703 003470
E-mail: tommy.alklint@fk12.sfa.se

Knut Erik Andersen MD

Dr Knut Erik Andersen is a specialist mentor and tutor in occupational medicine, currently working for the Jotun A/S company as Chief Medical Adviser to HSE Group Staff. He was Norway's governmental representative to the International Labour Organisation (ILO) in the spring of 1980. Following clinical postgraduate training, he has held posts as an occupational physician in Svalbard, Norway, in Greenland, and within the Directorate of Labour Inspection, Oslo.

Contact information
Office address: Jotun A/S, HSE Group Staff, Post Box 2221, N-3248 Sandefjord, Norway
Tel: +47 33 457410
E-mail: knut.erik.andersen@jotun.no or knut-erik.andersen@c2i.net

Olivia Carlton MB, BS, DRCOG, FFOM

Dr Olivia Carlton is an occupational physician who has worked for London Transport, later London Underground, for 14 years, and now acts as adviser to the London Underground Board on occupational health policy and strategy. She heads a multidisciplinary occupational health team that includes medical and nursing advisers, a counselling and trauma service, a drug and alcohol advisory service, and a physiotherapy service. Since 1997 she has been seconded to the Department of Health to provide policy advice on occupational health to the Minister of Public Health. She was closely involved in the development of the British government's 'Healthy Workplace' initiative and the occupational health strategy for 'Securing Health Together' and in developing the conceptual framework for 'NHS Plus' standards – the vehicle through which the National Health Service (NHS) provides occupational health services to non-NHS employers. She was elected as Registrar of the Faculty of Occupational Medicine in May 2003.

Contact information
Office address: London Underground Limited, 280 Old Marylebone Road, Griffith House, London NW1 5RJ, UK
Tel: +44 207 918 1973
E-mail: olivia.carlton@tube.tfl.gov.uk

David Coggon OBE, MA, PhD, DM, FRCP, FFOM, FMed Sci, MRC

David Coggon has been Professor of Occupational and Environmental Medicine at the University of Southampton in the UK since 1997. He studied mathematics and medicine at Cambridge and Oxford universities and has also received clinical training in internal medicine. He has been an epidemiologist at the MRC Environmental Epidemiology Unit since 1980 and Honorary Consultant Occupational Physician, Southampton University Hospitals Trust since 1987.

Contact information
Office address: MRC Environmental Epidemiology Unit, Southampton General Hospital, Southampton, SO16 6YD, UK
Tel: +44 23 807 77624

Niki Ellis PhD, MBBS, FAFOM, FAFPHM

Dr Niki Ellis is an occupational and public health consultant, currently working as research associate at the Wellcome Trust Centre for the History of Medicine, University College London, UK. She was Director of Health Risk Management, PricewaterhouseCoopers, Sydney, Australia (2000–01), Principal of NE&A, Sydney and Melbourne (1990–2000) and Head of Preventive Strategies, National Occupational Health and Safety Commission (1985–90). She was Inaugural President of the Australasian Faculty of Occupational Medicine (1992–94).

Contact information
Office address: Flat 14, 1 Batemans Row, London EC2A 3HH, UK
Tel: +44 207 729 8640
E-mail: nikiellis@btopenworld.com

Stein E Grytten MD, Cand Med
Dr Stein E Grytten is a specialist in occupational and family medicine, currently working at the Spiggeren Health Centre in Mandal in Norway, which he established in 2002. He also works as a general practitioner and further specialises in orthopaedic surgery. He received his post-graduate training in Tromsö, Norway. He has great experience of major industrial and commercial operations in Norway and was a member of the Norwegian Medical Association's Board of Occupational Physicians (1996–2002).

Contact information
Office address: Spiggeren legesenter, Sandskargata 6, 4515 Mandal, Norway
Tel: +47 382 71933
E-mail: segrytt@online.no

Kit Harling MD
Professor Kit Harling was appointed as consultant in the UK National Health Service in 1984, where he continues to work as a clinical occupational physician. He is currently seconded to the UK Department of Health to direct a national occupational health service. He has been an examiner with the Faculty of Occupational Medicine at the Royal College of Physicians of London for 10 years and was Dean of the Faculty (1996–99). He has been a member of the Faculty's Ethics Committee for eight years, the last three as chair, and is currently editing the sixth edition of the Faculty's *Guidance on Ethics for Occupational Physicians*. Following undergraduate training in Oxford and London, he undertook specialist training in occupational medicine in the diving, aviation, chemical and coal-mining industries.

Contact information
Office address: Department of Health, Room 330b, Skipton House, 80 London Road, London SE1 6LH, UK.
Tel: +44 207 972 3830
E-mail: kit.harling@doh.gsi.gov.uk or kit.harling@doctors.org.uk

Peter Hasle PhD
Dr Peter Hasle is an associate professor, in organisation, management and working life, at the Department of Engineering Manufacturing and Management, Technical University of Denmark. He has held assignments as a consultant in the occupational health service of the Municipality of Copenhagen. He acted as adviser on work environment during the UNDP/ILO project for the establishment of a national institute for work conditions and environment in Bangkok, Thailand (1985–87). Previously, he was research manager at the Centre for Alternative Social Analysis (1990–2002), and a trainer at the Danish TUC School.

Contact information
Office address: Department of Engineering Manufacturing and Management, Technical University of Denmark, Building 303, DK-2800 Lyngby, Denmark
Tel: +45 45 256056
E-mail: pha@ipl.dtu.dk

Carel Hulshof MD, PhD

Carel Hulshof is a certified occupational physician and epidemiologist. He has held posts as an occupational physician in Nijmegen and Amsterdam, Netherlands. From 1984 onwards he has combined work as an occupational health physician with scientific research in positions at the Coronel Institute of the Academic Medical Centre in Amsterdam. Since 1998 he has also been affiliated to the Foundation for Quality in Occupational Health Care (SKB). He is a member of the International Advisory Board of the *Scandinavian Journal for Work, Environment and Health*, a member of the Executive Board of the ICOH Scientific Committee on Health Services Research and Evaluation in Occupational Health and Vice-Chair of the Dutch National Complaints Committee for Pre-employment Medical Examinations.

Contact information
Office address: Academic Medical Center, University of Amsterdam Coronel Institute, PO Box 22700, 1100 DE Amsterdam, Netherlands
Tel: +31 20 5 665333/5325
E-mail: c.t.hulshof@amc.uva.nl

Bengt Järvholm PhD

Bengt Järvholm is Professor of Occupational and Environmental Medicine at the Department of Public Health and Clinical Medicine, Umeå University, Sweden. He is a consultant in the Department of Occupational and Clinical Medicine at the Northern University Hospital in Umeå. He worked previously at the Sahlgren University Hospital in Gothenburg, Sweden. He acts as an expert in legal cases involving compensation for occupational diseases, and is editor of a recently published Swedish textbook on insurance medicine.

Contact information
Office addresss: Occupational Medicine, Department of Public Health and Clinical Medicine, SE-901 85 Umeå, Sweden
Tel: +46 90 785 2241
E-mail: bengt.jarvholm@envmed.umu.se

Juhani Juntunen MD, PhD

Professor Juhani Juntunen is Medical Director of Etera Mutual Pension Insurance Company, Finland. He is a specialist in neurology, with special competence in insurance, addiction and traffic medicine. He was Chief Medical Officer for clinical neurosciences at the Institute of Occupational Health, Helsinki (1979–89) and has been Acting Professor of Neurology, University of Tampere, Professor of Alcohol Diseases, University of Helsinki, and Professor of Occupational Health, University of Bergen, Norway. Since 1986 he has specialised in insurance medicine at the University of Helsinki and in neurotoxicology at the University of Tampere.

Contact information
Office address: Etera Mutual Pension Insurance Company, Palkkatilan-portti 1, FIN-00240 Helsinki, Finland
Tel: +358 10 553 3324, +358 (0) 400 441 330
E-mail: juhani.juntunen@etera.fi

Marja J Kelder

Marja J Kelder is a certified occupational physician and jurist currently working for Arbo Unie, an occupational health service in the Netherlands. She was course manager for occupational health training at the Netherlands School of Public Health for seven years. She is secretary of the Ethics Committee of the Dutch Society of Physicians in Occupational Health and member of the Pre-employment Medical Examinations Complaints Committee.

Contact information
Office address: Arbo Unie BV, Houtlaan 21, 3016 DA Rotterdam, Netherlands
Tel: +31 10 417 7500
Alternative address: Jeroen Boschlaan 60, 3055 NR Rotterdam, Netherlands
Tel: +31 10 418 2011
E-mail: markeld@knmg.nl

Lisbeth Ehlert Knudsen PhD

Dr Lisbeth Ehlert Knudsen is associate professor at the Institute of Public Health, University of Copenhagen, Denmark. She has trained in toxicology and occupational health, specialising in genetic toxicology and biomonitoring and their ethical aspects. She has held assignments in the Danish Environmental Protection Agency, the Danish Working Environment Inspection Service, the National Institute of Occupational Health and the Danish Medicines Agency. She is involved in a number of EU projects and European networks, such as Children's Susceptibility to Environmental

Genotoxicants, Evaluation of Medicinal Products, Validation of Alternative Methods (ECVAM) and the Implementation of the EU Data Protection Directive in Relation to Medical Research and the Role of Ethics Committees.

Contact information
Office address: Environmental Medicine Institute of Public Health, University of Copenhagen, c/o Dept of Pharmacology, Panum Blegdamsvej 3, DK-2200 Copenhagen, Denmark
Tel: +45 353 27653
E-mail: l.knudsen@pubhealth.ku.dk

Hans Jørgen Limborg PhD

Dr Hans Jørgen Limborg has been research co-ordinator and senior work-environment consultant at the Centre for Alternative Social Analysis (CASA), Copenhagen, Denmark since 1994. He has been an occupational health hygienist at Midtsjællands Bedriftssundhedscenter and an occupational health work-environment planner at Bedriftssundhedscenter København Vest. He was educational adviser at Denmark's Work Environment Fund in charge of programmes aimed at occupational health staff (1990–93). In his present position, as senior research consultant at CASA, he is responsible for the development and implementation of occupational health and safety projects and for programmes aimed at third world countries.

Contact information
Office address: CASA, Linnésgade 25, III, DK-1361 Copenhagen, Denmark
Tel: +45 33 320555
E-mail: hjl@casa-analyse.dk

Kari-Pekka Martimo Lic Med

Kari-Pekka Martimo is a specialist in occupational healthcare and occupational medicine, and has been Chief Physician at M-real Corporation in Finland since 1998. He has previously held assignments as an occupational physician in the Kruunuhaka Medical Centre, Oy Lohja Ab, and the Neste Oil Refinery. He was trained as a specialist physician at the Finnish Institute of Occupational Health. He has been appointed as EU Pre-accession Adviser in Estonia during 2003–04.

Contact information
Office address: Corporate Human Resources, M-real Corp, PO Box 582, FIN-33101 Tampere, Finland
Tel: +358 50 566 5797
E-mail: kari-pekka.martimo@m-real.com

Noks Nauta MD

Dr Noks Nauta is an occupational health physician and psychologist (specialising in work and organisation), and has worked at the Netherlands Expert Centre for Work-related Musculoskeletal Disorders, Erasmus Medical Centre, Rotterdam since 2001. She has previously held posts as a school doctor in Veenendaal and worked within the Dutch Governmental Occupational Health Service, The Hague, as an occupational health physician and specialist in occupation-related infectious diseases. She was earlier course manager for occupational health training in Leiden and co-ordinator for the training of general practitioners at Erasmus University.

Contact information
Office address: Netherlands Expert Centre for Work-related Musculo-skeletal Disorders, Erasmus Medical Centre, Rotterdam, Nieuw Hoboken, PO Box 2040, 3000 CA Rotterdam, Netherlands
Tel: +31 10 46 32012
E-mail: a.nauta@erasmusmc.nl or Noks_nauta@hotmail.com

Ian S Symington MB, ChB, FRCP, FFOM

Dr Ian Symington is an occupational physician. He is currently Director of Glasgow Occupational Health, based at Glasgow Royal Infirmary in Scotland, with responsibility for occupational health services covering a population of more than 20 000 healthcare workers. He holds honorary appointments at the University of Glasgow and Strathclyde University and is actively involved in research related to blood-borne viruses and the prevention of infection between patients and hospital staff. A former President of the UK Society of Occupational Medicine, he has recently completed a term of office as Chair of the Scientific Committee on Occupational Health for Health Care Workers under the auspices of the International Commission on Occupational Health (ICOH).

Contact information
Office address: Director, Glasgow Occupational Health, Glasgow Royal Infirmary, Cuthbertson Building, 91 Wishart St, Glasgow G31 3HT, Scotland, UK
Tel: +44 141 211 0427
E-mail: ian.symington@northglasgow.scot.nhs.uk

Jos Verbeek PhD

Dr Jos Verbeek is a senior lecturer and researcher in occupational health at the Coronel Institute for Occupational and Environmental Health at the Academic Medical Centre in Amsterdam, the Netherlands. He has practised occupational medicine during various periods of his career. Evaluation of occupational health interventions is his main research field. He is secretary of the ICOH Scientific Committee for Health Services Research and Evaluation in Occupational Health.

Contact information
Office address: Academic Medical Center, University of Amsterdam, Coronel Institute, PO Box 22700, 1100 DE Amsterdam, Netherlands
Tel: +31 20 566 5333 or 5325
E-mail: j.h.verbeek@amc.uva.nl

Laurent Vogel
Laurent Vogel works for the European Trade Union Technical Bureau for Health and Safety (TUTB).

Contact information
Tel: +32 2 224 0555
Mail address and telefax numbers are available on TUTB website (www.e-tuc.org/tutb)

André NH Weel MD, PhD
Dr André NH Weel, born in 1947, has been working as an occupational health physician in a regional occupational health centre in the Netherlands for many years. He is also affiliated to the Foundation for Quality in Occupational Health (SKB, Amsterdam, Netherlands). In this capacity, he has been involved in the development of professional guidelines for occupational physicians. He has been working simultaneously as a teacher and tutor at the Netherlands School of Public and Occupational Health. He is currently Chief Medical Officer and Manager of Training Programmes in Mediforce, a Dutch network organisation for occupational health physicians. He is a board member of the European Association of Schools of Occupational Medicine (EASOM) and a member of the editorial board of *The Netherlands Journal of Occupational and Insurance Medicine.*

Contact information
Office address: Mediforce bv, PO Box 174, 3970 AD Driebergen, Netherlands
Tel: +31 65 357 6148
E-mail: FAM.weel@inter.nl.net

Stuart Whitaker RGN, RMN, OHNC, MIOSH, MMedSc, PhD
Dr Stuart Whitaker, born in 1955, is Director of Occupational Health, Safety and Rehabilitation Services at BMI Health Services in the UK. He trained initially as a registered nurse and later as a psychiatric nurse. At age 21, he was selected to work as one of the youngest ever appointed offshore medics for the North Sea oil rigs. He had been strongly influenced by earlier

experience of hand injuries in industrial machinery. He completed his occupational health nursing training at Manchester University. After completing his PhD, he became Senior Research Fellow and Head of the Health Services Research Unit at Birmingham University, before joining BMI Health Services in 2002. Stuart has worked with the World Health Organization, the UK Health and Safety Executive and the UK Department of Health and has been active in the International Commission on Occupational Health for a number of years.

Contact information
Office address: BMI Health Services, Box Tree House, Lupton, Carnforth, Lancashire LA6 2PR, UK
Tel: +44 1539 567869
E-mail: swhitaker@bmihs.co.uk

Acknowledgements

The preparation of this book – from a loose set of ideas through conception to implementation – has been a most challenging and educational experience. Its fulfilment was made possible only through the joint efforts of us, as editors, and the chapter authors. We all perceived the mid-term seminar for authors, organised in Borupgaard, Denmark, as representing a strategic point of departure that made us jointly aware of what we had to do.

Special thanks are due to the Labour Market Insurance Company of Sweden (AFA) for making the financial contribution that enabled us to organise the project on a realistic basis.

Thanks are also due to Jon Kimber PhD, Stockholm, for his skilful review of our draft texts – many of the authors not having English as their mother tongue – and for sub-editing the whole package, introducing amendments with a view to fluency and consistency in use of language.

Our thanks also to Mrs Gunilla Sandegård, Stockholm, for her technical editing of all the texts and for patient and skilful assistance throughout in working the final manuscript into shape for submission to the publishers.

CHAPTER 1

A changing life at work: ethical ramifications

Peter Westerholm

This opening chapter presents an overview of global trends in life at work. It focuses on the occupational health implications of work and thereby on the roles and functions of, and also the expectations placed upon, all the health professionals involved there. The aim is to provide a background to, and perspective on, issues of ethics in occupational health professions, which are described and discussed in greater detail and on a more concrete level later in this book.

We start with a review of the overarching trends in global development that have an important impact on life at work. By so doing, we are reminded of both positive aspects, such as significant improvements in material work conditions, and some negative aspects, such as significant inequalities in health and safety between and within regions and nations of the world. The United Nations *Universal Declaration of Human Rights*[1] and the *International Covenant on Civil and Political Rights*[2] are referred to as cornerstone documents with regard to ethical dimensions of conditions at work. Developments in Europe, with reference to the *European Social Charter*[3] and the framework directive on safety and health at work,[4] are commented upon in terms of their ethical implications. The changing horizon of occupational health hazards is described, in particular with respect to the emergence of work organisation as a carrier and source of health-determining factors. New conceptions of ethical implications in the arena of occupational health are introduced at this stage. In concluding the chapter, the implications of these changes for the roles of occupational health professionals are discussed. Examples are given of the kinds of ethical questions which arise.

Scope of the work–health relationship: an example

The company is a conference hotel establishment with half a dozen restaurants and bars, and other facilities. It has been reasonably successful on the market, but six months ago the company was taken over in a merger operation by a new majority owner. For many years, the new owner has been running a competing chain of hotels catering for tourists seeking action-holiday programmes. The consequences of the merger are not unexpected. There is drastic streamlining of the organisation, with reductions in staffing and increasing workload for practically everybody. Further cuts are advertised.

The company has a contract with an external health service organisation providing professional occupational health services. At the regular health examinations that form part of the service an increasing prevalence of ill health of many kinds is observed among staff. As well as increasing numbers of back and shoulder pain syndromes, many speak of a loss of meaning or motivation for work and a profound and lasting state of depression.

At the same time, complaints from customers about defects in service quality appear to be more frequent. There is a clear increase in sickness absenteeism in many parts of the new company.

The management of the new company, after consulting its internal bipartite safety and health committee, takes a decision to offer all personnel a programme of workplace health promotion. The programme consists of individual health counselling focusing on back pain control, stress management and lifestyle management (meaning smoking, alcohol, drugs, diet and physical exercise). The contracted occupational health service unit is asked to organise and manage the programme. Further, the stress management programme is to be integrated into training sessions in yoga offered by a specialised school recently established in the vicinity of the hotel.

This is a snapshot of a typical situation confronted by many occupational health professionals both in Europe and worldwide and will be recognised by many readers. It raises a number of substantial ethical questions.

> - How are occupational health professionals to position themselves with respect to the requests presented by a client company?
> - Do we know what to do?
> - Is it the right thing to do?
> - Are we the right ones to do it?
> - Do we have the requisite competencies?
> - What are the ethical implications?

Working life change

Over the last century, material working conditions have certainly improved significantly and this has led to a decrease in work-related diseases largely because of the implementation of technical and hygiene developments. The implication of this situation is that work is no longer necessarily seen as a biblical curse or something to put up with. Rather, work has turned into an important determinant of health, even seen by some as a fundamental human right, with potential for the development of human creativity, independence and health. We see how work can be used for the reintegration and self-sustainment of people with significant handicaps or health defects. This is the positive spiral.

But there is a negative spiral as well, consisting of the damage to health and work ability caused by work or work conditions. At the same time, an unequal distribution of workplace hazards and work-related health disorders can be observed between countries, and also between socio-economic strata in many countries. The life-expectancy gap between manual workers, on the one hand, and managerial staff and qualified professionals, on the other, is still considerable – and even increasing. Despite improving scientific and technological standards in practically all economic production, we still see examples of forced labour and inhumane exploitation. The initial statement of the International Labour Organization (ILO) *World Labour Report* from 1993 puts the matter starkly: 'At the end of the twentieth century many people assume that slavery has been eradicated. Unfortunately this is not so'.[5] *See also* the ILO report, *Decent Work*, presented to the XVIth World Congress on Safety and Health at Work, in Vienna 2002.[6]

Coping with change in workplaces and the organisation of work is the primary challenge facing nations and social partners on the labour market. This applies to public organisations, enterprises and people at work. For obvious reasons, the direction and pace of technological, social and structural change in working life differ between and within countries, regions and segments of the labour market. There are also many types of work and economic activity that do not change very much. The bottom line, however, is that occupational health professionals are confronted with new horizons concerning health hazards, priorities and expectations. They may also encounter new health objectives at work. That is, as well as health hazards, they must also take account of the health-promotional effects and health potentials of good quality of life at work. This can be seen as a public-health aspect of occupational health.

Changes in work design and management strategies occur at three levels.

1 There are socio-economic, political, technological and demographic forces operating at community, national and international levels (trade policies, and the introduction and implementation of information technology).
2 There are macro-level changes at industry, branch or enterprise levels (i.e. technical change, downsizing, outsourcing, etc.).
3 There are micro-level changes in the workplace (i.e. workload, hazardous exposures, participation and support).

And there is another important set of challenges in changing working life, which lies in demographic developments. The industrialised countries of the Western hemisphere face rapid ageing of the workforce, a growing number of migrants, a shortage of young workers and greater mobility of working people.

Globalisation

Globalisation as an economic process implies in essence a combination of the two macro processes of liberalisation of world trade and the introduction of new information and communication technology on a vast and ever-increasing scale (involving all production, distribution and finance). Globalisation as a sociological process involves social activities, such as in the fields of culture, communication and ideas. That information has become raw material, method and outcome in industrial and service processes makes for radical changes in the conditions of existence for enterprises and in the economic life of nations. There are benefits to be reaped in the economic globalisation process and the net effects are generally held to be conducive to wealth creation. There are, however, also effects that are regarded as adverse, such as widening economic gaps between wealthy and less privileged regions and segments of populations.

It is an oversimplification to see globalisation as something that transcends and marginalises nation states. A common misunderstanding is to see it as something that is best avoided. This is hardly possible. Indeed, even publishing this book is an 'act of globalisation'. Globalisation creates winners and losers, integration as well as fragmentation. It is, in itself, neither inherently good nor bad. There is, however, broad political and scientific consensus that there is an urgent need to strengthen global governance so as to balance its impact.[7]

The employer–employee relationship

Throughout history, a pervasive component of the relationship between employers and employees has concerned aspects related to its nature as a power equilibrium. The employment or contractual arrangement between an employer and an employed person is a bond that divides responsibilities and aims at achievement for the benefit of both parties. An enterprise cannot prosper without the co-operation of its employees. It is also a bond where there are differences in values and interests. One point of potential conflict lies in employees' rights to safety and health and the right of business to maximise production for reasons of competition. It is here that the most contentious issues arise. It is a *prima facie* interest of the employer to pay as little as possible in wages and to minimise other costs for the work to be done. But this applies only up to a point. Well-paid and well-looked-after staff perform better. If, however, pay and work conditions do not offer a competitive advantage, an employer accepting these costs will soon be driven out of the market. The nature of the power balance is subject to various, more or less developed, mechanisms of state control in most countries. The controlling mechanisms, commonly regulated by legislation, aim at maintaining the accountability of enterprise owners and the trust of workers and their representatives, the general public and the other stakeholders involved.

Work and human rights

In recent decades the moral principles underlying the concept of human rights have been canonised in universal instruments of an authoritative nature. Since some of them have implications for the relationships between human work, economics and health, reference will be made to some important ones. A document of distinguished importance is the *Universal Declaration of Human Rights*, adopted by the United Nations Assembly in 1948.[1] Paragraph 1 of Article 23 of the *Declaration* contains the following statement: 'Everyone has the right to work, to free choice of employment, to just and favourable conditions of work and to protection against unemployment'.

A document of almost equal strength and global prestige is the *Universal Declaration of Human Responsibilities*, proposed in 1997 by the Inter-Action Council, a body of 30 former heads of state and ex-prime ministers from all regions of the world.[8] The *Declaration* has been conceived as a basis on which the United Nations human rights declaration might be amended. The InterAction Council emphasised human obligations for several reasons. The primary motive of the Council was to achieve a balance between the notions of freedom and responsibility, both of which have important moral implications. Whereas rights relate more to freedom, obligations are associated with responsibility. Responsibility, as a moral quality, thus serves as a natural, voluntary control of or counterpoint to freedom. Freedom cannot be exercised without limits in any society. Unrestricted economic freedom may be abused and result in great social injustice, as observed by the InterAction Council.

Article 4 of the InterAction Council *Declaration* states: 'All people, endowed with reason and conscience, must accept a responsibility to each and all, to families and communities, to races, nations, and religions in a spirit of solidarity. What you do not wish to be done to yourself, do not do to others'. Thus, the principles of solidarity and mutuality are clearly embodied in these authoritative universal declarations.

In the context of this book, it is also appropriate to recall the *European Social Charter*,[3] a document agreed between member nations of the European Council in 1961, and the *Charter of Fundamental Rights of the European Union*,[9] proclaimed in 2000 by the European Parliament, Council and Commission as founding documents of occupational health ethics in Europe. These two political documents represent a solid manifestation and commitment on the part of European countries to safeguard the ideals and principles identified as their common heritage for the purpose of maintaining and further realising human rights and fundamental freedoms. They were agreed to provide a basis for the joint policy goals of economic and social progress in the European Union. It is significant that articles 1–10 of the *European Social Charter*[3] deal with the right to work, the right to just conditions of work, the right to safe and healthy work conditions and the right to vocational training. Article 13, under Chapter 1 entitled Dignity, of the *Charter of Fundamental Rights of the European Union* proclaims the right to integrity of the person. Under chapters on freedoms, equality, solidarity and citizens' rights, many articles deal with aspects pertinent to the life at work of citizens and to workplace conditions.

These statements, in international instruments of a normative character, make up the gist of the issues related to the ethical dimension of the work and health relationship. This association is itself of a multidimensional nature. It may be seen as paired with solid mutual interdependence, where one component part is a prerequisite for the other. It may, however, also be seen as a source of conflict in situations and contexts where work may actually have destructive effects on workers' health. These issues have abundant ramifications in the field of professional health ethics.

One aspect of the employer–worker–workplace–health relationships, as observed by Berlinguer *et al.*,[10] is the increasing use of scientific and expert knowledge in assessments and decision making. In the complexity of the changing world at work, occupational health professionals assume important roles. It is, thus, noteworthy that a European Commission White Paper from 2001, *Governance in the European Union*, makes the following statement: '. . . scientific and other experts play an increasingly significant role in preparing and monitoring decisions. From human and animal health to social legislation, the institutions rely on specialist expertise to anticipate and identify the nature of the problems and uncertainties that the Union faces, to take decisions and to ensure that risks can be explained clearly and simply to the public'.[11]

So, the subject matter of the work and health relationship has come of age. It concerns human biology and economics and the interface between these two realms. The question to address is whether and in what regard the various paths of development in life at work have had or can be seen to have an impact on the ethical positioning of health professionals in issues relevant to the classic coupling of work and health.

The European Union framework directive on occupational safety and health

The new approach to occupational safety and health management in the European Union, as represented by the adoption of the framework directive (89/391/EEC), comprises a shift of regulatory emphasis away from prescriptive technical requirements on duty holders, primarily employers, towards more process-oriented measures.[4] It has two major general implications. First, it emphasises the duty of employers to implement a broadened and comprehensive concept of occupational health; this is a move towards self-regulation, which also implies changing roles and shifts in responsibilities for the law-enforcing and inspecting agencies of the state (labour inspectorates or their equivalents). Second, it implies a requirement for the systematic management of occupational health and safety matters. As well as specifying these basic steps, the framework directive includes requirements for: a hierarchical approach to preventive measures; risk assessments; participation of workers and their representatives; and preventive services and competence.

The adoption of the framework directive marks a cornerstone in European Union policies in that it serves the twin purposes of: establishing free movement of capital, goods and labour between member states; and supporting the development of working and living conditions for citizens in the member states (the 'social dimension' of a good life in Europe).

This move towards self-regulation in the management of health and safety matters in workplaces should be seen as linked to the wider social and economic policies of the European Union, which also embrace human rights at work, work conditions and socially responsible business. It should also be observed, following this extended and broadened health agenda, that, during the late 1990s, the notion of 'employability' came visibly closer to a wider conception of health and safety – embodying organisation and conditions of work as well as its traditional technical features. Thus, in practice, the conception of 'health' has been re-appraised in order to bear a new, much broader connotation of employability. Such a conception of health is no longer defined by health professionals on the basis of uncontested authority. It has just as much become a form of 'account-ability' and thereby a legitimate interest for responsible employers. As pointed out by Walters (2002), employers are unmistakably responsible agents as regards matters of safety and health in the legislation of practically all European countries.[12]

The changing organisation of work

In many industrialised countries throughout the world there are key changes in the organisation of work, brought about by economic, technological, legal and other forces. Manufacturing tasks are steadily decreasing and giving way to work in service and knowledge sectors of the labour market. Trade and computer technologies enable companies in many industries to operate globally in markets under intense price and product competition. In many branches of economic activity, pressures for increased ownership control can be discerned. There are also pressures from client systems for high quality and customisation in all manufactured products and service performance. There is increasing specialisation of personnel and the general trend is towards more qualified labour.

At a corporation or enterprise level organisational practices have changed to cope with these trends. To compete more effectively, destructuring is often undertaken – with downsizing of the workforce and outsourcing of all but core functions. The use of contract labour and temporary workers has increased. Menial tasks and support functions are not regarded as core functions. They are simply outsourced. Organisations adopt new and flat management structures with downwards transfer of responsibilities and decentralised control. Flexibility, quality and lean or just-in-time production have become key concepts in the production of goods and services.

In many Western European countries the role of the state in the organisational governance of production of goods and services has changed visibly. The trends toward deregulation, decentralisation and ways of organising manufacturing and services so as to satisfy clients' and customers' freedom of choice have been jointly referred to as new public management – as described by Rose and Miller,[13] Power[14] and Pollitt and Bouckaert.[15] The motives were, from the very outset, to diminish the economic commitment of state organs, to improve political governance of public sector organisations, to strengthen leadership and management, to contain costs and – at the same time – to effect improvement in quality of services and the benefits of a broadened freedom of choice for consumers.

In organisational thinking two main streams of ideas seem to have emerged and remained relatively constant, sometimes co-existing in an enterprise or groups of enterprises. Basically, they can be seen as competing themes. Broadly speaking, one emphasises cost-effective production, the other quality of working life (implying the life quality of people at work). There is a transition to flexible organisations – marked by specialisation – in both European and other Western economies. New functional demands are faced by enterprises and organisations. As well as efficiency, markets increasingly demand quality, flexibility and the capacity to innovate. Cost-efficiency pursuits aim at development of quality control, shop-floor management strategies, continuous improvement, just-in-time production, kaizen and lean production – to mention just a few of the popular and still-surviving conceptions of our time. The concept of lean production lies very close to that of cost efficiency.

The other mainstream current, referred to here as quality of working life, has taken another direction (at least in part). This policy foundation was underpinned by another set of values – democratic dialogue, the importance of developing skills and craftsmanship, participation, an awareness of the importance of motivation, teamwork arrangements and the meaningfulness of work. In a work organisation permeated by such values, the responsible autonomy of employees has come to be regarded both as a key prerequisite for efficient production and as an ideological basis on which to take the moral high ground in dealing with the labour force, often referred to as human capital. Also, it has been argued for as a strategy of health promotion. The implications of these developments in the countries of the European Union have been described and analysed by Totterdill et al.[16]

The general trends in the labour market and in life at work in the European Union, with their implications for occupational safety and health, have also been described in a document entitled *The Changing World of Work*, published by the European Occupational Safety and Health Agency (2003).[17] The major trends described include an increase in small business operations, changes in management methods, increased use of contractors and temporary staff, changes in working hours and the increasing practice of working at a distance from a fixed worksite or at home, the introduction of new working practices (such as just-in-time production) and the use of casual labour for temporary work.

One trend in enterprises and corporations observed in several recent research reports is the significant managerial transfer of problems and decisions, including workplace health hazards and issues, from the centre of organisations to their periphery. *See*, for example, Larsson[18] and Härenstam.[19] Such transfers go from corporations to subcontractors, from strategic senior management to operational levels of middle management, further on to individual staff members and still further to contingent and substitute workers. The changes within organisations have been described as processes of flexibilisation and individualisation. The rhetoric supporting this type of change as a strategy of human resource management often emphasises the positive aspects of individualised responsibility. One of the topical questions in today's working life is whether such individualisation has contributed to employees driving themselves to excessive work intensity and overload.

The introduction of remote-control mechanisms of work performance in public sector organisations has been one of the features of new public management. Such deregulation has resulted in tight requirements for 'management by objectives', where managers are pressed to achieve economic targets – no matter how – if they want to keep their jobs and preserve their programmes. This may leave many personnel overworked, undersupported and over-regulated. Indeed, many are burnt out and simply leave.

To sum up, surveys within the European Union and in other European countries suggest that while traditional hazards in the workplace prove to be persistent causes of both short-term absence and permanent withdrawal from work, the new forms of work and work conditions are also associated with major losses to society and the economy, especially through ill health caused by high-intensity jobs and work stress.

Health and work conditions

From the perspective of health, ongoing technical, economic and societal developments have resulted in stressful and hazardous work conditions. These include reduced work stability, precarious employment and an increasing workload. The features of development commonly held as most important are as follows.

- The transition from stable employment to precarious employment. Unemployment is known to be associated with increased mortality, morbidity and lowering of life quality. The changes referred to above imply a gradual shift for many segments of the labour force from full employment to various forms of flexible contracts or informal work with lower economic compensation and poor work conditions.
- The transition from safety and hygienic hazards at work to psychosocial strain. This refers to a gradual shift in emphasis, since many physical, chemical and ergonomic exposures still remain potential health hazards in the workplace. Pressures for higher productivity, mediated by new management systems, cause mental strain and a broad range of stress-related disorders. The interface between the work and non-work spheres of individuals' lives becomes blurred, implying that work is brought home with an impact on quality of life away from work.
- The transition from hazardous workplaces to social inequalities in health at work. Evidence indicating social inequalities in health and healthcare and their impact on health outcomes is generally recognised in European research communities. Work conditions play an important role in the explanation of such inequalities.
- The emergence of a new labour force composition, with an increasing proportion of older workers. This raises new questions concerning essential reviews of preventive practices and adaptations of programmes for occupational health education and training.
- The increasing incidence of violence and harassment, which affects older employees and women in the labour force in particular.

There is good reason to regard such developments as having a negative impact on public health.

Health outcomes and their implications

Looking in the late 1990s at the new occupational health horizon for changes in the panorama of workplace health hazards and health disorders in diverse ways associated with work, Rantanen[20] came to the conclusion that the following items had obtained more prominent positions in recent times:

- musculoskeletal disorders arising from physically light work and lack of mobility
- stress-related disorders
- hypersensitivity and allergies

- age-related disorders
- indoor air-quality problems
- HIV or AIDS
- alcohol and narcotic drugs
- socially destructive behaviour
- violence and harassment
- terrorism
- sickness absenteeism and early retirement exits from the labour market.

This last-mentioned item is an outcome variable, observed as an increasing and costly phenomenon in many European countries – in both the public and the private sectors. Clearly, this trend reflects, at least in significant part, perceived quality of life at work, including health characteristics of the workplace.

The implications of these changes are that occupational health professionals may be confronted with new issues of professional ethics. The following question arises.

> - Do occupational health professionals possess the requisite know-ledge of facts and experiences of new health challenges in life at work to be in a position to give adequate professional advice?

Conceptions of occupational health

As mentioned above, the definition of health is no longer a matter to be determined by the judgements of health professionals alone. In consequence, the conception of health deserves revisiting from a health professional point of view with regard to its ethical implications. The seminal World Health Organization (WHO) definition of health as a 'state of complete physical, mental and social well-being and not merely absence of disease' is now commonly regarded by health professionals not as an operational definition but rather as an abstract and broad indicator of direction. As to the term 'occupational health', the ILO and WHO adopted (in 1950) a shared definition. This was revised in 1995[21] and indicated strategies for the pursuance of specific objectives: the maintenance and promotion of workers' health and working capacity; the improvement of working environment and work to become conductive to safety and health; and development of work organisations and working cultures in a direction which supports health and safety at work.

In 1996, the WHO adopted its *Global Strategy on Occupational Health for All*,[22] within which the concept of health was referred to as follows: 'According to the principles of the United Nations, WHO and ILO, every citizen of the world has a right to healthy and safe work and to a work environment that enables him or her to live a socially and economically productive life'.

It is important to note that these statements of the WHO and ILO do not actually contain any definition of occupational health. It is also worthy of note that, in essence, they have a biomedical frame of reference. Accordingly, it deserves mentioning that, in the discourse of recent years within the disciplines that apply modern philosophy to the sciences of biomedicine, new types of definitions of health are emerging. One example lies in a definition of health based on action theory. A person's health, according to this school of thinking, consists of his or her ability to achieve vital goals. It rests on two fundamental assumptions: (i) the relation of the human individual to his or her environment, and (ii) the relation of the human individual to the self. In these types of definitions, no reference is made to presence or absence of disease. *See* Nordenfelt[23] and Pörn.[24]

The renewed scientific discourse on basic elements in the conception of health – this time coming from philosophically oriented researchers – has obvious ethical implications. The conceptions and operational definitions selected as a policy basis for the management of occupational safety and health issues are pertinent in determining the roles and responsibilities of occupational health professionals. Thus, the concept of 'occupational health' remains ambiguous. The term is used abundantly, but it is rare for much thought to be devoted to what it actually stands for.

- What definition of health is adopted by occupational health professionals and which operational health objectives are to be pursued in workplace settings?
- What is the mandate and role of the occupational health professional in such a context?
- What competencies are required?

Health as a human right

A key aspect and point of departure in the emergence of welfare states in Northern Europe during the second half of the last century has been the notion that it is a duty of governments to secure the well-being of the populations for which they are responsible. Over the years, as observed by Shaw and Crompton,[25] this has developed into the parallel idea that it is a civil right of the population to be provided with healthcare. In some countries it has also been extended to encompass the expectations that professional health services are provided in the workplace. At the same time, however, it is generally recognised that it is simply not possible to institute a right to health. The conceptualisation of health, including occupational health, is problematic and, as referred to above, widening in scope and increasingly indeterminate. National governments have no powers to guarantee the health of a population. They can, at best, set up healthcare systems and organisations that provide services for cure and prevention, which take care of problems and counteract health inequities. For life at work they can impose obligations on other agents, such as employers, to assume the roles of accountable social agent. As was argued by Foucault: 'Health – good health – can not derive from a right; good or bad health, however crude or subtle the criteria used, are facts – physical states and mental states'.[26] The bottom line is, in consequence, that the concept of health is difficult to operationalise in precise terms as a human right. This applies equally, by association, to the concept of occupational health. They both remain, however, the overriding visions and objectives of the healthcare provided by occupational health professionals.

The issue of competency

The shift of emphasis in the health disorder panorama – from well-known diseases, through clinical diagnostic techniques for identifiable occupational diseases, to the domination of less easily defined stress disorders and health disturbances – implies a need for new approaches to dealing with individual personnel and organisations. The basis for assessments of work conditions and determinants of health disorders often derive from perceptions and experiences of staff members. This has obvious ethical implications.

> - What competencies do occupational health professionals need to possess to deal with the subject of risk assessments and the taking of preventive action?
> - Is it ethically defensible for occupational health professionals to provide counselling to clients or customers on subjects or issues in which they lack relevant knowledge or competencies?
> - If so, under what conditions?

Knowledge and evidence

Health hazards at work are often complex – with many factors both at work and outside work contributing to their causation. This implies a need for structured approaches to problem identification and needs assessment by occupational health professionals. It also implies a need to utilise knowledge and experiences in other professional and client systems. And it is also necessary to involve clients in active participation. Clients in an enterprise operate at both employer or management and employed or contracted-staff levels. There has been a tradition of not questioning the views and judgements of health professionals. It is, however, increasingly observed that patients and customers of all kinds are becoming less disposed to take professional opinions 'on trust'. Health professionals must be prepared to explain not only what they advise but also the reasons why the advice given is appropriate and the expected efficacy of what is proposed. Creating and maintaining trust make up a core strategy for all the pursuits of occupational health professionals. In 2002, O'Neill[27] provided an exhaustive review of the issues of trust involved in bioethics.

The definition of evidence offered by the *Oxford English Dictionary* – 'the available body of facts or information indicating whether a belief or proposition is true or valid' – should be borne in mind. For an elaboration of the idea of evidence-based practice, *see* Chapter 2 in this book.

- What is entailed in the conception of 'evidence' with regard to the knowledge base for preventive action in occupational health?
- What facts are needed and what efforts need to be made by occupational health professionals to satisfy the objectives of evidence-based occupational health practice in giving competent advice to clients?

Recognition of occupational disease

In many countries of the world there is currently new interest in reviewing systems for the identification and recognition of and economic compensation to, via insurance payments, workers who have contracted an injury or a health disorder caused by their work. In 2002 the International Labour Organization reviewed its official list of occupational diseases.[28] Occupational health professionals have become increasingly involved in assessing claims for recognition of occupational disease. The context of such assessments and the features of insurance or social security systems for payments of compensation show large differences between countries. There are public social security insurance systems that operate on the basis of solidarity under a no-tort principle, implying that the causal nature of workplace factors can be accepted on the basis of presented evidence with no requirement to demonstrate the negligence of the agent responsible (usually the employer). In other types of insurance programmes payments of damages or benefits to claimants are conditional on demonstration of negligence.

Assessment of individual claims for insurance compensation payments is a professionally demanding field. It is at its most awkward when it comes to health disorders prevalent in the working population, regardless of work. Musculoskeletal disease and mental disorders of many kinds are well-known examples. Occupational health professionals often become involved in assessments of the 'work-relatedness' of diseases and health disorders. There are increasing demands for improved visibility of social justice in such assessments and also enhanced pressures for greater retribution aimed at those held responsible for injuries caused by or contributed to by workplace conditions.

- What efforts should be made to collect valid information for making reliable decisions in recognising a health disorder as occupationally related?
- Are there potential conflicts between stakeholders in relation to insurance policies?

Corporate social accountability in working life

Corporate social accountability is a concept adhered to by an increasing number of companies throughout the world. It is encouraged in the countries of the European Union[29] and implies in essence that companies decide voluntarily to contribute to a better society and a cleaner environment. It carries the vision of a company having a mission that goes beyond making its shareholders wealthy. In brief, socially responsible practices relate to issues such as investing in human capital, health and safety and human rights and also the management of change. The external dimension includes management of environmental impacts, responsible practices related to the use of natural resources in production and the effects of the company on the external world in general. Normann,[30] in discussing the features of organisations and institutions capable of long-term sustainability, observed the maintenance of consonance between the organisation and its environment to be a distinctive characteristic. A successful organisation, according to Normann, understands the values in that environment and its value-creating logic. Social accountability is one of these values. (For a more detailed discussion of corporate social accountability, *see* Chapter 20, in this book.)

- In view of the professional ethos of occupational health professionals – by virtue of their training and their qualifications – what expectations can be laid on them and what roles can be assumed by them in contributing to corporate social accountability?
- Is the task of occupational health professionals limited to and subservient to the objective of making enterprises more profitable?
- Or does the professional agenda also include, as well as health, the objective of improving life quality at work and in the societal setting of the client enterprise?

The professional profile of the occupational health specialist

Occupational health professionals commonly have an advisory, counselling role in relations with people who specifically ask for advice. In the world of occupational health the employer bears the responsibility for safe and healthy work conditions. The occupational health specialist seeks to give such advice in a professional and disinterested judgement, which is best from the recipient's point of view, and also within the remit of competencies of the specialist. It is to be borne in mind that the health needs perceived by clients are not necessarily identical to demands or requests for service. What are the professional's criteria of reasonable certainty in this regard? For example, the role of the occupational health counsellor may be framed in different ways according to the task and mandate given by the customer. The role may be one of a technical expert who puts 'all cards on the table', presenting the best available knowledge on a particular subject. It may also be one of an activist profoundly involved in processes of change or one of a mediator between employer or management and the workers.

And who is the client? In an enterprise occupational health professionals may be consulted by:

- individual staff members on personal health matters
- groups of employees on health matters, involving several people at the same time
- the employer on health matters related to one individual staff member or groups of employees or to issues associated in a more general way with work conditions or work environment.

All this implies that occupational health professionals must 'wear more than one hat' at one and the same time. Medically trained occupational health professionals have the additional challenge of having a relationship with individual staff members of a company while providing curative services to them and at the same time being accountable for health assessments aimed at ill health prevention and providing advisory services at group or company level. In recent decades the professional cadres of occupational health specialists have been reinforced by occupational nurses, physiotherapists, ergonomists, psychologists, therapists, health promoters, work organisation experts and many others. All these professional categories have been educated and trained for their roles on the labour market in academic institutions, in schools for health professionals and in the institutes for occupational health research set up in most countries of Europe. This development represents an expansion of and growing professionalisation in the arena of occupational health.

It is, on the other hand, commonly recognised that much of the work performed by occupational health specialists falls within the intellectual and practical capacities of many managers, workers, personnel administrators and other staff. Thus, a fundamental question concerns the added value contributed by occupational health specialists and the best ways to devise roles and tasks for them. One answer often heard to this question is that the core value of the responsibilities of occupational health professionals lies in broadness of scope rather than in depth of substance matter. Broad scope is a prerequisite for capturing a full perspective on the problems and issues arising in the realm of occupational health. At the same time, it leads to difficulties for managers, workers and others directly involved in keeping up to date with pertinent knowledge. Well-trained occupational health specialists can do this and, as a consequence, be attractive on the market for health services. Truly profound knowledge in narrow specialised fields, as increasingly experienced in occupational health, is needed only occasionally. The expert can then be hired or purchased on an *ad hoc* basis.

- Does professionalisation within the occupational health arena carry a risk of rivalry, with ethical implications, between different categories of health professions?
- Is there an inherent risk of pressure being exerted to provide services that are not really needed?
- What implications for professional ethics arise out of this?
- What is the accountability of occupational health experts in their advisory role?
- Who is the client?
- To whom are occupational health professionals accountable?
- What counselling role is appropriate?

Occupational health professionals in a market setting

Occupational health professionals and units in many European countries now operate as commercial organisations on a free health market. Under such circumstances, there is a duality to the role of occupational health professionals – in their capacities as health specialists and, at the same time, as partners in business transactions.

Basically, the occupational health professionals are, like most professionals in the health sector, expected to be committed to their profession and to act at least relatively independently of financial reward. It is envisaged that tasks are carried out primarily in terms of professional judgement on what needs to be done, not because they are paid for. This is at least the role model that prevails for health professionals within the public sector. Evidently, however, the remunerative aspect cannot be ignored. Professionals have to be paid by somebody. It costs money to use professional time and professionals must be allowed to earn their living. Indeed, on a free market, characterised by competition and with consumer choice as a driving force, health professionals may operate in organisations that are highly profit driven. Under such circumstances, occupational health management and client systems may set the priorities and the work agenda without paying attention to, even to the point of ignoring, the values and views of the health professionals. To this may be added a reminder that, as part of the currently ongoing transformations in many European countries of public healthcare institutions into privatised organisations, health professionals are often assigned to managerial posts. Again, this involves the assumption of a dual role. The professionals may find themselves in a combination of the health specialist role and the managerial role by having responsibility for the survival of their organisation on the market. As has recently been pointed out by Pollock and Price,[31] the workings of markets, by their nature, conflict with equity. Market logic in healthcare implies a risk of introducing incentives for selection of customers and shifting service performance towards the aim of financial gain.

The customer of an occupational health service unit is commonly an enterprise or an organisation, doing its best to achieve excellence, productivity and efficiency with a view to defending and expanding its market position. The enterprise is prepared to pay for the costs of business transactions in relation to external expert bodies, but is as a rule less interested in agendas other than its own. Unless satisfied with the services provided by the contracted occupational health service unit, the customer is likely to turn elsewhere to get the job done. Proposals by occupational health professionals that are judged to be too expensive may be turned down by the client. In order to ensure a contract with and commitment on the part of the customer, occupational health professionals may be tempted to offer proposals well aligned to clients' wishes but not consistent with professional ethics. The bottom line concerns the identity of the occupational health professional in a world undergoing change. We witness reconfigurations of systems in societies and businesses and also technical transformation. Accordingly, the boundaries of task identity are hazy. There is also among occupational health professionals an increasing awareness of the importance of a sense of professional identity and direction. As pointed out by Normann,[30] this is a general phenomenon, which also applies in the world of commerce. So, in a world undergoing change, we are all on board. The more features of the physical world become obscure, the more a professional sense of identity needs to come from reflection, from activity in the conceptual world. Only then can we compensate for the haziness involved.

- Where occupational health service organisations operate under commercial market conditions, is there a possibility that they offer services based more on the need to stay in business than the health needs of client enterprises?

'Take some more tea,' the March Hare said to Alice, very earnestly.
'I've had nothing yet,' Alice replied in an offended tone: 'so I can't take more.'
'You mean you can't take less,' said the Hatter: 'it's very easy to take more than nothing.'

Alice's Adventures in Wonderland
(Lewis Carroll, 1832–98)

References

1 United Nations (1948) *Universal Declaration of Human Rights*. UN General Assembly Resolution 217 A (III), 10 December 1948.

2 United Nations (2003) *International Covenant on Civil and Political Rights*. (www.hrweb.org/legal/cpr.html).

3 Council of Europe (1961) *European Social Charter*. ETS 035 (1961) with amendments ETS 42 and as revised ETS 163.

4 Council Directive 89/391/EEC (12 June 1989) on the introduction of measures to encourage improvements in the safety and health of workers at work. *Official Journal L 183*, 29/06/1989: 0001–8.

5 International Labour Organisation (1993) *World Labour Report 1993*. ILO, Geneva.

6 International Labour Organisation (2002) *Decent Work – Safe Work*. Introductory report to XVIth World Congress on Safety and Health at Work, Vienna.

7 Sörensen G (2002) Globalisation, values and global governance. In: G Bexell and D-E Andersson (eds) *Universal Ethics – Perspectives and Proposals from Scandinavian Scholars*. Martinus Nijhoff Publishers, The Hague.

8 InterAction Council (1997) *A Universal Declaration of Human Responsibilities*. Proposal of 1 September 1997. (www.asiawide.or.jp/iac/UDHR/EngDecl1.htm).

9 Charter of Fundamental Rights of the European Union (2000/C 364/01). *Official Journal of the European Communities*, 18 December 2000.

10 Berlinguer G, Falzi G and Figà Talamance I (1996) Ethical problems in the relationship between health and work. *International Journal of Health Services*. **26**: 147–71.

11 European Commission (2001) *Governance in the European Union: a White Paper*. European Commission: Brussels COM (2001) 428 final. (Available with supporting material via europa.eu.int/comm/governance/white_paper/index.htm).

12 Walters A (2002) *Regulating Health and Safety Management in the European Union – a study of the dynamics of change*. Peter Lang, S.A. Presses Inter-universitaires Européennes, Brussels.

13 Rose N and Miller P (1992) Political power beyond the state: problematics of government. *British Journal of Sociology*. **43**: 173–205.

14 Pollitt C and Bouckaert G (1992) *Public Management Reform – a comparative analysis*. Oxford University Press, Oxford.

15 Power M (1997) *The Audit Society – rituals of verification*. Oxford University Press, Oxford.

16 Totterdill P, Dhondt S and Milsome S (2002) *Partners at Work? A report to Europe's policy makers and social partners*. Report of the High Road Concept as a Resource funded by the DG Research of the European Commission. Nottingham Trent University, Nottingham.

17 European Agency for Safety and Health at Work (2003) *The Changing World of Work – trends and implications for occupational safety and health in the European Union 2002.* (Available on the EU Agency's website agency. osha.eu.int).

18 Larsson T (2000) The diffusion of employer responsibility. In: K Frick, P Langaa-Jensen, M Quinlan and T Wilthagen (eds) *Systematic Occupational Health and Safety Management – perspectives on an international development.* Pergamon Press, Oxford.

19 Härenstam A *et al.* (in press) Different development trends in working life and increasing occupational illness requires new environment strategies. *Work: A Journal of Prevention, Assessment and Rehabilitation.* **24**(3).

20 Rantanen J (1999) Research challenges arising from changes in worklife. *Scandinavian Journal of Work and Environmental Health.* **25**: 473–83.

21 Joint ILO/WHO Committee on Occupational Health. Proceedings of 12th Session of Committee (1995) (www.ilo.org/public/english/protection/safework/papers/asiachem/ch3.htm), August 2003.

22 World Health Organization (1995) *Global Strategy on Occupational Health for All.* WHO/OCH/95.1, Geneva.

23 Nordenfelt L (1987) On the nature of health: an action-theoretic approach. In: Philosophy and Medicine. No. 26. D. Reidel Publishing Company, Dordrecht.

24 Pörn I (1993) Health and adaptiveness. *Theoretical Medicine.* **14**: 295–303.

25 Shaw I and Crompton A (2003) Theory, like mist on spectacles, obscures vision. *Evaluation* **9**: 192–204.

26 Foucault M (1988) *On Problematization.* In: M Foucault, P Rabinow, M Feber and R Hurley (eds) *The Essential Works of Michel Foucault 1954–1984.* Vol. 3. Penguin Books, Harmondsworth.

27 O'Neill O (2002) *Autonomy and trust in bioethics.* Cambridge University Press, UK.

28 International Labour Organization (2003) Internet website for International Labour Congress Proceedings 2002 on recording and notification of occupational accidents and diseases. (www.ilo.org/public/english/standards/relm/ilc/ilc90/comreps.htm).

29 Commission of European Communities (2001) *Green Paper – promoting a European framework for corporate social responsibility.* Document COM. 366 final, dated 18.7.2001. Office for Official Publications of the European Communities, Luxembourg.

30 Normann R (2001) *Reframing Business – when the map changes the landscape.* John Wiley & Sons, Chichester.

31 Pollock A and Price D (2003) *In Place of Bevan. Briefing on the Health and Social Care Community Health and Standards Bill 2003.* Public Health Policy Unit, University College London. (www.catalystforum.org.uk).

CHAPTER 2

Ethics, research-informed practice and quality improvement

John Øvretveit

Introduction

Most of this book addresses ethical issues in professional practice, but two chapters specifically address ethics in occupational health management, namely this chapter and Chapter 23. Occupational health managers have direct responsibility for running an occupational health service and are often also professional practitioners for some time during their working week. The message of this chapter is that occupational health managers have an ethical duty to promote research-informed practice and quality improvement. This will enable them to respond to growing and conflicting demands (on them and their service). It explains why occupational health research and improving quality help to create a more ethical service and also provides ideas that will help in the work involved.

The aim is not to make managers feel guilty that they are not meeting ethical standards, but to show how ethics and other tools can help occupational health managers to create a better service for both personnel and the employees of the client companies they serve. Jointly, this and Chapter 23 present a view of 'ethical occupational health management', which is both a way of managing and a set of tools that enables managers to improve their service so as better to meet the demands of different groups.

Like the managers in the industries they serve, occupational health managers need continually to improve their service in an increasingly competitive environment. But what has this to do with ethics? Managing an occupational health service can be a lonely and thankless task. On occasions managers are accused of putting costs or other considerations before employees' interests and of 'being unethical'. One message of this chapter is that improving services is not just a requirement of a competitive market but an ethical imperative. Even if there were no payer demands or competition, there would still be an ethical obligation for managers continually to increase the efficiency, effectiveness and quality of occupational health services.

Ethics and evidence-based practice

As described in Chapter 23, a key ethical principle governing occupational health practice is beneficence – to do no harm and to do good. Practitioners who deliberately intend their diagnoses or treatments to harm a patient are hard to find. Most believe that the interventions they have learned to make will benefit the patient. Yet, we are all likely to be making interventions that have been proven to be either ineffective or of little effect. And we do not actually know how many of us are *not* using interventions that research has found to be effective. But, since we operate as in other branches of medicine, it is likely that we fail to use effective methods every day. There are many reasons for this, including lack of resources and client organisation preferences. However, one specific reason is a lack of awareness of research. The amount of research becoming available is difficult to keep up with. It is even more difficult to change our practices when we have become familiar with traditional methods and have a high workload. We will return later in this chapter to the challenges and 'implementation strategies' involved in the evidence-based practice that research itself has shown to be effective.

> Doctors cannot continue to fail to use treatments which we know are effective and inflict ineffective or harmful treatments on patients.
>
> Angela Coulter, Picker Institute Europe (personal communication)

Examples

There are many examples of newly gained knowledge about treatment effectiveness that have been slow to be applied in clinical practice. Research has shown some treatments to be ineffective for depression, but also some others to be of benefit (at least for certain patients). Appropriate prescription of aspirin or warfarin has been found to prevent strokes in patients with atrial fibrillation. Antithrombolytic treatment within two hours of certain types of chest pain can avoid serious heart muscle damage and the ventricular fibrillation that leads to cardiac arrest.

Elevated serum cholesterol and LDL cholesterol are major risk factors for recurrent cardiac events after myocardial infarction. Experiments with statins (HMG Co-A reductase inhibitors) have shown a reduction in mortality and cardiac events as a result of lowering serum cholesterol levels by 20–30% – both in primary prevention and afer myocardial infarction. Such research has been known for some time, but hospitals have been slow to use this preventive measure in relation to risk patients.[1,2] The new 'Best Treatments' website presents research showing that a number of treatments for anxiety are ineffective. The most effective – cognitive therapy – has been available for some time, but is often not prescribed when clearly needed.

These are examples from clinical practice and it would be surprising if occupational health clinicians were much different from others in their application of new knowledge. But what of the many other interventions made by occupational health practitioners, such as assessment methods, organisational interventions or health promotion programmes? Are there examples of research that has shown any of these interventions to be effective or ineffective?

There are, of course, some – but far fewer than in the case of clinical practice. Some pre-employment tests have been shown to be poor predictors of future job performance, but the tests continue to be used. And a review of research into return-to-work interventions after low back pain produced some evidence for the effectiveness of behavioural treatments and physical exercise, and also of multicomponent interventions.[3] The effectiveness of physical activity programmes at worksites is questionable with regard to work-related outcomes.[4] Is it worth spending resources on counselling at work to encourage physical activity and healthy lifestyle changes? Proper et al.[5] found evidence that it was. Further, another recent review has suggested that a number of interventions for reducing sickness absence and work-related psychological ill health are effective.[6]

Generally, for all occupational health interventions, the principle of beneficence requires that, from an ethical perspective, practitioners need to transform research into effectiveness. We cannot do this with the many non-clinical interventions that either have not been evaluated or are difficult to evaluate and fail to generate clear conclusions. This presents a technical and ethical challenge to occupational health researchers. No evidence of effectiveness is not the same as evidence of no effectiveness. However, the general principle still holds; there is an obligation to search for and act on the basis of evidence of effectiveness in order properly to serve patients and clients and avoid wasting resources that could be used for other beneficial purposes.

- How then might an occupational health manager develop a more evidence-based approach to practice?

What is evidence-based practice?

The simplest definition of evidence-based practice is that it is 'the process of systematically finding, appraising and using contemporaneous research findings as the basis for clinical decisions'.[7] The key ideas[8] are that:

- the best available evidence should inform clinical decisions
- the type of evidence you seek should be determined by the clinical problem
- epidemiological and statistical methods should be used to find the best evidence
- this evidence is only useful if put into action in treating patients
- practice should be evaluated continually.

Does this mean that clinical experience and judgement are now irrelevant? Sackett *et al.*[9] allow for flexibility in the approach when presenting it as 'the conscientious, explicit, and judicious use of current best evidence in making decisions about the care of individual patients . . . . The practice of EBP means integrating individual clinical expertise with best available external clinical evidence from systematic research'. Grey[10] also offers scope for the patient's views and other considerations when determining the nature of an intervention; being 'judicious' signifies that clinicians must take into account patients' condition, values and circumstances.

Such flexibility is important because many proponents of evidence-based practice have strict views on what is evidence of effectiveness and how to assess research. One version (adapted by Dixon *et al.*[11] from the US Task Force on Preventative Health Care) of the 'hierarchy of evidence' runs as follows.

I) Systematic reviews of published research into effectiveness.
II) Randomized controlled trial (RCT).
III) Non-random RCT.
IV) Quasi-experimental studies.
V) Non-experimental descriptive studies.
VI) Published opinion.

However, there have been criticisms that the 'traditional science model' of evidence-based practice is infeasible both in everyday practice and as an ideal. Black[12] argues that uncritical acceptance of the randomised controlled trial as the 'gold standard' might stifle professional actions in the absence of evidence and lead to a loss of self-confidence. One problem is that in occupational health there are a number of interventions that are difficult to evaluate by use of randomised controlled trials or even quasi-experimental designs. Does this mean that occupational health cannot become evidence based? Here, we need to remember the value of the considerable body of literature providing 'good practice guidance'.[13–15] This is based on evidence, but little of it meets randomised controlled trial standards and is unlikely ever to do so. Recognition of the uncertainties of such knowledge, and the need for it to be revised continually whilst being cognisant of its value, is the proper scientific and ethical approach.

Why is it so difficult to be evidence-based in occupational health service?

There are a number of challenges in creating an evidence-based occupational health service. First, the service is not simply clinical, aimed at individual patients. Occupational health services provide a range of preventive, consulting, advisory and training facilities to groups and populations, and also to managers. There is little research into the effectiveness of such non-clinical interventions. Where research has been performed, the findings are often not as clear-cut as those derived from clinical research evaluations. It is difficult to evaluate preventive programmes. Controls and randomisation are not possible; time is needed for outcomes to be studied, and there are many alternative explanations for any particular set of findings.

In individual clinical practice there is greater opportunity to use published research to determine more effective interventions. However, there are problems in applying research to many occupational health clinical services. Often, the patients in a clinical study group are not similar to patients seen in occupational health. Research findings are often published in many different places. Practitioners do not have time for educational programmes concerned with how to use the ideas or to search for and assess the research. There is also the challenge of changing clinical practice. Research has shown that many interventions, such as traditional, ongoing medical training, are ineffective. It is costly to change practice, even if there may be savings in the future.

Challenges in developing evidence-based occupational health practice

- There is a limited amount of evaluation research; many occupational health interventions have not been evaluated or are difficult to evaluate; it is hard to determine which outcomes to study or draw clear-cut conclusions about effectiveness.

- The research is published in different places and is not always easy to access or apply to a local service.
- Occupational health units are often small and not linked to universities and other centres that can help to apply research knowledge.
- There is little time for updating or learning new methods.
- There is uncertainty about effective ways of implementing evidence-based practice, and ineffective traditional educational methods continue to prevail.

How do managers promote research-informed practice?

The ethical argument for making greater use of research evidence in treatment decisions is clear. It avoids harm and increases the benefit to individual patients and others. This is not, however, just a matter for individual occupational health professionals. Managers of occupational health units have a professional and ethical duty to:

- make use of research about effectiveness, so as to set general policies about which tests and interventions should be used in the service
- ensure practitioners report the evidence base and the degree of certainty with regard to likely results when advising clients about tests and interventions, so as to allow informed decisions by clients
- work with practitioners to find ways of making greater use of research in clinical and policy decisions.

The challenge for managers and professionals is how to make their services more evidence based. Such a challenge does not mean that evidence-based practice is not relevant to occupational health services, but rather that managers need to be creative and selective in how they apply this approach to their own service.

The approach proposed here is for managers to promote 'research-informed' rather than 'evidence-based' practice. That is, they should make more use of research when deciding which treatments to use and how to use them, and also when determining which other interventions to use for other types of occupational health services. How then might occupational health managers generate changes to create more 'research-informed practice'?

Research into implementing evidence-based practice gives guidance to managers, although it is better at showing what does not work rather than what does. It demonstrates that managers, alongside practitioners, need to develop a plan that is suited to their local circumstances.

The most common approach is to use research to develop clinical guidelines about which diagnostic and treatment interventions to use and about how to use them, and then to find ways to get practitioners to follow these guidelines. We know that guidelines developed elsewhere need to be shaped to local circumstances. If they are simply imposed on practitioners, they are rejected. Traditional dissemination of information and education alone is ineffective.

Using guidelines requires professionals to take time to learn and adopt new behaviours with regard to the ways in which they diagnose or treat patients. They require support and special conditions if they are to change their practices. Research has revealed the barriers to the use of such guidelines, as experienced by practitioners. There are competency barriers such as a lack of knowledge, social barriers such as negative attitudes and organisational barriers such as a lack of clinical support;[16] and also, there is simply a lack of time.[17]

Interventions for implementing guidelines are educational, epidemiological, market oriented, behavioural, social-interactive, organisational and coercive. Research has investigated the effectiveness of these interventions. One review of 'research-informed practice' concludes that a combination of interventions, implemented in a planned manner, is the most likely to be successful. Thus:

- effectiveness of the method depends on the target group, the subject of the guideline and the situation
- passive dissemination (e.g. lectures and written information) alone is ineffective
- social science and behavioural knowledge are useful in designing appropriate and more effective interventions.[18]

Ethics and quality improvement

Quality is about giving the best service with the resources available – as most of the companies and other organisations served by occupational health will tell us. The quality of an occupational health service to them and others is how well it meets the wants of those most in need of the resources available. A poor-quality occupational health unit is one that is not available to those most in need, and one that causes harm to those who do actually use the service. When effective services are not provided, resources that could be used to do good are wasted. Thus, quality improvement is a way of realising a number of ethical principles in an occupational health service, not just a technique for making the service more competitive.

Often, it is easier to understand what we mean by the quality of an occupational health service by thinking of the features of a poor-quality service. A poor-quality occupational health service does not respect its users or the personnel providing it. This is not just a matter of giving a bad 'service experience'. The relationship between providers and 'users' in an occupational health service is deeper than in a fast-food outlet or a travel agency, and people have higher expectations of the human relations involved. A poor-quality occupational health service fails to enhance trusting relations and damages people's respect for others: 'If the doctor in our company acts like this, what else can we expect?'. Also, the service may be the only option available for some service users. Every practitioner has a duty not to put his or her own needs above the needs of those being served. Focusing on quality is one way of keeping the needs of patients and other service users in the forefront and promoting ethics in practice.

Using the latest research is one way to improve quality. It is a way of better meeting needs and of ensuring that resources are not wasted. Another is to use one or several of a variety of quality methods. (Such methods will be briefly summarised after defining quality more precisely.)

What is a quality occupational health service?

There are three dimensions to quality in an occupational health service: the client, the professional and the management. A quality occupational health service:

- gives patients and clients what they want and what they ask for (*customer quality*)
- gives patients and clients what they need – as assessed by the occupational health professionals, and according to best practice (*professional quality*)
- meets the most important patient and client needs safely, without errors or wasting resources (*management quality*).

The final dimension – management quality – is one that is most often forgotten in health services. It is the dimension that makes the quality concept realistic, since it emphasises making the best use of resources and recognising the waste that exists in all services.[19]

The definition above raises questions about conflicts and ethical issues. As occupational health managers are well aware, there are conflicts between the competing demands of different types of 'customers' – individual patients, client organisation managers, one or more trade unions and possibly the general public. There may also be conflicts between what clients want and what professional assessment shows them to need. Many occupational health services are multiprofessional, so there may be conflicts between different views about which interventions to make.

Ethics is about recognising conflicts and the choices available, and also about using principles to find a satisfactory solution or accommodation. Quality improvement emphasises processes that encourage professionals to be more responsive to clients' wants, without abandoning their professional views. It involves methods for facing conflicts and determining priorities. It emphasises 'client and professional in dialogue' to find a way forward. This can take time in the short term, but will save time in the long run.

A further potential conflict is between the need for efficiency and the need to give time to clients. Experience of quality methods, however, shows that these are not necessarily incompatible. The best quality improvement methods make it possible to improve each aspect of quality at the same time, for example by using process enhancement methods.[20]

Getting personnel interested in quality, however, is rather like raising their interests in ethics. We all like and need to believe that our service is of high quality and ethical. Highlighting quality and ethical weaknesses and issues, but always in the interest and spirit of improvement, is the starting point for change. Managers' experience of implementing changes ethically in their own service gives them greater insight into how changes can be carried out more ethically in the organisations they advise or serve. Then, there is the gain in terms of practical experience on which they and their staff can draw when advising on changes in client organisations.

How can we ensure and improve quality?

Quality improvement is a service in itself; it is a way of fulfilling the ethical principles of avoiding doing harm and helping to do good. Using research is one way to improve quality. The more common approaches can be categorised as follows.

Customer service-based approaches

These include:

- a statement about what patients and users have a right to expect from the service

- user participation, giving feedback about quality, working with providers to make improvements and helping with or carrying out public health interventions
- surveys of patients to discover what they like and do not like about the service, determining priorities for action from these surveys and using problem-solving methods to improve services from patients' perspectives.

Although appropriate for a service in a highly competitive situation, the disadvantages of such approaches are that they neglect professional quality, might not receive support from personnel and often use methods that do not deal with the deep-rooted organisational causes of poor quality.

Standards-based approaches

On these approaches, standards of how to provide effective and safe care are defined and communicated, often as guidelines. Personnel are helped to follow standards through training, job aids and supervision. Where standards are not followed, this is documented and supervisors and managers have responsibility for taking corrective action. In addition, standards are defined for management activities and service performance.

There are three phases to carrying out a standards-based approach:

- develop standards that will ensure effective and safe care that are feasible given the resources available
- implement standards, communicate and supervise the standards, and document where standards are not met
- take corrective action where practice falls below standard, using problem-solving methods.

Many occupational health services adopt this approach, but some do not have systems for the last part of the cycle – corrective action and problem solving. The advantage of the approach is that it is easy to understand. A disadvantage is that such 'top-down' management may not be accepted in the professional cultures of some services. In other services the occupational management and supervision structure might not be strong enough to communicate and uphold standards or there may not be resources for supervision or effective action if practice is below standard. Making it obvious that care is below standard when nothing can be done damages morale and raises anxiety.

The modern approach to quality improvement is to change the ways in which care is organised or service is given and to recognise the organisational causes of poor quality rather than focus on the deficiencies of individual practitioners. This idea is often implemented as described in the sections below.

Assessment- or accreditation-based approaches

These approaches employ a framework that specifies the standards to be met by many aspects of an occupational health service, such as standards for documentation, operating procedures, dealing with complaints, and management and organisation of the service. Examples of such frameworks are the ISO 9000 standard for a quality system[21] and the European Foundation for Quality Management (EFQM) framework.[22]

The approach can be applied by educating personnel in the standards, carrying out a self-assessment and then deciding which areas need most attention. The approach may be just to perform a self-assessment and regular reviews or to use a peer assessment approach and invite colleagues from other occupational health services to use the framework to assess a particular service. In some countries an external and formal assessment or accreditation is necessary for some services or is required by some employers (e.g. according to ISO 9000).

TQM and CQI project-based approaches

Total Quality Management (TQM) and Continuous Quality Improvement (CQI) are organisation-wide approaches to improving quality. They often concentrate on setting up quality problem-solving teams that work on specific problems using simple methods ('quality tools'), which they have been trained to use.[23] The 'plan–do–study–act' cycle to test small changes provides one example. Other examples include a team of occupational health practitioners working on over-prescription of antibiotics or improving medical records.

The main advantage of these approaches is that they allow services to solve prioritised quality problems quickly. They might benefit patients rapidly if their problems are selected by the team. They could also improve personnel morale and pride, and develop professionals' ability to work in teams. The disadvantages are that they may not benefit many patients and affect only a few problem areas; also, teams need time to learn the methods before producing results. Experience elsewhere shows that regular facilitation and management support are needed for the teams to be successful; otherwise, the training and time spent by the team are wasted.

The evidence is that there is not a large difference in effectiveness between different approaches to ensuring and improving service quality, although there are strong supporters of each approach.[24-26] It appears that what is more important is for managers to continue consistently to apply just one approach, and that they adapt it to their local circumstances in collaboration with their personnel.

The quality of an occupational health service is not only the responsibility of each practitioner, but also the responsibility of the manager of the service. The manager is more responsible than anyone else for a poor-quality service that harms patients or fails to help them, and also for a service that fails to alert others to health hazards for workers. An ethical occupational health service is one that is aware of quality, measures quality and works to improve quality. Making more use of research is one way of improving quality, but there are also other methods (such as those entailed by the four sets of approaches noted above). Such activities are practical ways of realising ethical principles in occupational health services.

Conclusion

Managers have an influence on whether practitioners experience ethical practice as being in conflict with other demands or whether ethical practice is a means by which the increasing demands of the service can be met. Managers can also take specific and tangible actions to promote an ethical approach. These include introducing research-informed practice and quality improvement. In this chapter, it is proposed that this will not only support ethical practice but will also help managers to meet their primary responsibility of running an efficient service. Chapter 23 explains how ethics can help occupational health managers in everyday management issues.

References

1 The Scandinavian Simvastatin Survival Study (4S) (1994) Randomised trial of cholesterol lowering in 4444 patients with coronary heart disease. *Lancet.* **344**: 1383–9.

2 Dutta D and Ognunnaike B (2002) Lipid lowering after myocardial infarction in hospital practice. *British Journal of Clinical Governance.* **7**: 154–7.

3 Staal J *et al.* (2002) Return to work interventions for low back pain. *Sports Medicine.* **32**: 251–67.

4   Proper K *et al.* (2002) Effectiveness of physical activity programmes at work-site with respect to work-related outcomes. *Scandinavian Journal of Work Environment and Health.* **2:** 75–84.

5   Proper K *et al.* (2003) Effect of individual counselling on physical activity fitness and health. *American Journal of Preventative Medicine.* **24:** 218–26.

6   Michie S and Williams S (2002) Reducing work related psychological ill health and sickness absence: a systematic literature review. *Occupational and Environmental Medicine.* **60:** 3–9.

7   Rosenberg W and Donald A (1995) Evidence-based medicine: an approach to clinical problem-solving. *British Medical Journal.* **310:** 1122–6.

8   Davids F, Hayes B, Sackett D and Smith R (1995) Evidence based medicine. *British Medical Journal.* **310:** 1086–9.

9   Sackett D, Rosenberg W, Gray J, Haynes R and Scott-Richardson W (1996) Evidence-based medicine: what it is and what it isn't. *British Medical Journal.* **312:** 71–2.

10 Gray M (1997) *Evidence-Based Healthcare.* Churchill Livingstone, London.

11 Dixon S, Booth A and Perrett K (1997) The application of evidence-based priority setting in a district health authority. *Journal of Public Health Medicine.* **19:** 307–12.

12 Black D (1998) The limitations of evidence. *Journal of the Royal College of Physicians of London.* **32:** 23–5.

13 Ministry of Social Affairs and Health Finland and Finnish Institute of Occupational Health (2001) *Good Occupational Health Practice – a guide for planning and follow-up of occupational health services.* FIOH, Helsinki.

14 Norwegian Institute of Occupational Health (2000) *Good Occupational Health Service – workbook with audit matrix.* Oslo. (www.stami.no/hotell/baltic/pdf/OHS00.pdf).

15 WHO/Euro GOHP (2002) *Good Practice in Occupational Health Services – a guide to workplace health.* (www.euro.who.int/document/e77650.pdf).

16 Wensing M and Grol R (1994) Single and combined strategies for implementing changes in primary care: a literature review. *International Journal of Quality Health Care.* **6:** 115–32.

17 McColl A, Smith H, White P *et al.* (1998) General practitioners' perceptions of the route to evidence based medicine: a questionnaire survey. *British Medical Journal.* **316:** 361–5.

18 Bero L, Grilli R, Grimshaw J *et al.* (1998) Closing the gap between research and practice: an overview of systematic reviews of interventions to promote the implementation of research findings. *British Medical Journal.* **317:** 465–8.

19 Øvretveit J (2000) The economics of quality – a practical approach. *International Journal of Health Care Quality Assurance.* **13:** 200–7.

20 Øvretveit J (1992) *Health Service Quality.* Blackwell Scientific Press, Oxford.

21 ISO 10011 (1990) *Guidelines for Auditing Quality Systems.* British Standards Institute, London.

22 EFQM (1992) *The European Quality Award.* European Foundation for Quality Management, Brussels, Belgium.

23 Langly G, Nolan K, Nolan T, Norman C and Provost L (1997) *The Improvement Guide.* Jossey Bass, San Francisco.

24 Walshe K and Freeman T (2002) Effectiveness of quality improvement: learning from evaluations. *Quality and Safety in Health Care.* **11**: 85–7.

25 Øvretveit J and Gustafson D (2003) Evaluation of quality improvement programmes. *British Medical Journal.* **326**: 759–61.

26 Øvretveit J (2002) *Action Evaluation of Health Programmes and Change: a handbook for a user focused approach.* Radcliffe Medical Press, Oxford.

CHAPTER 3

Ethical analysis

Tore Nilstun and John Øvretveit

'Tut, tut, child!' said the Duchess. 'Everything's got a moral, if only you can find it.'

Alice's Adventures in Wonderland (Lewis Carroll, 1832–98)

Most issues in occupational health do not require any sophisticated ethical analysis. The problems are easy to recognise and the solutions often uncontroversial. But some problems give rise to so-called 'ethical conflicts'; that is, situations in which occupational health professionals might feel obliged to take two or more incompatible actions.[1] Occupational health professionals have at least three forms of contact with employees. They are involved in a traditional health professional–patient relationship, are impartial medical examiners reporting to a third party (commonly the employer) and are also research workers. In some situations, there might be conflicts of interest between two or all three roles. Under practical circumstances, however, it is usually not possible to fulfil more than one of these roles at one time. But under all conditions, it is vitally important to make unmistakably clear the particular role assumed by all the stakeholders involved.

The main purpose of this chapter is to describe how ethical conflicts in occupational health may be dealt with in a systematic manner so as to achieve better outcomes. In accordance with this aim, we shall introduce and apply a model for ethical analysis. But first, we make some comments on the concepts of 'ethics' and 'morality' and also say a few words about moral philosophy.

Ethics and morality

There is no general agreement about the definition of the two words *ethics* and *morality*. Moral philosophers, however, usually define *ethics* as 'the philosophical study of morality', whereas *morality* denotes 'the subject matter of ethics'.[2,3] In this sense, ethics is one of the main branches of philosophy – alongside epistemology, logic and metaphysics – whereas morality consists of the conceptions about right and wrong – good and bad, just and unjust – that actually influence the actions of individuals and groups. Accordingly, the morality 'of a person or a group is indicated by their actions'.[4]

But this way of defining *ethics* and *morality* remains controversial. *Ethics* comes from the Greek *ethos*, which means 'having to do with character', whereas *morality* derives from the Latin *mores*, which means 'character or custom and habit'. In everyday language, the two words are often used interchangeably, but they are not quite synonymous. The word *moral* is often used to imply conformity with generally accepted standards of conduct, whereas the word *ethical* implies conformity with an elaborated, ideal code of conduct – specifically with the code of a particular profession.[5]

Since the word *morality* has to do with situations in individuals' private lives, there is a potential conflict between people's private morality and their professional ethics. For example, how much time and resources should occupational health personnel devote to collective health promotion programmes and how much to individual care? Occupational health professionals may adhere to a personal morality that emphasises protecting health and promoting the well-being of the entire population they serve. In practice, this means all personnel in an employing organisation or company. However, the rules of professional ethics may require them to focus on individual employees.

Moral philosophy

It is useful to distinguish between the motive or motives for an act, the act itself, the consequences of the act and the situation in which the act is performed.[6] Indeed, praise or blame is often bestowed on agents depending on whether or not they have the right motives. It is to be observed, though, that motives for an action may be more or less generally held as 'right' within the confines of a community or society. The theory underlying this perspective is sometimes called 'virtue ethics'. Questions such as 'Why did the agent act (or not act) in a particular way?' are answered with reference to motives.

Other moral philosophers adhere to so-called 'deontological ethics' and emphasise the importance of the act itself. They maintain that some acts (or omissions) are right or obligatory, regardless of motives or consequences. The acts themselves differ in such a way that some are right and some are wrong.

There are, however, moral philosophers who question deontological ethics. They maintain that for an action to be right, its consequences must be as good as any other action or set of actions that might have been performed instead. On this position, founded in so-called 'consequential ethics', no other considerations are relevant. For the consequentialist, the ethical value of an act is determined purely by its consequences.

In yet another group, the context or circumstances of an act are of decisive importance. According to the position called 'situation ethics', ethical principles, which usually emphasise an act and its consequences, are only rules of thumb. An ethical actor should be prepared to set them aside, according to the situation he or she happens to be in. The key concepts underlying these four perspectives are illustrated in Figure 3.1.

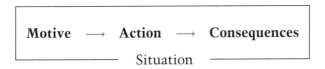

Figure 3.1 Ethical positions as expressed by one or a combination of four perspectives: virtue ethics (motive), deontological ethics (action), consequential ethics (consequences) and situation ethics (situation or context).

But one more distinction is relevant here – that between substantive and procedural issues.[7] Substantive questions are rooted in ethical principles, most of which have their basis in moral philosophy or in religious precepts. Substantive moral questions concern 'What is the ethically right thing to do?'. Procedural questions, by contrast and despite their critical importance when decisions have to be made and actions taken, rarely have a basis in ethical theory. Procedural questions concern 'Who should decide in troubling cases with moral implications?'. Most ethical questions in occupational health have both a substantive and a procedural dimension.

There are many examples of ethical issues in occupational health. They are all more or less directly related to action of some kind. For example, how are medical records to be dealt with? Assuming that informed consent has not been obtained from the patient, should a physiotherapist have access to a patient's case notes? Laws and regulations do not always give a clear answer to questions of this kind. Another set of issues relates to conflicts of interest. If a patient says that her illness is caused by her superior's harassment but the latter describes the patient as incompetent and lazy, how is the professional to deal with this conflict in an impartial way? Or a patient requests sick leave for several months but after a month or two, the occupational health professional concerned feels that the patient is well enough to go back to work. Is honesty always required in such situations?

Problematic ethical situations

There would be no need for ethics if there were no choice. In occupational health practice there are many choices and more-or-less predictable situations that give rise to ethical considerations. Some of these are mentioned in *Guidance on Ethics for Occupational Physicians*.[8]

- The confidentiality of medical information. Managers have no automatic right to know anything of a medically confidential nature about employees. They do have, however, a right to know whether their employees are fit for the purpose for which they are employed.
- The need for informed consent of the subject before the release to others of any information passed in confidence to the occupational health professionals. Consent is only informed if the subject understands what information is being released, the purpose for which it will be used and the possible consequences of that use. Consent must be given freely, under no duress or threat of coercion, and applies only for the time and event for which it is given.
- The extent and scope of the occupational health professional's duty of care towards the employer, the individual and other employees or members of the public, including job applicants.
- The conflicts of interest which may arise over safeguarding the rights of the individual and those of the employers, other employees and the general public.
- The need for care in the handling, storage and transfer of confidential occupational health records, which differs from that needed for clinical records made by other occupational health professionals.
- The need for occupational health professionals to maintain their expertise not only in health sciences and their application, but also in health and safety and in relevant employment legislation, if employers and employees are to be advised effectively.

There are, however, also other situations requiring consideration. Ethical codes cannot prescribe for all situations and even in the ones mentioned above, there are choices within the code about how to act. New situations arise that were not considered or contemplated by the formulators of the code. For example, there have been fundamental changes to the organisation and management of occupational health practice in recent years. Ever fewer healthcare workers are employees of the company to which they provide services. The following example utilises this situation to show how to make an ethical analysis.

A physician working in an occupational health service has been asked to provide medical examinations for new employees in a large company. The employer is enthusiastic. When the physician discusses the idea with the employer and describes the procedure and the service that she could provide, she realises that the employer's interest might be based on unrealistic expectations. He seems to be convinced that health examinations will be able to identify individuals with an increased risk of long-term absence caused by illness.

But the physician doubts very much that pre-employment examinations will be useful in making any such predictions. There may be 'false-positive' results (labelling a healthy person as sick) and 'false-negative' results (labelling a sick person as healthy). Thus, cost-effectiveness for the company is doubtful. Nevertheless, the physician hesitates despite her scepticism. Her occupational health service needs the income; the pre-employment examinations would pay an occupational health professional's salary for several months and she would very much like to return to her superior with a successfully negotiated contract.

To illustrate an ethical analysis, we can pose the question of how specific she should be in stating the doubtful predictive value of pre-employment examinations.

Ethical analysis

Many approaches to such questions have been suggested in the specialised literature. Here, we shall present one model to show how the physician might employ a systematic ethical analysis to help in deciding what to do. The model has two dimensions. The first dimension identifies the different people involved in or affected by the ethical conflict (what are now popularly called the 'stakeholders'). The second dimension formulates the ethical principles to be used as value premises in the ethical analysis. To avoid misunderstanding, it is important to bear in mind that the model, or matrix table, should only be used as a checklist – as an instrument for the identification and analysis of an ethical conflict – not as a decision model.

People involved or affected

The first task is to identify the stakeholders involved in or affected by the ethical conflict. These vary from one situation to another, but in this particular case, with the occupational health professional negotiating with an employer about pre-employment tests, the most important people involved or affected are potential employees, the employer, the negotiating occupational health professional and the management and personnel of the occupational health centre.

Choice of ethical principles

The second task is to identify and formulate relevant ethical principles. These should jointly constitute a set of principles that are intellectually and emotionally satisfying to the people involved or affected in the situation to be analysed. The principles should be 'stable' – in the sense that they do not 'bend' in response to further information (old or new) or to emotional adjustment on the part of any of the stakeholders involved.[9] Several ethical principles are required to satisfy these conditions, but for the purpose of occupational health services, three are sufficient in most cases. These are the principles of 'beneficence', 'autonomy' and 'justice'.

- The principle of *beneficence* entails that all people have an obligation to prevent, avoid and eliminate harm, and to promote good. The infliction of harm on others can only be justified in certain cases by the pursuit of some other value of moral relevance – principally benefits to those involved or affected that are sufficient to outweigh the harm.
- The principle of *autonomy* (or *respect for people*) can mean different things. At an individual level, the principle entails that all people have an obligation to respect others' right to self-determination (to make their own choices and decisions) and to protect people who are dependent or vulnerable. At community or societal levels, the principle gives expression to the arguable democratic requirement that the opinion of the majority should always be considered in an ethical analysis, while those of minorities should not be neglected.
- The principle of *justice* implies both non-discrimination and solidarity. All people have an obligation of equality (non-discrimination), entailing that circumstances such as ability to pay, age, education, ethnicity, nationality and sex are not ethically relevant. Solidarity requires that dependent and vulnerable people have a right or claim to obtain satisfaction of needs if their own searches or efforts fail to achieve this. Justice can also entail equity, meaning that people with different needs are not treated equally according to some general rule that 'all must get the same', but that attention is also paid to recognising and responding to different needs. This is what some refer to as 'fairness'.

The word *justice* is often used to refer to the legal system but – to avoid misunderstanding – the term 'legal justice' should be employed in such a context. From the point of view of beneficence, breaking the law is an ethical cost – at least to the occupational health professional – but it might be of ethical benefit to someone else.

Beneficence, autonomy and justice are three fundamental ethical principles that provide guidance in many situations and they may be regarded as underpinning secondary principles or derivative rules – such as those concerning confidentiality, fidelity, honesty, privacy, trust or veracity. For example, the rule of honesty should be subordinate to the fundamental ethical principle of beneficence; in some cases, telling the truth can be harmful and of little benefit to others. Some of these rules specify a single principle, whereas others specify more than one.

Note that the principle of beneficence is consequential (emphasising what is good and bad for people). The principle of autonomy is deontological (concentrating on self-determination, independent of consequences). The principle of justice is either deontological (when equity is in focus) or consequential (when equality or solidarity is in focus). The fact that issues related to motive and situation are almost invisible in ethical principles and professional guidelines do not entail that such considerations are less important. But it is far more difficult to formulate rules related to motive or situation.

Ethical costs and benefits

The next step in applying the model to a situation is to formulate the alternatives. Ethical analysis only makes sense when alternative choices are compared. If there is only one option or line of action and no choice, there is no need for ethics. The alternatives in the example are whether or not the health professional has an obligation to inform the employer more precisely about the uncertain predictive value of pre-employment examinations. In some situations, there may be more than two options.

The task is to identify the ethical costs and benefits to those involved in or affected by each option. Since the words *benefits* and *costs* are used in a broad sense, some clarification is needed. To identify and assess rightness or wrongness with reference to the principle of beneficence is to determine the good or bad consequences of the alternatives. Within the utilitarian tradition it is usual to refer to 'fulfilment' of the principle of beneficence (i.e. the good consequences) as ethical benefits and 'violation' of the principle (i.e. the bad consequences) as ethical costs.

However, the words *benefits* and *costs* are not commonly used in connection with the principle of autonomy. To assess the costs and benefits of alternatives with reference to this principle is not to determine any good or bad consequences. The rightness or wrongness of alternatives is assessed with reference to the obligation to respect the right to self-determination of the persons involved or affected (no matter what the consequences might be). In order to facilitate comparison in this context, however, the term 'ethical costs' will be used to denote violations of the principle of autonomy and the term 'ethical benefits' to denote its fulfilment. In the same way, we will refer to violations of the principle of justice as 'ethical costs' and cases of its fulfilment as 'ethical benefits'.

Application of the model

Here, we will employ the model simply as a checklist. A matrix of 12 cells (A–L) represents combinations of four groups of people and three ethical principles (Table 3.1). Later chapters will illustrate the utility of this simple model in practical situations.

Table 3.1 Combinations of four groups of people and three ethical principles, used as a checklist for ethical analysis of proposed pre-employment tests

People involved or affected	Ethical principles		
	Beneficence	Autonomy	Justice
Possible employees	A	E	I
The employer	B	F	J
The occupational health professional	C	G	K
People at the occupational health service	D	H	L

The principle of beneficence

First, we will apply the principle of *beneficence* (columns A–D in Table 3.1). To go through a pre-employment test is an 'ethical cost' to most people who want a job. Note that in some countries, for example Denmark, the law prohibits such tests. Here, we will assume that the occupational health professional is not in a country that bans the test. Also, if the employer is informed and understands that the tests are not cost-effective, they are unlikely to be carried out in any case. Thus, for the employer it would be an 'ethical benefit' to be informed. In the short run, however, honesty would probably be a disadvantage – both to the occupational health professional and to other people in the occupational health service in question. New contracts are needed to continue the business. In the long run, the benefits are more doubtful. When the employer understands that his expectations are unrealistic, his relation to the occupational health professional in particular, and the occupational health service in general, is likely to be negatively affected. Thus, we have clarified some of the issues but, as yet, there is no clear indication concerning what action to take.

The principle of autonomy

According to the principle of *autonomy* (columns E–H in Table 3.1), the preferences of all stakeholders should be taken into account. It is not difficult to say what the employees would prefer in this case. Most of them would reject any pre-employment test. However, they are probably not informed about specific plans for the test. The employer would like to be adequately informed. As regards the occupational health professional and her colleagues in the unit, it is difficult to guess their preferences. We imagine that their opinions would be divided. A difficult financial situation may also negatively affect the occupational health professional's willingness to check with the employer whether or not he has understood all the relevant information and drawn reasonable conclusions.

The principle of justice

In performing an ethical analysis it is best to stick to the two simple requirements of the principle of justice (columns I–L in Table 3.1) – namely, no discrimination and solidarity. It might be argued that pre-employment tests (to avoid future sick leave) could lead to discrimination against some job applicants. But equally important is that occupational health professionals also have an obligation to show some solidarity with vulnerable groups in society. Accepting participation in such tests seems to be inconsistent with this obligation – to the extent that job applicants assessed to have health shortcomings or defects are rejected on these grounds. The principle of justice, as an ethical principle (of fairness), is scarcely relevant to the others involved in this particular situation. However, interpreted as 'legal justice', it may well be.

Standards of intersubjectivity when balancing ethical costs and benefits

All costs are not equally serious and all benefits are not equally important. Some costs may be so serious that they outweigh minor benefits to other people or vice versa. However, our approach thus far has been simple, descriptive and analytic, and the ambition has been to meet a minimal standard of intersubjectivity. This entails that competent people, asking the same questions and using similar methods, should reach similar conclusions. Choosing ethical principles and using a checklist to identify ethical costs and benefits to stakeholders are intersubjective in this sense. But when costs and benefits are to be ordered with respect to degree, implying a quantitative assessment, it is more difficult to satisfy the requirement of intersubjectivity.

This does not imply, however, that ethical principles are useless. To the contrary, there are two important benefits in formulating such principles and in identifying – on the basis of these principles – the ethical costs and benefits to those involved or affected. Such an approach increases understanding of the alternatives and their probable consequences. It also counteracts the human tendency to 'forget' ethical costs or benefits. Our ability to provide an unbiased assessment of counter-arguments is easily lost if we believe that the right solution to an ethical conflict has been found.

We need to emphasise also that any attempt to solve ethical conflicts hinges on both personal values and factual assumptions. Different people may come to different views about what physicians ought to do because people have different values (especially on how they should be balanced in a particular situation). Also, some of the factual assumptions (especially those related to the consequences of providing information) are questionable. This means that the requirement of intersubjectivity is often not satisfied in an ethical analysis. Competent people, facing the same ethical conflict and using similar methods to solve that conflict, do not always reach similar conclusions.

It is, in this example, reasonable to assume that the long-term effects of giving supplementary information to the employer will probably determine the issue. The employer has to be more fully informed. Such a choice of alternative also finds support in *Guidance on Ethics for Occupational Physicians*[8] and in the *International Code of Ethics for Occupational Health Professionals*.[10] The former states that 'employers and employees have a right to competent and complete advice: failure to provide appropriate and timely advice is as reprehensible as providing poor and incorrect advice'. The latter requires that 'the objectives and the details of health surveillance must be clearly defined', and that employer and employees should be informed. However, both guidelines also emphasise a duty to safeguard the health of workers. But this latter aim, at least in this case, can scarcely be used to justify a violation of the former requirement.

Concluding remarks

Professional guidelines on ethics for occupational health professionals are sufficient in many situations. The choice between options is obvious and the decision is taken more or less routinely without any ethical analysis. But this is not always the case. Where there are ethical conflicts, a more systematic ethical analysis is necessary, and performing such an analysis also has the advantage of sensitising us to ethical issues in all situations. One way of doing this is to make the basic ethical principles of beneficence, autonomy and justice explicit, to identify stakeholders and to try to map out the ethical costs and benefits. There is no guarantee that the best solution as seen from the vantage point of professional ethics will be arrived at in this way, but the approach will help to identify and reject ethically unacceptable courses of action.

References

1 Gowans CW (ed.) (1987) *Moral Dilemmas*. Oxford University Press, Oxford.

2 Moll A (1902) *Ärztliche Ethik. Die Pflichten des Arztes in allen Beziehungen seiner Thätigkeit*. Verlag von Ferdinand Enke, Stuttgart.

3 Sumner WG (1907) *Folkways. A study of the sociological importance of usages, manners, customs, mores, and morals*. Ginn and Company, Boston.

4 Hermerén G (1996) Ethics, epidemiology, and the role of ethics experts. *Nordic Journal of Psychiatry*. **50** (Suppl. 36): 5–14.

5   *Webster's New World Dictionary of the American Language* (1970) The World Publishing Company, New York.

6 Beauchamp TL and Childress JF (1979) *Principles of Biomedical Ethics*. Oxford University Press, Oxford.

7 Macklin R (1987) *Mortal Choices. Ethical dilemmas in modern medicine*. Houghton Mifflin, New York.

8 Faculty of Occupational Medicine of the Royal College of Physicians (1999) *Guidance on Ethics for Occupational Physicians* (5e). Royal College of Physicians, London.

9 Halldén S (1995) *A Socratic Approach to Morality*. Thales, Stockholm.

10 International Commission on Occupational Health (1996) *International Code of Ethics for Occupational Health Professionals*. ICOH, Geneva.

CHAPTER 4

The ethics of risk assessment

Kit Harling

Risk assessment

The process of risk assessment, that is, an attempt to estimate the likelihood of an adverse outcome if a specified course of action is followed, is inherent in all human activity, not only in respect of tasks undertaken in the course of work. The concept of risk assessment is not new. The hunter gatherer of prehistoric times had to consider the risk to himself when hunting large animals capable of harming the hunter, and the wider population was at risk if poisonous berries were mistakenly gathered for the evening meal.

The term 'risk assessment', as used in contemporary occupational health, is to some extent misleading. The term implies not merely an assessment or attempted quantification of the risk, but the concept incorporates elements of managing the risk by risk reduction processes and consideration of the tolerability of the residual risk. Above all, the process of risk assessment in the workplace is meant to be a guide to action. No activity can ever be risk free and, in our societies, risk assessment is generally about making judgements as to whether or not to accept a given level of risk. Effectively, the question is whether or not the risk is low enough to be acceptable to the risk-taker specifically, other persons who may be affected by the work activity and society more generally.

Risk tolerance and acceptance

The level at which a risk is tolerable to an individual varies with a variety of factors. Although the precise numerical value of the probability of the adverse event occurring cannot be given in all circumstances, an estimate based on experience or calculation can be provided in most cases. Consideration of the mathematical magnitude of the risk is combined with the concept of voluntariness of the risk, immediacy of the adverse consequence and easy identification of an individual or body who might be blamed for the adverse event. It is this combination that forms the basis of the individual's judgement of what is acceptable. A dread factor, incorporating ideas of horror of the particular nature of the adverse outcome (large numbers killed at once, lingering or unpleasant death, etc.) may also substantially affect the judgement of what is acceptable and what is not. Where no reasonable estimate of risk can be given, for example with exposure to a radically new chemical substance, further uncertainty is added to the consideration; uncertainty itself is normally an adverse factor for most people

These factors are seen at work in two very different examples of risk taking. A mathematically large individual risk, which is accepted by those who smoke cigarettes, may be contrasted with the lack of acceptability for many of a low mathematical risk of injury arising from residence near to a nuclear power plant. Even within similar human activities such as transport, perceptions of risk and the acceptability of that risk are rarely based solely on the mathematical description of experience and vary markedly between different modes of travel.

Acceptance of a particular level of risk begs the question of 'acceptable to whom?'. Decisions about what is an acceptable risk for an individual are not taken in isolation. A smoker does not make his decision in an abstract setting; rather, his decision is strongly influenced by the addictive nature of tobacco smoke. It is rare for the harm arising from the adverse event to be manifest solely in the individual. Family and colleagues may be directly influenced by the harm, and society – to which we all contribute – may be called upon to rectify the harm.

In our societies, judgements about the acceptability of risk levels are often institutionalised by governments; regulatory authorities are established to set 'acceptable levels'. The courts, by their decisions, set a framework for such considerations. Internationally, explicit accident-risk levels are used in the design of aircraft and aviation operating systems; and, in the UK, the Health and Safety Executive (HSE) has published a document[1] setting out how to approach the decisions about the management of risk that are required under health and safety legislation, including explicit numerical examples. This includes the differing tolerability of levels of risk to general classes of people, such as 'people at work' and the 'general population'.

These then are the essentially pragmatic guidelines against which tolerability of risk is judged on a practical, day-to-day level. What, however, does the study of ethics tell us about the process of risk assessment? Does the ethical approach commonly accepted, in our societies at least, support the pragmatic outcomes produced by the application of our health and safety legislation?

Ethical theory and principles

Ethics is a generic term for various ways of understanding and examining the moral life. The term morality refers to social conventions about right and wrong human conduct that are so widely shared that they form a stable (although usually incomplete) communal conscience.[2]

Thus, a study of ethics and the application of ethical theory should provide action guides for human behaviour. Therefore, consideration of ethical theories and their application to the work environment should help us in the practical application of risk assessment in various settings.

The application of ethics to healthcare work – usually termed 'biomedical ethics' – is not an entirely abstract issue, but nor is it unchanging dogma. Whilst there is a strong logical and academic base to the study of biomedical ethics, the practical application of such ethics ought to build upon a consensus from within the society, expressed by democratically elected government. This leads to laws, professional rules of behaviour and collective agreements, which in turn can be analysed in an ethical manner, leading to a complete cycle of development

There are many competing ethical theories that may be applied to the study of biomedical ethics. This chapter is not the place to describe each theory in full and debate their strengths and weaknesses. Readers interested in a more general discussion and critical analysis of ethical theories as applied in the biomedical field are referred initially to the account by Beauchamp and Childress.[2] See also the British Medical Association overview of 1993[3] and Campbell.[4]

Here, we will base our analysis on the common morality-based ethical values that use three (or possibly four) main principles or shared moral beliefs. These were considered in detail in Chapter 3.

Respect for the *autonomy* of an individual has been at the centre of medical ethics for decades. This is more easily seen within the traditional treatment aspect of healthcare. Here, it is accepted that competent adults have the right, for example, to decline treatment even where that decision may cause them serious harm or even death. There is no doubt in English law that followers of the Jehovah's Witness church may decline a blood transfusion even though their death may result.

A further ethical principle, possibly better described as two closely related ethical principles, is that physicians should do no harm (*non-maleficence*)

and should do good for their patients (*beneficence*). The principle is commonly applied in a healthcare context and can readily be identified in the Hippocratic Oath. It or they remain fundamental to the modern delivery of healthcare.

Lastly, the concept of *justice*, or more properly of distributive justice, involves the ideas of fairness and the equitable distribution of both rights and responsibilities within a society. The emergence of the importance of this principle is a relatively modern development compared with the acceptance of the previous two. It allows us to balance the rights of the individual, which are to some extent pre-eminent in our society, with corresponding responsibilities when analysing biomedical ethical issues.

These principles are further illuminated or specified by ethical rules such as truthfulness, privacy, fidelity and confidentiality. For example, health professionals are expected to be honest in what they say and do. In many societies, higher standards of behaviour are expected of doctors than the general public. Although there may be a pragmatic justification for such rules, they are still founded in ethical analysis. Thus, these rules help us in the application of the principles to practical activity, and hence to derive moral action guides from our shared moral principles.

Let us consider a relatively simple risk assessment.

Case 4.1: a simple risk assessment and ethical analysis

An individual is working in a factory and is required to handle a substance containing one of the isocyanate group of chemicals in such a way that his airway is exposed to the active ingredient. A risk assessment is required and the occupational health team is called in.

The team considers the work involved, the chemicals handled and the nature of the exposure. After discussion with the workforce, the occupational health hygienist lists the appropriate environmental measurements. The results are reviewed by the team with a view to making a recommendation to the company and its staff.

In this case, there are clear, explicit standards of permitted exposure that have been set by the regulatory authority to protect employees from developing occupational asthma. Indeed, so overwhelming is the evidence linking respiratory exposure to isocyanate to the development of occupational asthma[5] that the process of risk assessment may be thought of as being largely mechanical. After all the necessary control measures have been put in place, exposure to isocyanate is measured in an appropriate way. Should this exposure exceed a predetermined level, set by the regulatory authority, the work activity may not continue. See also recent guidance on management of occupational asthma given by Snashall[6] and Sym[7] in 2003.

We must, however, question the assumptions. Does the application of an exposure limit protect all individuals in all circumstances? The duration of the sample collection may mask excursions of isocyanate concentration over short periods that may pose a risk to workers. The exposure standard must be written with these factors in mind, and the importance of the competence of the risk assessor cannot be stressed too highly. Individual variations in susceptibility may mean that not all workers are protected; concentrations of isocyanate below the level of detection may be harmful to some people. The work environment on the day the measurements were taken may not be representative. Thus, even an apparently simple risk assessment may not be entirely straightforward.

The occupational health professional wishes procedures to be put in place to protect the health of the worker; unnecessary restriction on work practices that are not required for health protection, or banning the work altogether, will prevent workers from earning a living. The risk assessment and the action that will flow from it need to be balanced against the interests of the players involved: the workers and the factory owner. The ethical analysis provides a way to balance the interests of the parties. The fact that the evidence base for the link between exposure to isocyanates and the development, in some people, of occupational asthma is so overwhelming makes it easy to conclude that an ethical consideration is not required. However, the relative simplicity of this risk assessment makes it useful to test out our ethical principles in a circumstance where the pragmatic answer is clear.

At first consideration, the disadvantage – developing occupational asthma – and the high likelihood of this disadvantage being expressed in the presence of excess exposure to the chemical mean that the principle of doing no harm is such as to render consideration of the other principles unnecessary.

However, it is of interest to examine the application of the principle of respect for autonomy to the factory worker; the worker, as an autonomous individual, apparently has the right to choose whether or not to be exposed. Although we may say that the risk of developing occupational asthma is unacceptable, the worker has, under our system of ethical values, the right to act autonomously, making his own choice. In this case, if we say that at a particular level of exposure, the work must stop, do we deny the worker the ethical right of respect for his autonomy? Under this principle he could validly argue that he wished to do his work without the necessary protection. Although it may be difficult for a rational occupational health physician to conceive of circumstances where such a view would be held, the ethical principle of respect for autonomy does not allow for the paternalistic judgement that the worker cannot come to this view because a second party, the occupational health physician, finds the outcome illogical.

This is not to say that the denial of this principle of respect for autonomy is unarguable, but suggests that more careful consideration of what is meant by the term 'autonomy' is required. As we have seen earlier, application of the principle of respect for autonomy is very powerful in other areas of biomedical ethics. However, we can argue that what is meant by respect for autonomy or, put another way, freedom of autonomous action is that agents, or workers, while exercising this principle, act *intentionally*, with *understanding* and *without any controlling influence* over them.

In our particular case, the worker, choosing not to avail himself of protection, can clearly be seen to be acting intentionally. Assuming that he is conscious and competent, the oral expression of his wish is sufficient to satisfy this point. The question of whether he understands the decision he is making is more difficult to address. The subprinciple of acting with understanding does not mean that we must agree with the conclusion at which the worker arrives; rather, it only entails that the individual can collect evidence that has been provided in an intelligible way, can hold the information long enough to form a decision, and can adequately express that decision. This is a very similar principle to the concept of 'competence' used in UK law, which deals with the ability of an individual to make decisions autonomously about treatment options. Autonomous individuals are able to make their decisions for what others may consider good reasons, bad reasons or, indeed, no discernible reasons at all.

It is, however, in the area of freedom from controlling influences that the principle of respect for autonomy is most vulnerable in dealing with this scenario. It has long been recognised that there is a great disparity between the power and influence of an individual workers and their employers. Indeed, in nineteenth century English Common Law the term used to describe the relationship between an employer and employee was 'the master–servant relationship'. It is also a matter of common experience for occupational health professionals that in many circumstances the discussions and decisions reached between employers and employees are not as between two equal agents.

Hence, if we accept the condition that autonomous acts should be made without any external controlling influence, and that the relationship between the worker and the employer is unequal, the importance in the ethical analysis of the principle of respect for the autonomy of the worker is modified by the extra power or 'controlling influence' wielded by an employer in a free employment labour market. This must be reflected in the balancing of principles that is required in the conduct of an ethical analysis.

Let us now consider a more complicated risk assessment.

Case 4.2: a complicated risk assessment and ethical analysis

A new factory has been built and the occupational health team has been asked to contribute to a risk assessment for the proposed removal of the lining of a kiln as part of regular routine maintenance. The lining is made of refractory ceramic fibres and it is anticipated that the work will generate airborne fibres. The work is physically demanding and commercial pressures mean that the company has offered a bonus to employees if the work is completed quickly. Wearing cumbersome personal protective equipment will slow down the work.

Data from other plants owned by the company suggest that the work will generate dust levels just below the current exposure limit set many years ago by the national regulatory authority. However, the occupational health professionals are aware that the regulatory authority is currently considering tightening the limit. If the proposed changes were put in place, the proposed work would produce exposure levels well above the new standard.

It is considered that the fibres may cause cancer, but there is no direct evidence for carcinogenicity in humans. Some evidence from the USA suggests an increased prevalence of pleural plaques, related to the duration of exposure, in workers. Some animal experiments in rats show the development of both lung cancer and mesothelioma, but the significance of the data is disputed. The substance has been designated a Category 2 carcinogen.

The workers are exposed to a substance that has been categorised as a potential carcinogen on the basis of animal experiments,[8] but the work – using existing controls – will produce exposures within the existing maximum exposure limit. The work may legally be carried out and there is pressure on the workforce to get the work done quickly, with the promise of a large bonus if the work is completed quickly. The occupational health physician must review the evidence and produce a view for the company and its employees.

The ethical problem for the occupational health physician remains balancing the ethical rights of the stakeholders – the workers and the factory owners. Harm may affect one of them because of the actions of the other, but they both have an interest in seeing the work take place, albeit for their own reasons. The dilemma for the occupational health professional is that, in this case, there is great uncertainty around the information with which his team has to work (much more so than in Case 4.1). The factory owner can argue that he is legally entitled to undertake the work in the way suggested, and that such work is within currently accepted norms. But, for the occupational health physician, additional information does exist, even if the bureaucracy of the regulatory authority has not been able to turn this information into concrete standards.

There is inevitably considerable uncertainty in the meaning of the research data. Interpreting animal data and applying it to human experience is fraught with difficulty. People find dealing with uncertainty difficult and it is in this area that the expertise of occupational health physicians is most useful for the two stakeholders in Case 4.2. It is the role of the physician to produce a coherent and intelligible opinion that is free of bias towards one party or other; indeed, this is a professional duty.

The rules that we identified earlier in this chapter, which specify the ethical principles, aid occupational health physicians in the practical process of risk assessment. Thus, if the risk assessment is to be valid and acceptable, the physician will observe the rules of truthfulness and fidelity when dealing with both the worker and the employer. How then will the application of the main principles help in this task?

Looking at our first principle, *respect for autonomy*, which in the ethical analysis for Case 4.1 was reduced in importance because of the external 'controlling influence' inherent in the worker–employer relationship, is now further challenged because the requirement that the worker makes his decision 'with understanding' is also not met in Case 4.2.

There is uncertainty about the level of hazard of the substance and the occupational health physician cannot therefore give a clear explanation of the consequences of the proposed exposure. Any explanation must necessarily include a discussion of the uncertainties of experiments and the difficulty of extrapolating animal data to humans. A cursory examination of the literature and the different positions taken by the various protagonists shows the difficulty of putting the arguments into lay terms, let alone the problems of coming to a clear view of the evidence.

As with the analysis in Case 4.1, we must consider the relative weight to be given to the principle of autonomy for the different stakeholders. The principle of autonomy is specified by the requirements for the autonomous agent to act intentionally, with understanding, and without external controlling influences. In Case 4.2, the worker is unable to act with complete understanding because of the inherent uncertainty of the information. This is not to say that the occupational health physician should refuse to provide an opinion that workers can use to inform their decision. Indeed, the physician acting in this case, being best placed by his training to weigh up the competing arguments, must seek to produce a reasoned report. However, the uncertainty surrounding the opinion of risk must be stated explicitly.

Ethical analysis must lead to action, and uncertainty cannot be allowed to lead to paralysis. Some view of the evidence must be taken, and formulated into a recommendation, before an ethical analysis of the guidance given by the occupational health team can be performed.

There are many examples of uncertainty in occupational health practice and the 'precautionary principle' has been developed to help deal with such circumstances. Put simply, where there is uncertainty about the risk of harm to health, decision-makers should err on the side of caution and act to prevent potential risks to health. This principle, which is not a moral principle in itself, derives from consideration of the principle of non-maleficence – an expression of the Hippocratic injunction of 'firstly, do no harm'. It is widely accepted in European and North American societies – though interpretation varies, particularly amongst lobby groups. From a philosophical point of view, certainty about the future can never be proved. It can then be argued that such lack of certainty means that the precautionary principle should be applied on all occasions to every new development. Indeed, it can be misused to prevent all change if applied as an over-riding 'moral imperative'. However, as we have seen above, it is not an over-arching ethical principle in its own right but rather a development of one of the three (or four) main ethical values used in analysis. Its benefit is that it assists in weighing the evidence where uncertainty exists and ethical analysis is required

The ethical principle of doing good or 'beneficence' relates to the whole range of 'goods' that may emerge from the work activity. Thus, the worker has a job and earns a living, which is in itself a valuable good; the proposed work offers an increase in this good. The company in its turn is carrying on a business, offering employment and a return on money invested by its shareholders. Assuming that the company is successful and survives, and that markets are found for its product, society obtains a 'good' in the shape of economic activity. There are, therefore, *a priori* goods arising from the work activity that must be taken into account when applying ethical principles to the process of risk assessment, and the formulation by the occupational health physician of his report and recommendations. It cannot be the case that a simplistic, one-dimensional and often paternalistic view of the term 'doing good' gives a complete answer to the ethical dilemmas of physicians.

The principle of doing no harm or 'non-maleficence' is not simply the converse of the principle of doing good; the two often exist at the same. For the worker, the potential harm to health exists at the same time as the 'good' of having a job and receiving money. This dichotomy is not confined to the worker. The good for the company of having the work done with the minimum interruption to production may be balanced by the harm of future compensation claims if the current evidence does lead to a tightening of the exposure standard. Hence, the principles of doing good and doing no harm must be applied to all stakeholders in Case 4.2 without the use of *a priori* moral-sounding judgements.

The ethical principle of distributive 'justice' must also be considered, and in this case is particularly helpful. This principle requires that both the benefits and disadvantages of a particular course of action should be fairly distributed amongst the various parties. This principle would seem to be violated in Case 4.2 as the risks fall largely on the workers, whereas benefits are unequally shared amongst the different agents (worker, employer, shareholder) and society as a whole. The maldistribution of benefits and harms strongly suggests that the proposal to allow the work to continue would be inconsistent with a proper ethical analysis.

Thus, the application of our ethical principles does help guide us in making our risk assessment. In practical terms, it is very rarely the case that the risk of exposure to a chemical is completely unknown. Some testing will almost certainly have taken place, and judgements based on the nature and structure of the chemical can help us to decide on the likelihood of risk to human health.

However, the ethical principles help us to judge that information and suggest that only a low level of risk to the worker's health should be considered acceptable in these circumstances.

Discussion

Who should define the acceptability of a given risk? Where the risk is only taken by one person it might be reasonable to accept that the individual decides what is acceptable or not to him or her. Thus, the decision to accept a hazardous treatment, a question debated in traditional biomedical ethics, is clearly seen as belonging to individuals themselves.

For reasons illustrated given above, in the workplace it is rare for a risk to affect just one person, and for that person to be able to act autonomously. In the more complicated scenario we have described (Case 4.2), for example, it is clear that there are many stakeholders in the decision-making process.

In Western societies there are usually mechanisms for such decisions to be made. Regulatory authorities are established, with the legislature (Parliament) at least setting the boundaries of acceptable risk. Courts or other government bodies offer more precise advice in specific circumstances. What is clear is that the decision about the acceptability of risk is not one for occupational health practitioners or indeed any scientific specialists. The decision is one for all those involved and for society in general.

Occupational health professionals may say, under similar circumstances, that in the past a risk has been found acceptable. But occupational health professionals must, in fact, guard against saying, or appearing to say, from their professional position, that a particular risk is (or is not) acceptable. They should confine themselves to carrying out competent risk assessments.

The application and enforcement of risk assessment are not uniform throughout the world. Prevailing ethical principles vary considerably. Application of ethical theories, such as utilitarianism or communitarianism, to the performance of a risk assessment may produce very different answers.

A utilitarian would hold that an action is to be considered right or wrong simply on the basis of the sum of good or bad consequences for society. Thus, any action should produce an excess of good over evil. Although there are many types of utilitarian theory, one of the consequences of this approach is to deny the central role of the individual. It may be concluded that a course of action is right or 'moral' if it produces benefit for the majority in a society, even if an individual (say, a worker) is damaged by the process. Thus, workers would be expected to accept a risk for the benefit of management and society in general. It is the latter who draw the benefits from, but do not share, the taking of risk.

The communitarian would argue that a risk assessment should be judged in terms of communal values, whereby concepts of the common good and social goals would have a much higher priority in determining its outcome. Again, the individual position would be compromised if the community determined the 'correct' outcome of the risk assessment simply on the basis of the majority view. Such 'dictatorship of the majority' is evident in a number of societies, at least in some behavioural respects.

The approach to risk assessment in Europe is generally based on the prevalent ethical principles within our society. We can see that they give ethical and moral support for our day-to-day practical approach.

References

1 HSE (2001) *HSE's Decision-making Process: reducing risks, protecting people.* HMSO, London.

2 Beauchamp TL and Childress JF (2001) *Principles of Biomedical Ethics* (5e). Oxford University Press, New York.

3 British Medical Association (1993) *Medical Ethics Today: its practice and philosophy.* BMA, London.

4 Campbell AV (2001) *Medical Ethics*. Oxford University Press, New York.

5 Chan-Yeung M and Malo JL (1995) Occupational asthma. *New England Journal of Medicine*. **333**: 107–12.

6 Snashall D (2003) Occupational asthma – another fresh start in the UK (editorial). *Occupational and Environmental Medicine*. **60**: 711–12.

7 Sim M (2003) The continuing challenge to reduce the burden of occupational asthma – what is the best approach? *Occupational and Environmental Medicine*. **60**: 713–14.

8 IARC (2002) *Man-made Vitreous Fibres*. IARC monographs on the evaluation of carcinogenic risk to humans, no. 82. IARC, Lyon.

CHAPTER 5

The ethics of workplace intervations

Peter Hasle and Hans Jørgen Limborg

'Who are you?' said the Caterpillar.
This was not an encouraging opening for a conversation. Alice replied, rather shyly,
'I – I hardly know, Sir, just at present – at least I know who I was when I got up this
morning, but I think I must have been changed several times since then.'

Alice's Adventures in Wonderland (Lewis Carroll, 1832–98)

The most important objective of the occupational health service is the prevention of health risks in the workplace. But several other objectives can also be listed. The term 'prevention' in this context implies that something is changed in the workplace in order to avoid hazards from giving rise to health damage. Possible changes cover a huge spectrum ranging from more traditional technical prevention, such as ear protectors, safety screens and dust extraction, through to more extensive changes to technology and work organisation, such as substitution of hazardous chemicals and machines and the introduction of group organisation and skills development.

The traditional health-based occupational health service had its point of departure in medical check-ups of employees and subsequent advice to individuals and employers. The workplace was rarely visited and it was seldom that advice on preventive measures related to medical check-ups was relayed to employers. But, in recent decades, many – albeit not all – countries have experienced a tendency to expand the preventive activities of occupational health services. The Netherlands may provide an example of the counter-tendency. (*See* Chapters 8 and 9.) Nevertheless, the expansion that has taken place has gone in two directions, first broadening competencies in occupational health services in terms of including new professions, such as hygienists, safety engineers, ergonomists and psychologists. The second concerns involvement in the workplace. It has become ever more an integrated part of occupational health service duties to work closely with management and employees on the development and implementation of suitable preventive measures. In this way occupational health professionals have become agents of change.[1]

The ethical dimension has a major role to play in such development. Occupational health professionals have to take an interest in what their advice is being used for. It is, for example, not satisfactory from an ethical point of view to give best professional advice if such advice is not going to be used for preventive action of any kind. The reasons for not adopting advised proposals can be manifold. Maybe the recipient (management and/ or employees) does not understand the advice; maybe the advice is regarded as unrealistic from a technical point of view; maybe it is considered to be costly; or maybe it challenges the position of certain subgroups in the workplace. Whatever the reason, the logical consequence is that the occupational health professionals get involved in an attempt to secure practical preventive outcomes.

In turn, such involvement raises several concerns. First, new competencies on the part of various categories of occupational health professionals are required. It is no longer enough for occupational health physicians or ergonomists to have thorough knowledge in a specific field. It is also necessary for them to be qualified in how to control or manage change processes within an organisation. Such supplementary qualifications are multidisciplinary and require familiarity with organisation theory, group behaviour, project management and – not least – business economics. Further, there is the strategic requirement of being able to understand the goals and plans of the organisation. Finally, some basic qualifications regarding other occupational health service-relevant professions are demanded. It would not be helpful for either employers or employees for an ergonomist to introduce measures to prevent repetitive strain injury (RSI) while giving rise to an elevated risk of unintentional injury or stress.

The demand for new competencies has become an ethical issue for occupational health services. When are occupational health professionals sufficiently qualified to manage control processes and to understand what is important with regard to the practice of other professions? They can never acquire the same qualifications as a trained process consultant or a degree in another occupational health field. Nevertheless, practitioners will have to act to the best of their knowledge and qualifications.

Another important question concerns the extent to which best possible advice can or should be altered or the extent to which occupational health professionals should accept a compromise in order to ensure practical application. Most will accept shift work on the part of their clients, even though the health risk of this is well documented; accordingly, they will give advice to an employer on how to introduce shift work in the least harmful way. But, is it also acceptable to propose job rotation as a means of preventing RSI, even though occupational health professionals are well aware that real causes are not addressed and that the effects of job rotation are questionable?

Basically, workplace intervention will inevitably result in the 'dirtying of hands'. Occupational health professionals will be involved in processes in the workplace that they – even with the very best qualifications – can control to only a very limited extent. Quite often, the mandate provided in the workplace (typically by the employer) is narrower, in terms of priorities and economic resources, than desired from a professional point of view. In such a case, it can be difficult for occupational health professionals to take the necessary actions. Even if a broad mandate is provided, actors in the workplace may use the advice for purposes other than those intended or introduce other changes that remove the impact of the change or even worsen the situation. But nor is the alternative to involvement ethically acceptable. Occupational health professionals cannot be indifferent to the effect their advice is having on the workplace. When they know that certain hazards have to be prevented, they must be under an obligation to work for implementation of preventive measures to the best of their ability.

Two case histories may illustrate some of the ethical dilemmas in workplace intervention. The stories come from Denmark and are based on the Danish occupational health system, which is quite different from systems in many other European countries. Before the case histories, therefore, the Danish system will briefly be described.

The Danish occupational health service

The Danish occupational health service was developed at the beginning of the 1980s. Pursuant to legal requirements, it is now organised in occupational health service centres covering regions or specific branches of industry. The centres are non-profit organisations, with equal representation of employers and employees on their boards of directors. Certain business sectors – including manufacturing industry, construction, restaurants and hotels, and public welfare and health – are required to affiliate to an occupational health service centre and buy 0.6 hours of service per employee each year.

In Denmark, there was an initial emphasis on a specific professional approach designed to favour technical prevention. Accordingly, personnel were selected from engineers, physiotherapists, ergonomists and even architects. The aim was to cure the workplace, not the worker! But from the mid-1990s, psychologists and various professionals with degrees in organisation were included among occupational health personnel. At first, the demand for services in work psychology and organisation came from the public, social and health sectors, but nowadays Danish occupational health units provide preventive services to many industries with regard to both technical and psychosocial issues.

As a result of the European Union framework directive, the implementation of workplace assessments (referred to as risk assessments in most other countries) has played a key role in the relation between companies and occupational health services. The occupational health service in Denmark has been characterised by a diversity of approaches to workplace assessment. Development has included a strong emphasis on adaptation of methodology to concrete local context, and Danish legislation makes only few demands with regard to the specific form any workplace assessment should take.[2] It can be argued that workplace assessment focuses more on involvement of the actors within a company and on local commitment than it does on scientifically documented methodology and analysis. And, of course, such a situation creates problems for occupational health professionals. We will return to this point in the first case we describe.

In the late 1990s a system of quality certification for the Danish occupational health service was established, and the definition of quality was further reinforced through a revision of legislation in 2001. It is now required that each advisory task focuses on concrete preventive improvement, has an integrated approach and supports local empowerment. Such requirements highlight the possibility of establishing trusting and respectful co-operation between parties within a company, even before occupational health personnel activate their own professional knowledge.

Thus, there is a potential ethical dilemma in terms of what might go wrong if there is an imbalance in the relation between the judgement of the occupational health professionals and clients' ability and willingness to understand and implement improvement. Such an imbalance can be provoked if consultants – in order to gain at least some response from a company – bring up a proposal that is not based upon solid professional knowledge but, more or less, just rephrases what the company has been able to think up itself. Further, consultants must be able to foresee at what time in the development process support from the occupational health professional will be needed. Early feedback may close the eyes of company actors to problems that will arise later, for example when implementing new technology or work organisation. In order to prevent future occupational health service problems and to make improvements sustainable, occupational health professionals must facilitate the learning process. This will always be a part of any process of change and will ensure that health and safety considerations are integrated into the ongoing management of change and development.

Case 5.1: workplace assessment in a hospital laboratory

The first case history takes place in the laboratory of a hospital during the implementation of workplace assessment for the first time.[3] Danish implementation of the European Union framework directive has made it mandatory for all enterprises in Denmark to identify hazards, set risk priorities, prepare action plans and follow up any implementations. Enterprises are free to select any method as long as the four phases outlined above are followed and employees are involved. The emphasis is on local commitment to preventive action, which can be compared with a more systematic expert-oriented approach.[4]

The laboratory has 48 employees, the majority being laboratory technicians. Main tasks are sampling and analysis of blood, urine and tissue from patients, and taking blood from donors. The laboratory has a safety group, comprising the head laboratory technician and a safety representative. Such laboratories are now required to affiliate to a specific occupational health service. But, during the late 1990s, the laboratory was not affiliated and had chosen a local multipurpose occupational health centre. The safety group also participated in general safety organisation at the hospital, which comprised many safety units in different departments, a safety committee and a safety manager.

The safety committee advised all departments to carry out workplace assessments, and the safety group in the laboratory used the opportunity of membership of the occupational health centre to ask for assistance. An occupational health professional was appointed to help the workplace. The freedom of choice this entailed meant that several different methods could be used for workplace assessment. The safety group gave priority to methods based on local activities, with which the occupational health professional in question was fully in agreement. She presented several methods to the safety group, all of which were based on identification of risks by employees themselves. The safety group chose a Danish method, simply called 'Good Work'.[5] It is based on the idea of mapping both positive and negative aspects of work – selecting the most important on both sides – and then working on strengthening the good aspects and disregarding the negative ones. The mapping is carried out by each employee, who fills out an open-ended questionnaire; the results are then used at a subsequent meeting for all employees, with joint brainstorming concerning items in the questionnaires.

The occupational health professional planned the application together with the safety group, and chaired the most important brainstorming meeting. This consisted of a staff seminar for laboratory technicians, all of whom were well prepared for the meeting. In total, 40 positive aspects of the work and 140 problems were identified. Many of the problems were small, and also overlapped. Problems were grouped into ergonomic, psychosocial, indoor climate-related categories and an untraditional category for operations and management. The meeting was a good experience for personnel and they left in high spirits.

Afterwards, the safety group and the occupational health professional held a meeting to evaluate the seminar and to plan the next steps of the intervention. The three people involved used a checklist to assess whether all important risks had been identified and to prioritise the problems (as 'serious', 'less serious' or 'minor'). The head laboratory technician and the safety representative felt quite satisfied, but the occupational health professional regarded chemical and biological hazards as having been neglected. The two members of the safety group argued that chemicals and biological matters were old hazards in the laboratory, with which they had been dealing for years; they were quite certain that the risks were properly controlled. The occupational health professional felt that chemical and biological risks had never really been assessed – either at the seminar or by the safety group. In her opinion, it was quite possible that a 'blind eye' had been turned to chemical and biological agents; the possible health effects would be long term, with no acute symptoms, and the technicians believed that nothing could be done about the way chemicals were used in any case. However, she chose not to pursue this argument because she considered that the workplace assessment exercise had proved to be positive so far; there was a potential for improvement with regard to a number of other work environment problems and she feared that pressure on her part would be experienced as disqualifying local (workplace-based) decisions. It was further concluded, following the wish of the safety group, that the group should carry out follow-up themselves without additional assistance from the occupational health professional.

The safety group organised a follow-up meeting for all staff. They presented their priority proposal, which was basically endorsed by the participants. Nevertheless, working alone and assault alarm were given greatest priority. The safety group also asked the staff to make an analysis of causes of the problems. That exercise was carried out in a plenary session and it turned out badly. The laboratory technicians were not trained in this kind of analysis and the consideration of each problem was either too trivial or too complicated to carry through. Afterwards, the follow-up meeting participants felt disappointed, losing most of the high expectations they had obtained from the first seminar.

In their evaluation after the follow-up meeting, the safety group realised that they could not conduct workplace assessments at meetings of all personnel. Some of the larger (very costly) problems were forwarded to the safety committee in the hospital; for the rest of the problems, small working groups (of two to four people) were set up, each with the task of developing and implementing solutions. Each working group was given a number of problems to deal with, and each laboratory technician was free to choose a group of interest. The safety group co-ordinated enrolment to the groups.

The staff took a strong interest in the groups and six were formed, with the majority of staff participating. They resolved most of the problems commissioned over a period of six months. Examples of issues were:

- new procedures for the requisition of samples in order to avoid doctors' labelling most samples as 'emergency', which created stress
- organisation of samples in the refrigerator
- reduction in heavy carrying during sampling outside the hospital at homes for the elderly
- training of laboratory technicians in working alone on night watch
- improvement in communication
- a seminar about objectives and visions for the future, with participation of the head physician responsible for the laboratory.

In addition, the safety committee allocated funds for lighting, the reduction of noise in the protein laboratory and a lifting table for handling heavy equipment.

Both the safety group and the staff felt that the workplace assessment had been a valuable exercise. Although they felt more or less alienated from most of the work environment activities, they felt that the workplace assessment approach was relevant and they had realised their own ability to take responsibility and to take action; they had even overcome the temporary setback they had experienced at the plenary meeting.

Discussion

The workplace obviously gained at least two things. A number of problems were solved to great satisfaction and autonomous activities seemed to offer a sustainable foundation for future actions. But the course of events also left the occupational health professional with several ethical questions.

The chemical and biological hazards were never assessed properly and most professionals would expect that any laboratory would have certain problems in this field if they were not properly controlled. The question here is whether the occupational health professional should have acted differently. It is likely that a more expert-driven workplace assessment would have identified several health hazards related to chemicals and may have succeeded in controlling some of the risks. But, another likely result would have been limited local commitment, as a result of which respons-ibility for further action would have been left to professionals (the occupa-tional health professional and maybe the safety manager at the hospital). Consequently, fewer small problems would have been solved and the safety group and the staff would not have experienced their ability to take responsibility growing during the process. In this particular case, the occupational health professional had a long-term relationship with the company because of her permanent affiliation and she was able to use another opportunity to raise the issue. In other cases, where the relation-ship is more temporary, the choice is not so simple.

Another ethical question concerns whether the occupational health professional should have withdrawn midway, which may have spoiled the process. She did a qualified job in assisting with the planning and organisation of the first meeting, including adopting the role of chair. But the safety group wanted to maintain control and decided to continue alone after the first successful seminar. However, its members came close to spoiling the process at the follow-up meeting. The safety group asked staff to undertake an analysis of causal relations, which was too difficult, and the staff ended up rather disappointed. The process may easily have ended up with almost nothing after this disappointment. In the end, the safety group proved wise enough to change strategy and launch the small working groups, which turned out to be quite successful. But did the occupational health professional have a better alternative? Telling the safety group (more or less explicitly) that she was not certain whether they would be able to handle the process in the future would certainly not have empowered it. In many cases, budget constraints on the occupational health side will require the professional to withdraw; the opportunity to follow a case to its conclusion is an exception rather than the rule.

The occupational health professional lost some professional autonomy in accepting the safety group strategy for the workplace assessment, which entailed that chemical and biological hazards were given lower priority. But this was likely to have been matched by a compensatory gain in trust from the client, thereby improving the relationship and future prospects for preventive work. The autonomy of the client was unaffected. The safety group got its way as a representative body or as part of the client system. With regard to beneficence, the client gained in terms of a larger number of problems identified and solved. Other gains were increased competence in the client system and self-confidence. A possible loss of beneficence lay in missing opportunities to find long-term solutions for the biological and chemical hazards.

Case 5.2: workplace development in a food-manufacturing company

Case 5.2 concerns a small food-manufacturing company.[6,7] An entrepreneur established the company in the late 1960s for the production of frankfurter sausages. It was located in an abandoned dairy production facility in a small village. The company was quite successful because of high quality and successful marketing. The premises were extended twice and in the late 1990s the company employed 65 workers. Forty-five of these were women, who all worked on the production line, mainly sausage making and packing. The male workers did the meat processing and smoking and also performed technical service functions. The company had established a safety committee with a fluctuating activity level. This was very much due to the elected safety representatives, who tended to 'run out of steam' shortly after their election.

Being in the food-processing business, there were problems related to repetitive and monotonous work, noise (walls and floors covered with tiles without sound-damping materials) and a cold indoor climate (the temperature in the packing area not exceeding $12\,^{\circ}\mathrm{C}$). The company is affiliated to a local occupational health centre and has had one occupational health professional as a permanent contact. Over the years, small adjustments have been made, especially in relation to the height of tables and mats to soften the floor surface. It was nevertheless obvious to the safety committee and the occupational health professional that conditions were not satisfactory and did not fully comply with work environment legislation (although the situation was not extreme by the standards of the industry). Over several meetings the safety committee discussed how it should meet the demand for a workplace assessment. It was finally agreed that the occupational health professional should assist the safety committee in making a general workplace assessment, followed by a special plan to reduce the risk of RSI on the production line. The female safety representative on the production line favoured some sort of job rotation, whereas the male safety representative from the meat-processing group argued that technical improvements to the feeding machines and the production tables would be the most efficient set of measures.

At the same time, the founder of the company left the organisation. It was taken over by a food conglomerate, but continued as a separate production unit. A new manager was employed and he soon realised that the production goals set by the new owners would require a rise in productivity. The manager was inspired by the ideas of human resource management and he had visited other companies with a group organisation and various forms of lean manufacturing. The new owners also favoured such a management approach, but did not guide the manager directly with regard to the necessary changes. Through the union, workers' representatives participated in a programme focusing upon 'the developmental work'[8] and they supported the ideas of management.

The manager eventually established a development committee in the plant, which included an external organisational development consultant, the shop steward and a former active safety representative. The occupational health professional had co-operated with the company for several years, but it did not occur to the manager or the workers to invite her to join the committee. They considered the role of the occupational health professional as that of making certain ergonomic or technical adjustments and they did not foresee any particular health risks arising from an organisation development project. The professional was somewhat sceptical about the outcome of the project, but she did not have much experience of organisational development and was uncertain about what advice to offer. At the same time, she did not feel that she could take the liberty to force herself on to the committee. Further, the safety committee's workplace assessment project was put on standby, since the safety representative (from the production line) had become involved in the development committee.

The manager and the development committee decided to make radical changes to the work organisation, based on the concept of semi-autonomous groups. Responsibility for a wide range of issues, such as production quantity, hygiene, safety and quality, was delegated to the production groups and the employees in turn had to assume new roles, such as group co-ordinator, quality assessor and hygiene controller. Four out of five shop foremen left the company and were not replaced.

The organisational change started with a three-day seminar for all employees, which covered a range of important issues – such as formation of groups and definitions of codes of work. Opportunities and threats were considered. All the changes were implemented soon afterwards and the employees were more or less taken by surprise when they realised the scale of their new responsibilities. The employees had different reactions to the new demands. One group found the new conditions challenging and regarded the role of group co-ordinator as offering an opportunity for proving their own ability to organise the work. A second group looked upon the changes, and also their committed colleagues, with scepticism, feeling quite sure that things soon would fall back to normal. A third group felt insecure; some employees were afraid of not being able to meet the new demands and thus risk losing their jobs. Gradually, the social climate became more and more harsh, leading to cases of harassment and frequent misunderstanding of even simple messages.

The problem was addressed at a seminar organised by the occupational health centre at the request of the safety representative in the development committee. The 'house' occupational health professional wanted to re-establish the RSI project, but the members of the development committee, backed by a majority of employees, argued that problems related to the implementation of the production groups should be given first priority. The occupational health professional still refrained from involvement in the work organisation project. She proposed instead to engage an external consultant experienced in mediation. The proposal was accepted, but the consultant was not able to 'break the ice'. Later on, a local vocational training centre was hired to set up a programme on group work and co-operation, but this did not improve the social atmosphere either. In order not to obstruct production during the training programme, participants were picked from several different production groups. For this reason, it was felt that the courses did not develop co-operation between workmates and that the training programme had little effect. The expected rise in productivity failed to materialise and as a final effort, the manager introduced a productivity-related bonus scheme. The system revealed great differences in the productivity of the groups, which only intensified conflicts and still did not lead to the desired productivity rise.

Resistance to the organisational changes among employees increased as they ran into problems related to them. The first result of the resistance was the unseating of the shop steward. Then, following a quarrel about acceptable product quality, there was a meeting of workers where a large group pressed for a return to traditional work organisation. Eventually the change project was abandoned and the owners dismissed the production manager. A new manager returned to a more traditional style of work organisation.

Throughout the group organisation period, the safety committee had been on standby, with active employees being involved in either the development committee or the working groups. The new management decided to revive the safety committee, whose first assignment was to perform a workplace assessment. The professional from the local occupational health centre was asked to support the committee in this task. The first question posed to her was 'How could we have avoided all those psychosocial problems?'.

Discussion

Nobody had carried out a thorough risk assessment of the plan for extensive organisational changes, and it may not have been possible for the parties involved to foresee the problems. Looking at the chain of events, the employees did not experience an improved work environment as expected, but – to the contrary – encountered a number of new work strains that overshadowed more traditional work environment problems. Attempts to involve external consultants were never fruitful, since they were not fully able to comprehend the background to the conflicts. If any external consultant had the knowledge to question the development, it was the occupational health professional. It might be argued that the problems were very much related to a poorly planned process by the production manager, who proved incapable of effecting a potentially successful change process. But the case also shows that changes in work organisation and roles of employees give rise to risks with regard to social relations that – if they are taken into account – might be prevented or eased. The position of the occupational health professional was weakened by virtue of the fact that the implementation of the development project was carried out by a quite specific development committee. The safety committee, which was the usual medium through which she related to the company, was not involved. Nevertheless, the so-called development committee did discuss several psychosocial work environment problems.

In this context, it is important to consider the ethical implications of the role played by the occupational health professional in development of the project. On the one hand, the company did not have a clear notion either of the possible risks or of the potential benefits of involvement of the occupational health professional. On the other, she chose to abstain from involvement at two possible entry points – at the start of the project and during organisation of the seminar (in both cases resulting from limited qualifications and a fear of failure). Indeed, she never really considered the possibility of giving advice to the development committee. Looking at the course of events, it is obvious that qualified advice from an occupational health professional might have made a difference, and some of the obstacles in a poorly performed change process might have been overcome. But it also seems likely that the 'house' occupational health professional was not the appropriate person – lacking the necessary qualifications and also self-confidence. She might have referred to someone else in her occupational health centre, but that centre – at a general level – also obviously lacked the necessary qualifications (since, for example, it had to refer to an external consultant for the seminar). Further, it might be argued that the occupational health centre, as a professional service institution, failed to live up to its obligation to assess prevailing work-related problems and to develop its services and qualifications in order to provide the services needed by the company.

The case illustrates a possible conflict between the ethical principles of autonomy and beneficence. The mandate from the company was rather limited, leaving almost full autonomy within the company itself. The question therefore arises as to whether the occupational health professional should have intervened, and thereby reduced the autonomy of the client, in order to 'do good' by giving informed advice on the possible harmful effects of the change process.

Conclusion

Although it would be unethical for occupational health professionals to abstain from involvement in preventive activities in the workplace, the two cases illustrate the multiple ethical problems workplace intervention now raises for them. Quite new qualifications are required for successful interventions, often far away from the basic professional training of occupational health professionals. This is a challenge that must be taken up, both by occupational health service institutions and by the individual professionals.

But even with the very best qualifications, it may be difficult to follow a change or development to its conclusion. In both cases, the occupational health professionals were eventually excluded – in Case 5.1 after a successful start-up, in Case 5.2 because of problems that employees regarded as more important. Again, in both cases, the occupational health professionals could have made a difference, and some of the problems encountered in the workplace might have been avoided. It is one of the tasks of an occupational health professional to interpret a mandate that is only too often unclear. The client may not understand all the problems related to the case, and therefore all the implications of occupational health service involvement. The question of interpretation of an occupational health mandate is affected by the growing market orientation of the services. Clients may want a clear and limited mandate in order to control costs; occupational health professionals are dependent on what services clients will buy, and will have little opportunity to follow up and expand the mandate if payment is not secured.

The two cases also illustrate that involvement in workplace interventions inevitably creates many ethical choices as events develop. For each decision, advantages and disadvantages have to be carefully considered. However, even if the best possible choice is made, possible benefits will be lost – as when the occupational health professional declined to push for the assessment of chemical hazards (Case 5.1). And the outcome is never certain. The workplace assessment process stopped after a failed second seminar in Case 5.1. However, was the choice made by the occupational health professional in Case 5.1 ethically wrong? To the contrary, it now seems clear that the choice was morally correct. A decision not to intervene because of an uncertain outcome is by no means a better ethical solution. Case 5.2 clearly demonstrates that involvement on the part of the occupational health professional may have been of great help to the workplace.

Scientific evidence will not always give any clear guidance. Confirmed knowledge about psychosocial strain and organisational development may provide general advice to managers and representatives involved, but is not of much help unless a consultant can help to clarify or foresee the consequences of the very concrete choices that have to be made.

In fact, ethical principles may well offer the best guidance. The general principles of beneficence and autonomy can be expanded into three specific items, all of which are in accordance with current Danish legislation in the occupational health arena. Any workplace intervention should fulfil the following requirements.

- An intervention must result in a concrete improvement to the work environment (beneficence).
- A holistic approach must be applied in order to assure that the improvement is not creating new health problems (also beneficence).
- The result must be empowerment of the workplace to control future hazards (autonomy).

It follows from these items that simply to disregard facts about occupational health problems with the client would be unethical in most cases. Such an approach would not secure concrete improvements or empower the workplace. It follows that occupational health professionals have an ethical obligation to intervene. Such intervention might, in some cases, be rather limited, taking the form of recommendations, or it might be more extensive, involving intervention in the process. Nevertheless, in both cases, it implies that occupational health professionals – to a greater or lesser extent – assume responsibility for the consequences of their interventions. They can never be completely certain that their intervention will lead to the desired positive outcome, and they must accept that there is always a risk of doing wrong or even causing harm. There will inevitably be dilemmas involved. How can short- and long-term effects be weighed against each other? How is a best but costly solution weighed against a less effective but also less expensive solution? Occupational health professionals have to make their own judgements in each case, knowing that there will be drawbacks whatever choice is made. Guidance on judgement is to be found in the above-mentioned three principle-based items for workplace intervention, subject to the mandate provided by the client. And in cases with too narrow a mandate, there must also be an obligation to inform the client about the consequences – to the extent that even abstaining from providing the requested service is a possible option.

References

1 Westerholm P, Hasle P and Fortuin R (2001) Occupational health service as external agents of change. In: K Frick, PL Jensen, M Quinlan and T Wilthagen (eds) *Systematic Occupational Health and Safety Management*. Pergamon Elsevier Science, Oxford, 311–20.

2 Jensen PL and Langaa P (2001) Risk assessment: a regulatory strategy for stimulating working environment activities? *Human Factors and Ergonomics in Manufacturing.* **11**: 101–16.

3 Hasle P, Thoft E, Jan R. *et al.* (1999) *APV undervejs – om muligheder og barrierer i APV-arbejdet.* ('Workplace Assessment on the Way – possibilities and constraints in implementing workplace assessment'). Arbejdsmiljørådets Service Center, Copenhagen.

4 Jensen PL and Langaa P (2002) Assessing assessment – the Danish experience of worker participation in risk assessment. *Economic and Industrial Democracy.* **23**: 201–28.

5 Olsen PB, Hasle P and Thoft E (1995) *Idékatalog med metoder og redskaber til at gennemføre arbejdspladsvurdering.* ('Catalogue of Ideas, Methods and Tools for Workplace Assessment'). Arbejdsmiljøfondet, Copenhagen.

6 Limborg HJ (2002) *Den risikable fleksibilitet – på vej mod et nyt arbejdsmiljø.* ('The Hazardous Flexibility – on the road towards a new working environment'). Frydenlund, Copenhagen.

7 Limborg HJ (2001) The professional working environment consultant – a new actor on the health and safety arena. *Human Factors and Ergonomics in Manufacturing.* **11**(2): 159–72.

8 Hvid H and Møller N (2001) The developmental work. *Human Factors and Ergonomics in Manufacturing.* **11**(2): 89–100.

CHAPTER 6

Workplace health surveillance

Kari-Pekka Martimo

Background

Workplace health surveillance is based on the existence of known work-related hazards that might give rise to deterioration in heath among employees. Its central role is the primary prevention of occupational and work-related diseases and injuries.[1,2] Health surveillance serves also as a method to gain information on the safety of working methods, the correct use of protective devices and the working climate. If any flaws are noticed, additional information and counselling will be offered. If an employee has already developed a suspected work-related disease, further examinations and medical care must be embarked upon and any limitations concerning continuation of the exposure have to be dealt with.

One essential part of health surveillance is screening, which may include interviews, questionnaires, diagnostic tests, function measurements and biological tests of exposure to environmental agents in the workplace. The most commonly used method for health surveillance is medical examination, which aims to evaluate individual risk factors, to detect early signs of diseases and to assess fitness for work.

In addition to the health surveillance required by law, some employers offer their personnel an opportunity for health examinations that are not directly related to any specific occupational exposure. One basis for voluntary health examinations is age. For example, in Finland, employees are usually invited to examinations every fifth year up to 45 years of age, after which the interval may be shortened to two to three years. If work-related exposures do not require more frequent attention, statutory health surveillance can be combined with age-related health examinations.

Voluntary health surveillance is directed at all employees, including those without any evident health hazards in their work environment. In a general health examination, not only work-related issues are covered but also information on employees' lifestyles and other private factors. In non-statutory health examinations, an interest in 'measuring health' has led to the use of various screening tests for non-occupational diseases and their risk factors.

Case 6.1: an occupational health dilemma

As the head of an occupational health service unit, a Finnish occupational physician is going through the results of an annual client satisfaction survey. The questionnaire has been sent to every employee, first-line supervisor and manager in the company. Each year the personnel give very positive comments, especially on curative care and health examinations. Many of them even suggest that consultation hours should be increased and health examinations repeated annually.

According to the respondents, duties and the working climate have become more demanding and working days are now longer and more intense. All this requires good health, which – in their opinion – could be maintained with more comprehensive and frequent 'health checks'. Some employees think that 'all possible tests' should be taken automatically at least once a year in order to promote health and work capacity.

First-line supervisors regard health examinations and curative services as more important than workplace surveys, which are seen more as the responsibility of occupational safety personnel. 'Put them in order' was a comment of one of the supervisors, who wanted to get the health and work capacity of his employees improved in order to avoid sickness absenteeism and to increase work motivation.

Information on client satisfaction was also collected from the management of the company. The managers are willing to procure more information on the general level of health and work capacity of personnel and wanted to know if there are any employees who may have serious health problems in the near future. They would even invest more money in medical examinations if they received relevant information to support their human resources strategy. In future, more attention will be paid to the reduction of personnel costs, such as those caused by sickness absenteeism and early retirement, and there are many expectations for health surveillance in this regard.

When considering the practical implications of these results, various questions bother the occupational health physician. Even at present, health examinations are taking a substantial amount of time from occupational health personnel. Shouldn't the primary responsibility of occupational health services be to improve work conditions even before there are any health effects among personnel? Thus, is the division of resources concentrated too much on individuals instead of the workplace? Do clients have unrealistic expectations or do they recognise the realistic possibilities as well as the limitations of health examinations? Is there a risk that more attention is paid to lifestyle than to work-related issues? Can it be guaranteed that health surveillance, and voluntary surveillance in particular, do not endanger employees' health, well-being and quality of life?

The occupational health physician has two extreme options: to increase individual health surveillance in order to satisfy the expectations of the workplaces or openly to inform the managers and employees about the limits and actual possibilities of health examinations. The latter should be followed by maintaining or even decreasing their frequency and using other methods, with better outcomes in terms of health and safety promotion and workplace improvement, instead.

Ethical analysis

Health surveillance is very challenging from an ethical point of view because it is an intervention aimed at basically symptom-free employees to help them stay healthy. Health surveillance carries risks that have to be compared with its potential benefits, which must then be properly justified in order to avoid unfounded expectations on the part of both employees and employer. Defining quality as a capacity of services to meet client needs and expectations leads us to the dilemma of balancing between the hopes and wishes of clients, their actual occupational health needs (as assessed by professionals), the attainable outcomes of occupational health activities and occupational health professional ethics.

The aims of health surveillance can be broken down as follows:

- early identification of the health effects of work conditions
- early initiation of preventive actions
- early identification of declining or dysfunctional work capacity
- early initiation of rehabilitation or work reassignment and workplace adaptation
- improvement of individual health through counselling
- optimisation of healthcare for specific health disorders.

The ethical value of fulfilling these aims depends very much on who initiates the activity. When initiated by individual employees, many of the ethical ambiguities do not arise. However, health surveillance most commonly derives from an initiative of either the employer or occupational health services, not of individual employees. Sometimes, employees' participation is taken as a sign of them taking the initiative. However, in many workplaces individual employees are very much influenced by their colleagues and do not always follow their own minds; they may even be afraid to refuse an invitation to an examination from healthcare personnel.

Another dilemma related to initiative lies in the employees' and employer's impression of health surveillance. It might be that only a few of the above-mentioned aims form part of an employee's expectations, whereas the others are way beyond the range of his or her personal ambitions. As for employers, they may well give greater priority to aims at the level of individual employees rather than expect initiation of actions in the workplace. In such situations, the initiative for comprehensive health surveillance with broad aims comes solely from occupational health personnel.

The priorities that various stakeholders set in the above-mentioned situations, which involve multiple expectations, are influenced by their loyalties. Employers emphasise productivity and business efficiency, whereas employees have a primary loyalty to their own health and wellbeing. In certain situations, the occupational health physician may even have to handle a double-loyalty situation. As employees of the same company as the employees they are consulting, occupational health physicians have to consider both the health agenda of the workforce and of individual employees, on the one hand, and the productivity and efficiency agenda of the company, on the other. When an external consulting firm offering occupational health services to a company is hired, the situation of double loyalties is different. Recognising the challenges of varying situations is of paramount importance to the conception of professional independence of health expertise. If we claim to be professionally independent of health experts, physicians and others, we should know what we are doing and seeking!

The stakeholders involved in the decision-making process are primarily the employees, as the target group, and their employer as the commissioner of and payer for the service. Occupational health professionals themselves, their management (especially in commercial services) and society as a whole also need to be taken into consideration. Society is important for two reasons: first, because of the statutory requirements it makes and second, at least in Finland, because half the costs of occupational health services are reimbursed by society to the employer. This means that the services the employers are paying for must be conducive to better occupational health in the workforce.

Indirectly, other parties can also be regarded as involved. The results or consequences of health examinations can affect the families of employees.

Further, other employees and employers served by one and the same occupational health unit are involved because the resources of occupational health professionals are limited and therefore affected by priority setting.

In this ethical analysis, the value premises employed are beneficence, autonomy and justice. How is the decision made by the occupational health physician to benefit the various stakeholders and what are the threats that it will not benefit any or some of them? How is the autonomy of the stakeholders respected or violated? How does the final decision promote justice in the provision of occupational health services?

The ethical premises, the stakeholders involved and the aims of health surveillance can be arrayed in a three-dimensional matrix. To make any ethical analysis as thorough as possible, all cells in the matrix should be evaluated in order to obtain a profound understanding of the ethical implications of health surveillance. The following evaluation is made at a very general level. To make any analysis more suitable in a real situation, practical details should be added.

Beneficence

Since the target group of health surveillance is all employees, most of them basically healthy, the moral obligation of 'doing good and not harming people' is even more relevant than in curative services (where the patient is actively looking for information, medical care and support in relation to a diagnosed health problem). In health surveillance, employees are invited or even obliged to participate in health screening, most of them without any self-generated need for it.

Health examinations seldom cause any visible harm to the participant. This has led to a common belief that health examinations are beneficial *per se*, which has made it tempting just to follow the wish of clients to increase the frequency of such examinations. However, on the one hand, the most important ethical consideration in health surveillance concerns the potential direct and indirect harm that it may prompt us to induce. On the other, the option of not applying health surveillance at all, or doing it too seldom, can lead to potential harm for members of the groups involved. Late diagnosis of occupational diseases or of other work-related symptoms may lead to prolonged harmful exposure among personnel as a whole.

Let us consider first the health surveillance required by law. As mentioned earlier, both workers and their employers expect health surveillance to be based on possible harmful exposures at work. Thus, its effectiveness in identifying the health impacts of work conditions depends primarily on the adequacy and validity of risk identification and risk assessment in the workplace. Ideally, all work-related risks should be identified in advance and the detection of their effects on health encompassed by the health surveillance. But because of changes in the workplace, the frequency of and methods used for workplace surveys may be insufficient to bring to light all the harmful exposures that should be included in any health examination.

Health surveillance is highly valued by personnel and employers alike. Decreasing the frequency of health examinations, or even abandoning them altogether, would lead to insecurity, dissatisfaction and distrust among both employees and employers. This is due to the full confidence they have in such examinations and their capacity to screen for abnormalities. Accordingly, the essential role of relevant risk identification and risk assessment in the workplace prior to health surveillance has to be acknowledged.

Recording a normal value in health surveillance can easily lead simply to reinforcement of a current behaviour, despite the fact that this could sometimes mean continuation of inadequate protection and harmful exposure. Practical experience shows repeatedly that individual behaviour is influenced more strongly by the results an employee receives from health surveillance (a personal medical examination) than by counselling on safe working methods or healthy lifestyles. Obtaining a normal value on a cholesterol or liver test scarcely provides the motivation to diminish consumption of fatty food or alcohol!

The motivation of employers to improve their work environment can also be compromised if they take negative results as a confirmation of safety. This is especially dangerous when screening methods are not relevant to the hazards in question. There are ergonomic, chemical and physical risks (like carcinogenic agents, solvents or radiation), not to mention psychosocial risks, that do not have any valid screening method to show exposure before illness has occurred. In such situations, a misguided perception of safety can have severe consequences.

It is not always evident that work-related abnormal findings in health surveillance lead to improvements in the work environment. Possible improvements are especially likely to be disregarded in the cases of ergonomic and psychosocial exposures at work. The symptoms and disorders caused by these factors are usually not taken as seriously as those resulting from more traditional exposures. One difficulty is the large individual variation in responses to ergonomic and psychosocial conditions. Further, the work-related measures needed may be rather complicated or expensive, or lack scientific evidence with regard to their effectiveness. All this can lead to affected employees being moved to another job or, in the worst of cases, their employment being terminated – neither of which is a satisfactory solution.

Health examinations as health surveillance give occupational health personnel a good opportunity to discuss work-related issues more widely than when just questionnaires or biochemical tests are employed. Individual counselling gives more room for confidential issues, although – with suitable working methods – reliable information can also be collected in group discussions (in a less time-consuming way). If an occupational health service does not include curative care, work-related ill health among personnel might remain undetected if comprehensive health surveillance is lacking.

In statutory health surveillance, occupational exposures help to define the necessary screening tests. By contrast, in voluntary health examinations, the broader aim is to detect signs of any medical disorders, not only work-related ones. This brings us to the fundamental dilemma involved in screening tests. People are often curious to know as much as possible about their own health status, including the results of biochemical tests. Because of modern technology and reasonable prices, the possibilities inherent in 'health checks' are unlimited. Not only client expectations but also the financial interests of commercial producers of occupational health services may be expected to favour the application of a wide range of screening tests.

Rather disappointingly, however, the number of screening tests supported by scientific evidence of their utility is very low. Most diseases do not have a symptom-free phase that can be detected by screening or would enable the course of a disease to be altered. On the contrary, there is evidence showing that 'false-positive' results frequently lead to unnecessary medical examinations and may cause tremendous anxiety to individuals and their relatives.[3]

Using screening tests or other health-surveillance methods that are not supported by scientific evidence is unethical for two reasons. First, it is a violation of the professional obligation to adhere to evidence-based methods; second, it represents a waste of time and money that could have been invested in more effective methods. It is equally unacceptable to create unrealistic expectations of the attainable advantages of health examination.

Laws and regulations concerning health surveillance in the workplace aim at a reduction in the incidence of occupational and work-related diseases. The burden of these diseases on society can be reduced only if the methods applied in occupational health services are appropriate for exposing and preventing the negative consequences of work and work environments. There is also the precondition that possible economic support from society is used in an ethically acceptable manner.

When considering the negative consequences of screening tests, we are not talking about anything uncommon but rather the everyday screening methods that are in use today. An abnormal finding from a screening test can have severe consequences for any person. Since, in occupational health services at least, the likelihood of an abnormal finding in this kind of screening is low, it seldom guides our judgement. However, low probability is no excuse not to inform the participant in advance about the possible disadvantages of screening tests. Additional control testing, for confirmation purposes, needs to be taken into account in planning commitment to and resources for any such programme.

One example of a potentially harmful screening test measure is sedimentation rate, which, despite recommendations to the contrary, is still often used in health examinations. Its usefulness in an occupational context is very limited, especially because of its low specificity. Much anxiety can be caused in subjectively healthy employees when their sedimentation rate is found repeatedly to be elevated (which demands further examinations, usually in hospital). The outcome might be that the result cannot be explained or that the person is suffering from some incurable condition – but nothing can be done until other symptoms appear that require medical intervention.

Autonomy

As far as statutory health surveillance is concerned, the employee's right to autonomy is limited by legislation on safety at work. If a person chooses to work in a hazardous environment, he or she has to follow safety instructions – including working methods, use of protective devices and participation in health surveillance. All this is based on an agreement between the employer and the employee and responsibility for its implementation rests on the employer.

The situation is totally different in voluntary health surveillance. The autonomy and integrity of employees require that this kind of health surveillance will always lack any kind of coercion – from either occupational health professionals, the employer or colleagues. No one can be compelled to participate. If statutory health surveillance is part of a more comprehensive health examination, both the participant and occupational health professional have to be able to distinguish between the part required by law and the part that the employee is entitled to refuse.[4]

Indeed, coercion is not even needed if voluntary health surveillance has been designed in such a way that it attracts all potential participants. One prerequisite for this is to speak openly in advance about how individual information and results are managed. If any information is to be delivered to the employer, participants are entitled to know in advance what this comprises and how the confidentiality of individual data will be secured. This also applies to recommendations for improvement of the work environment based on individual results derived from health surveillance.

Sometimes, health surveillance can lead to a situation in which continuation of individual exposure at work has to be stopped. This easily causes a conflict of interests, where the right of the individual to work collides with that of the employer to prevent future sickness absenteeism and employees' potential claims for compensation. Even if the primary duty of the occupational health professional is to prevent work-related diseases, employees' right and need to work cannot be disregarded. Such a situation has already been discussed in the context of beneficence. Nevertheless, from the perspective of autonomy, employees have the right to know in advance how it will be handled in the context of health surveillance.

As far as screening is concerned, it can be asked whether people always want to know about their future disease as soon as possible (especially in a case where they are unable to do anything to alter its course). The other option is for people to remain unaware of disease until symptoms appear. Early knowledge might endanger quality of life before outbreak of the disease.

This leads us to the conclusion that screening can never be a standard procedure; rather, individuals have to be able to give informed consent before testing. Responsible professional conduct requires an assessment of individuals' needs and open information on the advantages and disadvantages of the procedures involved in health examination. These demands are strongly reinforced by the professional obligation to support the employee's right to self-determination.

Sickness absenteeism and early retirement because of ill health give rise to both economic costs and productivity losses for employers. This has led many of them to pay attention to the health status of their employees. An employer's aim usually is to receive information on the work capacity of his or her personnel and to maintain their fitness for work – which is related to lower absenteeism and payroll costs, as well as to better productivity and quality of products and services.

In such a situation, occupational health professionals have to be as competent as possible so as not to miss any opportunity to promote health, safety and well-being at work. On the other hand, they have to maintain strict professional standards in offering evidence-based methods for the purpose (if relevant methods exist), and also to sustain a high level of confidentiality related to individual data.

Early identification of declining or dysfunctional work capacity in health surveillance can be an aim of both the employer and the employee, provided that both parties benefit from the consequences of assessment. The employee might not always agree with the result of a health impact assessment, for example in cases of alcohol abuse or a psychiatric disorder. This is a very challenging situation, because without agreement no rehabilitative actions are likely to succeed. From the employer's and even the work community's perspective, it might be preferable to opt for work reassignment instead of workplace adaptation or rehabilitation. Again, adopting such a course of action might collide with the employee's expectations of being able to continue in the same position. Fear of coercive measures can compromise the reliability of the entire assessment of work capacity.

Sometimes, the contents of health screening are influenced by a wish to maintain the image of the company or to reach other targets that are not directly related to the well-being of employees. Examples of such screening include compulsory HIV, drug and genetic testing. In situations of this kind, occupational health professionals are required to pay special attention to the rights and duties of all the parties involved. I am happy to leave these subjects to the contributions of other specialists in this book. In particular, there is the issue of sickness absence monitoring, which can be regarded as one form of health surveillance.

One restriction on the autonomy of both employees and the employer is that occupational health services must be planned and delivered by competent occupational health professionals and not by their clients. This means that responsibility for the validity of activities always lies with the professionals alone. Clients can never dictate the content of occupational health services, because society and its expectations, and also the integrity of the professionals themselves, have to be taken into account. Accordingly, client expectation is only one of the factors influencing the decision-making process in occupational services – the others being scientific evidence, resources and good practices.

Justice

The ethical demands of non-discrimination and solidarity are of crucial importance in health surveillance. Health examinations aim at assessing employees according to their health status or fitness for work and also targeting appropriate measures at those who benefit from them. This calls for sensitivity and strict confidentiality in order to avoid discrimination against any disadvantaged groups (from the side of either the employer or co-workers). Revelation of confidential data need not be intentional, but conclusions regarding a person's work capacity may become public through the action in which he or she is invited to participate, such as rehabilitation, a recommendation for improvement to the workplace, etc. One responsibility of occupational health services is to safeguard the rights of the individual even after the process of health examination has been completed.

It may even be asked whether improving general health is an aim of occupational health services, and if so, whether it is justifiable to collect comprehensive health data in an occupational health context. Health promotion nowadays is mostly a process that enables people to exert control over, and improve, their health. In this setting, a community approach is seen as the most effective way of promoting health. Occupational health professionals serve both communities and workplaces. This gives them an ideal opportunity to support individuals in adopting more favourable lifestyles. Inevitably, health examinations also reveal flaws in the treatment of specific health disorders. In the case where an occupational health physician cannot take responsibility for the optimisation of medical care, the employee should be referred to another physician for further action to be taken.

After health counselling, employees are always entitled to decide to reject recommendations based on the results of their health examination. This is sometimes highly frustrating for occupational health professionals, especially when the same employees repeatedly receive the same information, and the health risks remain the same. This is why professionals should receive support and counselling – so as not to lose their compassion or persistence in finding new ways of directing individuals towards a healthier lifestyle.

Health examinations can focus on primary, secondary or tertiary prevention, concerning both occupational and non-occupational health.[5] Limited time resources oblige occupational health personnel to concentrate on a restricted number of areas. According to international recommendations, occupational health services should prioritise adapting the work environment to individuals, and not vice versa. Health examinations, however, are aimed at individual employees. This may give the impression that occupational health professionals are primarily trying to change individuals and adapt workers to the prevailing work environment, regardless of conditions that may be unhealthy.

Health surveillance cannot be the same to all employees. As mentioned earlier, work conditions constitute the primary determinant of the contents and frequency of health surveillance required by law. As to voluntary health surveillance, individual characteristics of employees and the contract between the employer and occupational health service provider are the most important elements in planning a suitable approach. In order to promote equity and fairness in occupational health services, possible – often concealed – threats in these situations have to be carefully analysed.

In the commercial production of occupational health services, one employer's greater willingness to invest more in health surveillance diminishes the resources of occupational health personnel to motivate other less eager employers to fulfil even the basic requirements of the law. If resources are consumed for irrational health surveillance programmes in one company, these resources are not available to meet the genuine needs of other clients. Such an uneven distribution might endanger the right of all employees to their statutory share of occupational health services.

One duty of occupational health professionals is to safeguard the health of all employees regardless of their employment status. Health hazards at work endanger the well-being of both full-time and part-time employees, and also both the permanently and temporarily employed. Temporary or part-time workers exposed to harmful factors at work are in danger of being excluded from continuous health surveillance. Occupational health services should cover all employees, including those in precarious forms of employment.

Health examinations are so much appreciated by personnel that they are even sometimes regarded as 'fringe benefits'. White-collar workers, in particular executives, can be 'rewarded' by comprehensive health examinations, even if their well-being at work and off work requires less support than blue-collar workers. We, as professionals, have to be careful in deciding to what extent this can be considered acceptable, and when equity and justice are endangered.

From a societal point of view, it is considered justified that the employer is responsible for preventive services that deal with work-related issues. In situations where occupational health services are non-existent or do not perform comprehensive health surveillance, the management of ill-health related to work is externalised to the general health service system (with concomitant costs to society). This may diminish the capacity of an employer to understand the consequences of poor work conditions, and hinder the possibility of improving health and safety at work.

Discussion

In Finland, as in some other countries, national authorities have issued a *Good Occupational Health Practice Guide* for the conduct of occupational health services.[6] The cornerstones of good practice are high quality, ethics and effectiveness of services. None of these three qualities can be effective without the presence of the other two. High quality means both ethical and effective processes; ethics include client orientation as well as meeting the promised targets; effects, such as improvements to the health of employees and safety at work and in its environment, are more important than the number of performed actions. Without high-quality and ethically sustainable processes, the services can scarcely achieve any acceptable results.

Health surveillance and health examinations can play an important role in promoting both health and well-being at and away from work. However, they can never replace other tools, including work environment surveillance. We have to remember, and remind our clients, that regular health-screening test results provide no guarantee of health in the future. This is especially true if the methods do not meet the targets of health surveillance.

A survey of Finnish occupational health physicians and nurses suggests that ability to critically evaluate one's own performance is rather limited.[7] This creates a clear need for further training and guidelines. We should learn to be more critical, even if it sometimes seems like an overestimation of the negative consequences of our activities. Only in this way can both employers and employees rely on our expertise and ethical standards, and we ourselves utilise the opportunities to develop as professionals.

In the case presented, the occupational health physician might have considered using other than a client satisfaction approach to collecting information for decision making. Only too often occupational health services are offered on a 'set menu', where clients have to choose between given product alternatives, and thereafter give feedback on their experiences. Current phenomena in working life are so complex that more innovative approaches are needed.[8]

Most certainly in the presented case, further information on the occupational health needs of the workplace and the possibilities of health surveillance to meet them needed to be gathered. Only after this would it have been possible to choose the way to proceed – in close collaboration between the professional and the workplace.

References

1 International Labour Organisation (1997) *Technical and Ethical Guidelines for Workers' Health Surveillance.* Report Geneva, 2–9 September 1997 (www.ilo.org/public/english/protection/safework/health/whsguide.htm).

2 Koh D and Aw TC (2003) Surveillance in occupational health. *Occupational and Environmental Medicine.* **60**: 705–10.

3 Stewart-Brown S and Farmer A (1997) Screening can seriously damage your health. *British Medical Journal.* **314**: 533–4.

4 Faculty of Occupational Medicine of the Royal College of Physicians (1999) *Guidance on Ethics for Occupational Physicians* (5e). Royal College of Physicians, London.

5 Bell JG, Bishop C, Gann M *et al.* (1995) A systematic approach to health surveillance in the workplace. *Occupational Medicine.* **45**: 305–10.

6 Taskinen H (ed.) (2001) *Good Occupational Health Practice. A guide for planning and follow-up of occupational health services.* Finnish Institute of Occupational Health, Helsinki.

7 Martimo KP, Antti-Poika M, Leino T *et al.* (1998) Ethical issues among Finnish occupational physicians and nurses. *Occupational Medicine.* **48**: 375–80.

8 Franco G (2003) Consensus on evidence or evidence of consensus? The evolving role and the new expertise of the occupational physician. *Occupational Medicine.* **53**: 79–81.

CHAPTER 7

Health examinations on new employment: ethical issues

Stuart Whitaker

Case 7.1: Kapfunde versus Abbey National

Mrs Kapfunde was employed as a clerical worker on a temporary basis by the Abbey National building society in the UK. She applied for a permanent post as a cashier at the branch where she was working. As part of the standard recruitment procedure Mrs Kapfunde was required to complete a medical questionnaire, which asked her, among other things, to give details of any absences from work for health reasons. Mrs Kapfunde completed the medical questionnaire and declared a five-week absence from work due to sickle cell anaemia.

The completed questionnaire was sent to Dr Daniel, a general practitioner who worked part time for the Abbey National as their occupational health adviser. A part of Dr Daniel's duty was to consider whether applicants for employment were likely to have a higher than average sickness absence level. Dr Daniel considered that this would be the case with Mrs Kapfunde and advised the Abbey National that she was not suitable for employment. The Abbey National accepted this advice and refused to appoint Mrs Kapfunde to the vacant position.

Mrs Kapfunde commenced legal proceedings, alleging negligence against Dr Daniel and economic loss. This case was dismissed at the County Court. Mrs Kapfunde then took her case to the Court of Appeal, and, in addition to the original claim, submitted that it was also just, fair and reasonable in the circumstances that the Court should impose a legal duty of care. In her opinion, there is a duty to exercise the skill and care to be expected of a reasonably competent occupational health physician carrying out a medical assessment of a job applicant.

The issues facing the Court were whether Dr Daniel owed Mrs Kapfunde a duty of care, based on the proximity of their relationship in law, and whether Dr Daniel had breached that duty of care in dealing with Mrs Kapfunde's case.

The Court of Appeal concluded that there was no doctor–patient relationship between Dr Daniel and Mrs Kapfunde, and that the relationship was not of sufficient proximity to create a duty of care. Therefore, there had been no breach of that duty. The Court went on to say that even if a proximity had been established it would not be fair, just and reasonable to impose a legal liability because of the potential conflict between Dr Daniel's contractual duty to the Abbey National and alleged duty to Mrs Kapfunde.

The Court said that, even if there had been a duty of care, Dr Daniel would have been required to exercise no more than the degree of skill and care to be expected of an ordinary competent occupational health physician. The trial judge had found that Dr Daniel had consulted with a specialist in sickle cell anaemia before reaching her decision; and later a specialist in occupational medicine, called by the defence, had said that the course of action taken by Dr Daniel was well within the range of reasonable responses.

The Court of Appeal dismissed Mrs Kapfunde's appeal and refused her leave to appeal to the House of Lords.[1]

Ethical analysis

There are many, and varied ethical dilemmas that can arise in relation to the use of medical standards, or health assessments, as part of a process of selecting people for employment. This is particularly true when, as in this case, there is no statutory duty to screen applicants for reasons of health and safety or clearly identified need to protect the individual or others from an increased occupational risk. Some of the ethical dilemmas that arise in relation to the use of pre-employment health assessments do so because of the very strong element of compulsion that exists for job applicants to disclose what is often a wide range of private medical information, which is sometimes not directly related to their ability to do the job, simply in order to secure employment. Also, because the majority of job applicants are relatively powerless in this situation, they can be exposed to unnecessary discrimination, without adequate means of protection.

The questions that might arise when examining pre-employment assessment from an ethical perspective include the following.

- Should society allow employers to have access to private medical information, through their occupational health advisers, for the purpose of reducing economic risks or should this be limited solely for the purpose of reducing risks to health and safety?
- Could the use of pre-employment health assessments, for the purpose of controlling economic risks, result in disadvantaged groups being unnecessarily discriminated against in the labour market, and what might be the consequences of this strategy for both individuals and groups within society?
- Is the selection of workers on health grounds to reduce sickness absence risks an ethical practice for healthcare professionals to be involved in or is this an abuse of their privileged position in society?
- What is the evidence base on which predictions of an increased risk of sickness absence can be made, when those who do declare medical conditions are compared with those who either do not have those conditions, but have other risk factors, or do not declare such conditions? Further, can any increased risk be mitigated through further action, other than rejection from employment?
- Are applicants equally informed of the risks that they may be exposed to in their potential employment – through, for example, hazardous exposures or poor organisational management – that have adversely affected other employees?
- Lastly, how are the professionals involved in undertaking this activity going to be held accountable, both to the employer and job applicants, for the advice they offer on suitability for employment?

These questions all have practical, scientific and ethical dimensions. Many of the screening methods and tools used for conducting pre-employment assessments have poor sensitivity and specificity. This leads to high rates of 'false-positive' and 'false-negative' cases, poor predictive value and a lack of consistency in the advice that is given, even by specialists in occupational medicine when reviewing the same cases. Therefore, there is serious cause for concern.[2] The use of scarce occupational health resources to perform this type of screening, when they could possibly be used in different and more effective ways to help, protect and promote the health of the working population, also raises serious ethical issues.[3,4]

In Case 7.1 just one context in which an ethical dilemma might arise is examined; that is, the collection and use of private medical information, gathered at the pre-employment health assessment stage, in order to protect the commercial interests of the employer. The Kapfunde case illustrates clearly that this did occur. Medical information, gathered at the time of assessment, was used to identify a person who, it was assumed, would have an unacceptably high rate of sickness absence. This is primarily an economic risk to the employer. The recommendations made by the physician did result in the individual being rejected from employment.

It should be noted that, at the time of this Appeal Court decision in the UK, papers were published both welcoming the ruling[5] and cautioning against its implications for occupational health practice.[6]

The question to be discussed here is whether or not the occupational health professional should be allowed to use private medical information, disclosed at a pre-employment health assessment, to advise the employer not to employ people who might pose an increased risk of sickness absence.

The relevant value criteria involved are:

- autonomy
- beneficence
- justice.

The important stakeholders are:

- the employer
- the occupational health professionals involved
- the workforce
- the applicant
- the society in which this occurs
- the occupational health profession as a whole (which functions within a particular society).

In most cases the value criteria, for each stakeholder, are reciprocally related. For example, as the autonomy of the employer is increased, by having access to private medical information, it is reduced for applicants, by having to disclose that information on themselves in order to secure employment.

Stakeholders' views

The employer

The employer may view the process of pre-employment screening, including that undertaken for the purpose of avoiding any increased risk of sickness absence in his workforce, to be a legitimate step to take in order to protect his commercial interests. The employer may view any interference with this activity, by legal or professional bodies, to be an intrusion into his right to autonomy in running his business.

The employer may view the occupational health professionals, whom he pays to carry out this work, to be working within reasonable legal and professional boundaries, and at the same time to be working in his best interests. The employer may also regard operating within reasonable legal and professional boundaries to be the limit to which he could be expected to act as a responsible employer within a competitive commercial environment. This may represent the extent to which he might wish to support a concept of social justice.

The employer may be able to advance a well-reasoned argument in favour of selection, based on his desire to succeed in a commercial enterprise that provides employment and job security, and also helps to build social capital within the wider community. The employer may advance the argument that the benefits to the majority of the selection of workers on health grounds outweigh any 'harm' that a minority may suffer.

The occupational health professionals involved

The occupational health professionals involved could be expected to be familiar with, and have an obligation to take account of, all of the value criteria – autonomy, beneficence and justice. The reason for this is that these criteria underpin the ethical standards that apply to each of the professions in occupational health service.

Occupational health professionals may view the pre-employment health assessment process, and its use to reduce economic risks to the employer, to be a legitimate activity. This may be, in part, because pre-employment selection, for this purpose, would appear to be widely accepted within their specialty. The ethical implications of such activity have been relatively rarely challenged in the professional journals or scientific literature.

The professionals may also not have considered all of the options that they might exercise in order to meet their ethical obligations (i.e. not only to avoid harm but to promote good). They may not have been educated, or socialised, into thinking in ethical terms about their professional practice or recognise their obligations to act in different ways.

In addition, in this case, Mrs Kapfunde was not seeking medical advice, nor had she chosen to consult with Dr Daniel of her own accord. Professionals involved in these types of situations may not consider that their relationship is one that carries the same ethical obligations as it would if a patient were seeking advice or treatment.

The occupational health professionals may have been employed to carry out the process of screening with an explicit instruction or implicit expectation on the part of the employer that the process would be used to reduce the risk of sickness absence. They might not be fully aware of the ethical implications of such an activity for an individual or, as in the case described, of the impact it may have on an already disadvantaged group in society.

The professionals involved in this type of work may view their relationship with the employer to be more important, both professionally and financially, than their relationship with any potential job applicant. They would appear to be supported in this by the legal ruling.

It may also not be clear to the practitioner involved in delivering the service how abstract ethical principles should be applied or how they might be used to shape or justify their behaviour. At what point does the obligation to behave in an ethical manner become 'supraobligatory', that is, go beyond what might reasonably be expected of the average practitioner?

In addition, professionals working in this field, especially those who have not trained as specialists, may not be aware of the limitations of pre-employment screening or of the controversy that surrounds the process.[3,4] They may not necessarily be aware of the very many factors, other than disease, that can contribute to an increased rate of sickness absence in working populations.[7] Or they may not be acquainted with the management systems that can be put in place to manage attendance at work more effectively, as an alternative to trying to screen out potential risks at the pre-employment stage.

Further, the non-specialist may not fully understand the ethical dilemmas that can arise in relation to carrying out pre-employment screening. In the absence of specific training, the non-specialist may not have been exposed to other, more experienced specialists in the field, who could provide them with good role models, and also demonstrate how the ethical principles described could be applied under the sometimes complex and difficult circumstances that arise in occupational health practice.

The workforce

The workforce, already employed and having passed through this type of screening process, may view the use of medical screening to reduce sickness absence as acceptable in order to exclude those who may not be at work as often as they are. They may welcome this process if it helps to reduce any additional burden being placed on them.

In the longer term the workforce may view the process of reducing sickness absence risks as helping to sustain the commercial success of the organisation, and therefore their continuing employment, again in the context of social justice where their rights and expectations are protected.

Alternatively, since the workforce will not routinely have access to the results of pre-employment screening or know why some applicants are rejected from employment, its members may not be aware that medical information, gathered at pre-employment assessment, is being used to reduce absence. Or if they are aware, they may not necessarily feel empowered to do anything about it.

It would seem that the predominant value criteria from the workers' perspective might be more strongly related to the concept of social justice, and to protecting their own rights, and less strongly related to the concept of solidarity and their ability or power in this situation to stand up collectively for those who may be disadvantaged.

It is probably only when labour is organised in a trade union or some other collective body, and is supported by others who take a wider view, that issues such as the rights of workers at point of employment are considered from a collective viewpoint.

The applicant

Individual job applicants may have very different views on the process of pre-employment assessment. This is likely to depend upon their previous experience of job applications where screening has been applied, their level of understanding of their own medical conditions, and any genuine impairments or losses of functional ability to which these have given rise.

Job applicants may feel uncomfortable about having to disclose private medical information at recruitment, particularly if it includes information that does not appear to be directly related to their ability to do the job. However, they may still feel that in order to secure employment, and avoid unemployment, often in competition with other applicants, they are compelled to participate in the process of medical selection, without raising any concern, for fear of being viewed as difficult.

The process of pre-employment selection may be viewed as a direct challenge to the autonomy of the individual and – when used for reasons other than risks to health and safety – as raising serious ethical questions about the fairness and justice of such screening, and of the role of the healthcare professionals involved.

In Mrs Kapfunde's case it would appear that she did in fact suffer injustice in this way. As a person with a health defect, she was discriminated against on that basis, and suffered a 'harm' in not being employed in a position for which she would otherwise have been considered. The consequence of this was that a disadvantaged person in society was further disadvantaged (through the actions of Dr Daniel) for the benefit of another.

Although this 'harm' may have occurred unintentionally, there is no evidence that Dr Daniel sought to do more to avoid any harm to Mrs Kapfunde or tried to promote good by pursuing other courses of action. It would appear that Dr Daniel did not contact Mrs Kapfunde to discuss her condition, its implications for her future attendance at work or the recommendation that she would be making to the Abbey National building society.

Job applicants may also be asked to disclose medical information at the time of pre-employment assessment, but be largely unaware of the true extent and nature of the decisions that may be taken on the basis of that information or of their rights within the process.

Job applicants are unlikely to have a sophisticated view of the role of occupational health professionals, and may not appreciate that their relationship with any such healthcare professionals is quite different from those which exist in other professional–patient situations. In particular, the former has an apparent lack of protection at law. Certainly, in Mrs Kapfunde's situation, this would have appeared to have been the case.

Society

The concept of 'society' implies more than a collection of individuals making the best of situations for themselves, but also a degree of social cohesion and social responsibility that includes taking care of those minority or disadvantaged groups that are a part of our society.

Sickle cell anaemia is a condition that is predominant in the black community. If many large employers were to discriminate systematically, without clear justification, against employing people with sickle cell anaemia, this would result in the black community being seriously disadvantaged in comparison with other groups who are less affected. Within the value criterion of beneficence, there is an obligation placed on professionals to try to promote good, not just avoid harm, and to promote social justice.

In Mrs Kapfunde's case, additional steps could have been taken to explain the nature of the condition to the employer. This would have involved advising him on how minority groups are adversely affected, and perhaps identifying the opportunity for the Abbey National to become an exemplary employer and demonstrate its commitment to the black community. The employer could possibly have used this example of positive discrimination, or sensitivity to the needs of the black community, to help him promote his services to this part of the community, as a strategy for business development that might help offset any additional costs incurred by adopting this higher standard of social care.

Ethical dilemmas raise unexpected questions. They create opportunities for professionals to make different choices, pursue different strategies, and to be innovative in the ways in which they respond to different circumstances in their professional lives. Society expects professionals to behave in an ethical manner, and to promote those standards in their professional lives. Not to take account of or try to promote these principles will almost certainly be regarded as unethical.

The occupational health profession as a whole and in society

The occupational health community, that is, those professionals from different disciplines who are involved in delivering occupational health services to the workplace, requires the trust and co-operation of the working population, and society more widely, in order to function effectively. Its members need to have the confidence of employers, managers and those who pay for services, and to be able to demonstrate to these groups that they are making a useful contribution to the success of the organisations that employ them.

The actions of a few within the occupational health community can affect the perception of both employers and employees, and the general population more widely, of the role and function of occupational health services. Accordingly, the autonomy of an individual profession needs to be tempered by its responsibilities to uphold the ethical values of the occupational health profession as a whole.

There may be variation, between different professions and between different professionals within the same discipline, and also between different employers, in what is perceived to be the extent to which the obligation of the 'ordinary competent occupational health professional' should be to promote good. How far must professionals go to meet the ethical obligations discussed before their actions become 'supraobligatory' (such as is the case with 'whistleblowing')? A greater degree of consistency between these various groups will only be achieved through more open and better informed debate, both within and between the professions. In this way, the situation that occurred with Mrs Kapfunde, which left many occupational health professionals feeling uncomfortable, might help members of the occupational health community to understand more clearly their ethical obligations and the basis for practice in their specialty.

Discussion

The first recorded selection of workers by some formal method of assessment can be traced back to the Han dynasty in China, around 200 BC,[8] where entrants to the Civil Service were selected on competence rather than, as previously, through social status or family connection. However, historically, the selection of workers who were considered to be fit for the jobs or tasks they were expected to perform has probably taken place, without any medical involvement, for as long as work has been organised. From the slave markets of the Roman Empire, where slaves could be highly valued and hold important positions in their owner's household, through the period of the African slave trade for the Americas, to Nazi Germany where people were selected to go to work or to the concentration camps, some form of selection of people for work has been undertaken. Such selection has been based on appearance, apparent health, physical capacity, mental ability and the possession of special skills, all of which would have been taken into account by those doing the selecting.

It is a sobering reminder that, as recently as in 1996, trade ministers at the World Trade Organisation conference[9] thought it necessary to endorse internationally recognised fundamental labour standards, including those that prohibited the use of forced labour and child labour, and advocated the elimination of unnecessary discrimination in employment. There are many examples, even today in highly developed countries, where the selection of workers – in poorly paid jobs, in the black economy and for unpaid work – is carried out in ways that cannot be justified in advanced nations. Such circumstances raise many important legal, moral and ethical questions.

The first recorded history of a physician's involvement in the selection of workers by some sort of medical examination was in 1795, at the time of the Industrial Revolution.[10] Before there was any legal requirement to do so, the records show that a physician was employed at Quarry Bank Mill in the UK to examine the health of orphans who were sent from around the country to work in the textile industry. It would appear that the mill owner wanted to avoid any financial responsibility for any child who, because of ill-health or mental impairment, was not fit to work.

The physician's records make sad reading. Children aged as young as seven were identified as being ill or having abnormalities that made their ability to work uncertain, and – without any attempt at treatment or care – the physician recommended that they should not be employed. One is left to wonder at the fate of those children who were accepted and of those who were rejected, both of whom, in reality, had only the freedom to choose between work, in the terrible conditions of the day,[11] and absolute poverty.

For the vast majority of workers in highly developed countries today, the selection of people for work occurs in a much more civilised and sophisticated manner. Modern-day human resources departments will attempt to use objective criteria in their selection processes, which are often governed by specific legislation that helps to protect individuals, and minority groups from unnecessary discrimination in employment. Nowadays, in many situations, workers also have greater freedom to choose between employers than in the past. In most countries today, there is stronger trade union representation and greater legal protection in relation to employment than in the past. However, in the context of paid employment, the legal status of a contract of employment is still based on the 'master–servant' relationship, where powers and responsibilities are not distributed evenly. In this context, many ethical dilemmas can still arise.

The involvement of healthcare professionals in the selection process is still common, although in some countries it is now much more closely regulated than in the past.[12] The health assessment process is usually directed at the application of medical standards for the reduction of risks to health and safety. In such cases, it is designed to help match workers to jobs that they are capable of doing – safely and without undue risk to themselves or others. Few would argue against the application of rigorous medical standards in the selection of workers who would be placed in high-risk situations, such as the armed forces, police and fire services, or to those whose work could place others at significant risk, such as airline pilots or drivers of heavy goods vehicles (where statutory medical standards usually exist).

However, the pre-employment health assessment, in some countries, is still widely used by employers for applicants to jobs that do not carry such significant risks to health and safety, and where there is no statutory duty involved.[3,4] The use of medical, pre-employment screening in this context raises many different types of ethical dilemmas.

By requiring job applicants to divulge private medical information, in order to secure employment, there is an element of compulsion on applicants to disclose. Such a process directly challenges the right of individuals to maintain their privacy, and their right to self-determination, and may affect their autonomy in a significant way. As in the Kapfunde case, the outcome of a health assessment can clearly affect whether or not a person will be employed. Those individuals who are rejected are placed at risk of suffering some kind of 'harm' as a result of the process. For example, they may suffer reduced earning capacity, opportunities for promotion or career development, self-esteem, confidence or motivation. There may also be other long-term consequences – as, for example, when they are applying for other jobs. Indeed, one of the questions frequently asked in pre-employment questionnaires is 'Have you ever been rejected from employment because of a health condition?'. There may also be additional future difficulties for individuals in trying to get a mortgage to buy a house, negotiate financial loans, obtain health insurance, etc. when their ability to secure or maintain employment is questioned.

Occupational health professionals have a duty to try to do good, not just avoid harm, and one could look more closely at the pre-employment assessment process to see if the judgements that are made are in fact based on good evidence and sound logic and in addition, if there are omissions on the part of clinicians, who might have taken additional steps to try to mitigate any harm that may be caused. In some countries there are already established mechanisms for job applicants who have been rejected from employment, or who feel that they have been unfairly treated, to have their case reviewed by an independent panel of experts.[12]

Conclusion

It would appear in the case considered that the actions of the physician, and the role that she fulfilled on behalf of the employer, and indeed those of the other specialists that concurred with her, do raise serious ethical questions. At that point in time the physician's actions were judged to be perfectly legal and defensible. Many occupational health physicians in the UK welcomed the Court ruling, and the Faculty of Occupational Medicine advised its members of the case. However, the Kapfunde case demonstrates that an action may be judged to be lawful, and enjoy some support within the profession, but still raise serious ethical questions and leave some professionals feeling uncomfortable about its implications. However, this is of rather academic interest, because unless the professional bodies – those with the power to determine acceptable standards – can or do take some sort of decisive action to set the standards of professional practice that should apply, or that help to influence the behaviours of its members, no change will result (regardless of whether or not an ethical dilemma exists).

Of course, if the professional bodies are going to provide more detailed, clear and definitive guidance on the ethical standards that are expected of their members, this does raise other important questions. For example, if ethical behaviour is to be an important part of professional life – but by its nature is open to interpretation and debate according to each situation – how is widespread interest in ethical practice to be advanced in the face of what would often appear to be ambivalence to ethical questions on the part of a significant number of professionals within any specialty?

Will efforts to educate, socialise and influence professionals towards higher standards of ethical behaviour only really reach those who already have sufficient interest to purchase and read books such as this or to read articles and attend lectures, and then to try to incorporate the ideas into their daily practice? Or should greater responsibility be placed on those who teach and examine various occupational health professionals? For example, should some test of understanding of ethical principles and their application in practice form part of professional training? If so, this would certainly imply that the people conducting the examinations should themselves be well versed in analysing complex ethical situations. But it would also entail that they should be prepared specifically to refer candidates who cannot demonstrate an understanding or commitment to the high standards of ethical behaviour that prevail in professional life.

Note

Since the Kapfunde versus Abbey National ruling, the UK has introduced the Disability Discrimination Act, which now makes it much more difficult for applicants with health problems to be rejected without the employer considering reasonable adjustments. However, pre-employment health assessment continues to be widely used by employers in the UK.

References

1 Kapfunde vs. Abbey National and Daniel (1998) *Industrial Relations Law Reports.* 583–9.

2 de Kort WLAM (1992) Agreement on medical fitness for a job. *Scandinavian Journal of Work, Environment and Health.* **18**: 246–51.

3 Whitaker S and Aw TC (1995) Audit of pre-employment assessments by occupational health departments in the National Health Service. *Occupational Medicine.* **45**: 75–80.

4 Whitaker SC (1997) A critical evaluation of pre-employment assessment in the National Health Service. PhD thesis, British Library, London.

5 Seabrook R and Collins B (1999) The duty of care of the occupational physician in assessing job applicants. *Occupational Medicine.* **49**: 189–92.

6 Barrie M (1999) Letters to the editor. *Occupational Medicine.* **49**: 474.

7 Whitaker SC (2001) The management of sickness absence. *Occupational and Environmental Medicine.* **58**: 420–4. (www.occenvmed.com).

8 International Labour Organisation (1993) *Conditions of Work Digest.* ILO, Geneva.

9 LaDou J (2002) Occupational health in industrializing countries. In: LaDou J (ed.) *Occupational Medicine in Industrializing Countries. State of the art reviews.* Hanley & Belfus, Philadelphia.

10 Murray R (1992) Peter Holland: a pioneer of occupational medicine. *British Journal of Industrial Medicine.* **49**: 377–86.

11 Hunter D (1974) *Diseases of Occupations* (5e). English University Press, London.

12 The Medical Examinations Act (1998) *Pre-employment Medical Examinations Decree and Pre-employment Medical Examinations Complaints Decree.* A complaints committee for pre-employment medical examinations, Holland (www.aanstellingskeuringen.nl).

CHAPTER 8

Work disability assessment in the Netherlands

Jos Verbeek and Carel Hulshof

Case 8.1: a personal case history

Working as a physician in an occupational health service in the Netherlands, one of my client organisations is a medium-sized computer firm with 250 employees. I have been working for the firm for five years, and I feel that most things are going well. I have a good working relationship with company management, and I think they trust me. This is what it means to be working in close collaboration with an employing organisation.

One of my tasks is the work disability assessment of sick employees. When they are off work because of sickness for more than two weeks or more than five times per year, they are summoned to me for consultation. Each month, I liaise with the personnel manager to discuss the state of affairs of workers on sick leave. These are called 'social–medical team meetings'. Usually, the supervisor of the worker in question also attends the meeting.

Last week, during our meeting, the personnel manager asks me, as the occupational health physician, if I can have a word with one of the employees, a Mrs van Dijk. She works as a receptionist, and is frequently on sick leave because of headaches. 'It sounds to me that she is not very motivated, and a straightforward assessment of her work ability might give her some incentive to be at work more regularly,' says the personnel manager. 'Then, we can discuss what her problems are at the next meeting.'

During the consultation hour, it emerges that Mrs van Dijk is suffering from migraine. She favours herbal medicine because 'natural products are better for the human body than the chemicals made by the pharmaceutical industry'. In her case, the herbal treatment is feverfew – a herb that is supposed to prevent migraine attacks. After some discussion, it turns out that she does not want to get regular medical treatment (from her GP), but wants to carry on using the herb. She says that if she is sick, this is a natural reaction of her body – something that just has to be accepted despite the lost days at work. My assumption is that the herbal treatment is ineffective, and I have no sympathy for the idea of natural healing. I think this is too much for the firm, and I know that her colleagues often have to take over her work because of a migraine attack, which they experience as an unpleasant surprise. Accordingly, I insist on better medical treatment, and warn her that if she does not get it, this will lead to problems with her supervisor or with the personnel department.

At the next social–medical team meeting I tell the personnel manager about what I regard as inappropriate treatment and the warning I have given. The personnel manager takes it upon himself to have a proper conversation with her.

Value premises

In work disability assessment we can use the same value premises as for any kind of medical treatment.

Usually, the first principle in treatment is that of the *autonomy* of the patient. This is clearly at stake here. The patient should have the right to make her own choices, such as not wanting regular treatment. Based on the principle of autonomy, there is an issue of confidentiality in this case.

Next, there is the combined principles of *beneficence* and *non-maleficence*. Physicians should do no harm to the patient, and also should do no harm to others. Here, compared with regular treatment in curative care, there are more parties involved who can benefit or be harmed by the decisions of patient and physician. So, we should also consider the principle in the light of co-workers and the organisation. This principle also implies that the physician should do his best to provide optimal treatment and guidance to the patient. This involves a correct diagnosis and knowledge of the proper treatment and best possible assessment of work ability.

Lastly, the principle of *justice* applies, according to which we should consider equity and solidarity in relation to the people involved.

Work ability assessment

In the Netherlands, there is a strongly held belief among healthcare professionals and the general public that it is unethical for treating physicians to be involved in sickness certification. By sickness certification people usually mean that patients obtain a written statement from a doctor which legitimises their absence from work on medical grounds. In general, it is not very clear what the differences are between sickness certification, work-ability assessment, disability evaluation, sickness absence control, assessment of fitness for work and return-to-work assessment. Here, we will use work-ability assessment in the sense of disability evaluation. According to the definition under the medical subject heading (MeSH term) in MEDLINE, this involves determination of the degree of a physical, mental or emotional handicap. The result is applied to legal qualification for benefits and income under disability insurance, and to eligibility for social security and workers' compensation benefits. Cox et al.[1] define fitness-for-work assessment as a medical skill balancing the demands of a job and the medical abilities of a person. This seems equivalent to the first part of a disability evaluation.

Because it is not clear which statements of a physician could be used for qualification for a benefit, most treating physicians in the Netherlands refrain from any advice about return to work. Therefore, they usually do not make any work-ability assessments. Behind this is the idea that involvement in the assessment of work ability could lead to a conflict of interests. Patients could be afraid that information they reveal to their doctors could be used for work-ability assessment with the possible consequence of withholding sickness benefit. This in turn could harm patients by inappropriate diagnosis or treatment. Even though the practice in most other countries is the opposite, and there is no scientific evidence that this is problematic, practice in the Netherlands is not likely to change very quickly.[2]

About 80 years ago, a lengthy political discussion in the Netherlands led to the so-called 'separation' of treatment and sickness control. Until the 1990s only insurance physicians were entitled to make work disability assessments in order to provide a legal basis for sickness or disability benefit. After 1996 occupational health physicians became involved in disability assessment, because the law was changed to combine all occupational health and safety issues and sickness absence issues within occupational health services. Occupational health physicians have always opposed the idea of being responsible for work-ability assessment or sickness certification. And they have been partly successful in their opposition in the sense that, formally, there is no law that states that occupational health physicians are the ones to perform work-ability assessments. Nevertheless, because it is not clearly stated to the contrary, it has become, implicitly, an additional task for them. Nowadays, the general notion is that only occupational health physicians make a work-ability assessment, and it is on the basis of this assessment that employers will or will not provide wage or salary payments during sickness absence.

Work disability assessment in the case of migraine

The assessment of work ability is still the subject of debate in the medical literature. There is no evidence or general consensus on the best method to evaluate work ability. The closest is the model of functioning offered by the World Health Organization (WHO), formerly called the model of impairment disability and handicap. The model states that disease can lead to loss in abilities, which in turn can lead to problems in participating in society. This chain of problems is influenced by healthcare, by personal characteristics of the individual (such as beliefs or attitudes) and by environmental factors. Basically, work ability lies in a balance between loss of capacity and the role in society the person wants to occupy. This implies that disability assessment leaves ample room for professional judgement.[3]

It is generally recognised that migraine can be a seriously disabling disease. The indirect costs of days lost from work and productivity greatly exceed the direct costs of medical care. In the USA alone, they are estimated at $5–17 billion per year.[4] Clinicians are showing a much greater interest in migraine-related disability than previously. The development of a migraine disability questionnaire has been helpful in this respect, where five simple questions are used to assess extent of disability.[5] Clinical epidemiology has also been helpful in specifying diagnostic criteria.[6]

All this implies that a physician can make use of several clinical tools to make an assessment of work disability. Further, there is some research on the effectiveness of feverfew that indicates that the herb might be helpful in preventing a migraine attack.[7] When adopting the approach suggested by evidence-based medicine, there is a recommendation that the medical literature should be reviewed to find answers to clinical questions that arise out of practice. The effectiveness of feverfew is one such question.[8]

Patient autonomy

The value that is most at stake in this case is that of patient autonomy and how an occupational health physician might deal with it. Autonomy on the part of a patient entails that he or she has the basic right to deny treatment or to choose treatment in the domain of alternative medicine. This is usually a difficult situation for physicians because they cannot easily imagine that a patient would deliberately, out of free will, refuse what they regard as effective treatment. However, effectiveness of treatment is a relative and not an absolute matter. In particular, it is necessary to explain the consequences of no treatment at all. In the case of migraine, there is only symptomatic treatment, which means that causal treatment is not available. Accordingly, the ethical problem is much less severe than in the case of a life-saving treatment or of a treatment that was capable of eliminating the cause of a particular symptom.

In a work setting, autonomy of the patient is constrained – because treatment concerns not only the patient but also the employer and colleagues at work. The employer is affected by the financial consequences of patient behaviour. In order to encourage employers to be more active in decreasing sickness absence, the Dutch government has created many incentives for action to be taken. Sick leave has to be paid by the employer for up to one year of sickness absence, which could easily lead to the bankruptcy of a small firm that has no adequate insurance cover against this kind of risk. The legislator has stated that employees have to contribute to their own recovery. If this contribution is not sufficient, sick pay can be stopped. So, it seems that there is a limitation to full patient autonomy in a work setting. For an occupational health physician, who is a company doctor in the sense of being committed to the well-being of a firm as a whole (including co-workers and employer), restriction of autonomy of the patient is easier to acknowledge than for a GP or other treating physician.

For the occupational health physicians, patient autonomy creates a real dilemma in this case. Treatment may not contribute much to elimination of the cause of the disease, but there is evidence that disability is decreased by proper medication, and thereby most probably the length of sickness absence periods. This means that taking medication is of special interest to the employer, and possibly also to work colleagues who have to take over the tasks of people on sick leave. Not collaborating with proper treatment potentially carries a high penalty for the patient. But, in this case, this is also a penalty on the employer, in the form of burdening him or her with the high costs of sickness absence.

How far does patient autonomy extend? Does it also apply to inadequate illness behaviour? By the latter, we mean behaviour that does not help in relieving the symptoms, and possibly even reinforces symptoms and disability. Occupational health physicians should be able to make an assessment of whether a patient is deliberately obstructing work resumption or whether it is a matter of undesirable but uncontrolled illness behaviour on his or her part. Obviously, such an assessment would be difficult. Offering counselling to the patient might be an effective way of changing illness behaviour, and thereby solving the problem.

For Dutch society the costs of sickness absence and occupational disability have become so high that there is an ongoing discussion about simplification of the system and possible restriction of entitlement to an allowance. There should be a balance between being generous to people genuinely in need of benefit and restricting the access to benefit of those who still retain earning capacity. In the light of scarce resources, an unnecessary benefit for a fit person deprives an unfit person of an income. This would harm people who are so disabled that they are totally dependent on sickness or disability benefits. Thus, patient autonomy can be in conflict with the value of doing no harm to others (however indirectly). Also, the principle of equity would be at stake, since the amount of money that can be spent on sickness and disability benefits is not infinite. The principle of equity, which might be expected to be pursued in the granting of benefits, would imply that those in greatest need would be assured of benefit.

Confidentiality

For all the stakeholders involved, the principle of confidentiality regarding any information that the patient has given to the occupational health physician is an important item. Confidentiality is regarded as a key principle, with a foundation in at least three arguments. First, if the patient is not able to divulge all necessary information, this could harm treatment. Second, autonomy of the patient would require prior consent before any such information is released. Third, the physician's loyalty is supposed to be with the patient in the first instance. Also, legally, occupational health physicians in the Netherlands are bound to confidentiality of patient information – although such confidentiality is restricted, since statements about fitness for work (described in terms of tasks that can be performed) are exempted. In all codes of ethics strong statements about confidentiality can be found.[9]

It is interesting to note that where there is close collaboration with personnel managers, confidentiality is sometimes difficult to maintain. Personnel managers often complain that occupational health physicians hide behind their code of confidentiality. Even though it must be clear to them that confidentiality is a strong principle from both a legal and an ethical point of view, managers often try to persuade physicians to divulge confidential information about their patients. The structure of consultation between occupational health physician, personnel manager and the other professionals involved often makes it difficult to comply strictly with requirements of confidentiality. Such consultation takes the form of the parties involved striving to solve a communal problem on the basis of equal involvement. The occupational health physician who appeals to confidentiality can easily be accused of not being committed to the solution of a troublesome sickness absence problem on the part of the company. From both a legal and an ethical point of view, such a dilemma can only be resolved by requesting prior consent for discussing a patient's problem with third parties. In practice, there will be many occasions on which there will be a breach of confidentiality. However, this is usually difficult to prove for an employee because the flow of information will be difficult to trace.

From the point of view of the employer, medical confidentiality can sometimes give rise to powerlessness. The patient can conceal unwillingness to work behind medical reasons. The employer has to rely on the physician making a proper assessment of the employee's medical condition, and – in the meantime – salary payments have to continue. Especially in the case of somatisation, employers or colleagues can get suspicious about the real reasons for the patient's absence. Most of these patients have other problems in addition to their ill-defined medical problem. Others might see these problems as the real reason for sickness absence, but – if the patient does not give consent to divulge information – the physician has no option other than to remain restricted to a statement about fitness to work.

Beneficence

Work-ability assessment can be easily regarded as an activity that operates at the interface between the interests of employer and employee. It would be a caricature to state that it is in the interest of the employer to have employees return to work as quickly as possible, and that it would be in the interest of the employee to stay off work as long as possible. In practice, this conflict of interests seldom exists. In most situations it is in both employee's and employer's interest that the employee recovers as quickly as possible, and that the timing of return to work is optimal. In addition, in the Netherlands, workers on sick leave are legally quite well protected from unfair treatment by employers or occupational health physicians. They have the right to a second opinion from an insurance physician in case of differing opinions. It is also virtually impossible to dismiss a worker for reasons of sickness absence. Guidance on return to work advised by an occupational health physician is usually phrased in terms of a suggestion for rehabilitation, which would support the employee in recovery and return to normal functioning. This would be totally in line with the principle of beneficence.

But, in extreme situations, a conflict of interests can exist. Usually, in such cases, the employer is unwilling to improve work conditions, and the employee does not want to return to work that is unhealthy. Even today, we can easily envisage the exploitation of workers at the turn of the nineteenth century, which brought about the first basic laws on health and safety. The role of the occupational health physician would then have been to force the employee back to work, which would be detrimental to his or her health. Clearly, this would now be regarded as unethical, and in conflict with the principle of beneficence. Accordingly, the International Commission on Occupational Health (ICOH) *Code of Ethics*,[10] the International Labour Organization (ILO) and the professional statute of the Dutch occupational health physicians' association all state that occupational health physicians should not be involved in both sickness certification and prevention at the same time.

This is meant to avoid conflict with the principle of beneficence. However, it can be argued that workers are still in the same situation as they were 100 years ago. Nowadays, employees in the Netherlands are entitled to a second opinion in case of disagreement with the judgement of the occupational health physician. And they also have a right to appeal to the courts. This means that they are well protected against any arbitrary decision made by an occupational health physician. On the other hand, there are many arguments against combining work disability assessment with preventive occupational healthcare. Occupational health physicians experience work disability assessments as a heavy burden – largely because they are so much dependent on a good working relationship with the employer. Some argue that work disability assessment is performed at the expense of other preventive tasks because of scarcity of time and resources. There is also some research showing that patients are less satisfied with physicians who are associated with the interest of the employer. But however important these arguments might be, they are not ethical ones.

Nevertheless, it remains the case that promoting the good of one stakeholder can be damaging to that of another (as mentioned above). Certifying sickness for a worker who is not really incapacitated may sound like doing good to that worker, but it endorses wrong illness behaviour in the worker and deprives benefit from those in need. It may lead to a deterioration in relations at work and increase the financial burden on the employer. In addition, it will undermine the trustworthiness of the occupational health physician and the occupational health service. All this implies that the principle of beneficence should lead to good professional conduct and compliance with professional guidelines. In the case at issue, this would mean a proper diagnosis and disability assessment, and conferring with the treating physician or the primary care physician to obtain a proper medical picture.

Discussion

In the case at issue, ethical principles have a role to play in relation to all stakeholders. It is self-evident that the occupational health physician breached the rule of confidentiality, because there is no mention of patient's consent. And the personnel manager's behaviour was in conflict with the principle of beneficence by giving precedence to confidentiality of the information provided by the physician.

The case description does not contain sufficient information to make any judgement about the professional conduct of the physician in terms of diagnosis and disability assessment. However, this does not seem to play any major role. But being loyal to the firm seems at odds with proper professional judgement in making a diagnosis and assessing disability. Apparently, the word of the personnel manager is taken for granted, in that the employee is not motivated to take appropriate treatment and requires some cautioning words from the occupational health physician.

In this case, there is no way of knowing how much there is at stake for the employer and the employee's co-workers. The behaviour of the worker with migraine – of not wanting to have regular treatment that might lead to lesser disability – should be balanced against the interests of other stakeholders (such as the employer and co-workers). If there is a great deal of damage in financial terms for the employer, and in terms of additional effort made on the part of co-workers because of the absence of a sick colleague, the sick worker's behaviour is less tolerable. Autonomy of the patient may be at odds with the principle of justice for other sick people (in terms of the solidarity on which the social security system is based) and the employer in terms of financial demands imposed upon him.

Judgement on the way the occupational health physicians view their job is difficult in this case. However, loyalty to the firm goes beyond what is acceptable though the breaching of patient confidentiality. Being loyal to the firm to which you provide services may be in the interests of employer, employees and society. But in many cases, not only extreme ones, these various interests collide. Then, occupational health physicians suddenly find themselves in a difficult position. They cannot breach confidentiality, which makes them easily disloyal in the view of the firm. But legitimising sickness absence for which there is no reason makes them untrustworthy to both their patient's colleagues and the employer. The easiest way to avoid such conflicts would be to act fully in accordance with the various codes of ethics, and – more specifically – to avoid the combination of rehabilitation (or return-to-work management) and sickness certification. In the Netherlands, however, this will not be possible in the foreseeable future, and Dutch occupational health physicians will have to continue to maintain a balance between conflicting ethical principles.

Conclusion

For occupational health physicians, the combination of work-ability assessment and sickness certification can lead to collision between the ethical principles of beneficence or non-maleficence and justice. The easiest way to avoid such principled conflicts would be simply to refuse to accept that combination. In general, there are likely to be only a few cases where the ethical principles will be at stake, and there are also many non-ethical arguments involved.

References

1   Cox RAF, Edwards FC and Palmer K (2000) *Fitness for Work: the medical aspects* (3e). Oxford University Press, Oxford.

2   Reiso H, Nygard JF, Brage S, Gulbrandsen P and Tellnes G (2000) Work ability assessed by patients and their GPs in new episodes of sickness certification. *Family Practices.* **17**: 139–44.

3   Jette AM and Keysor JJ (2003) Disability models: implications for arthritis exercise and physical activity interventions. *Arthritis Care and Research.* **49**: 114–20.

4   Warshaw LJ and Burton WN (1998) Cutting the costs of migraine. Role of the employee health unit. *Journal of Occupational and Environmental Medicine.* **40**: 943–53.

5   Stewart WF, Lipton RB, Whyte J et al. (1999) An international study to assess the reliability of the Migraine Disability Assessment (MIDAS) score. *Neurology.* **53**: 988–94.

6   Lipton RB, Cady RK, Stewart WF, Wilks K and Hall C (2002) Diagnostic lessons from the Spectrum Study. *Neurology* **58**: 27–31.

7   Ernst E and Pittler MH (2000) The efficacy and safety of feverfew (*Tanacetum parthenium L.*): an update of a systematic review. *Public Health and Nutrition.* **3**: 509–14.

8   Verbeek JH, van Dijk FJ, Malmivaara A et al. (2002) Evidence-based medicine for occupational health. *Scandinavian Journal of Work, Environment and Health.* **28**: 197–204.

9   Mitchell CS (2002) Confidentiality in occupational medicine. *Occupational Medicine: State of the Art Reviews.* **17**: 617–35.

10 International Commission on Occupational Health (1996) *International Code of Ethics for Occupational Health Professions.* ICOH, Geneva.

CHAPTER 9

Sickness absence management

André NH Weel and Marja J Kelder

Introduction

In the Netherlands, the employer is obliged to continue wage or salary payments to an employee in the case of sickness absence. Since 1996 this obligation has applied to the full first year of sickness absence. Because of this, employers nowadays are much more concerned about the financial consequences of sickness absence than has been the case in the past.

Usually, an occupational health physician will give advice about an employee's work capacities and rehabilitation possibilities. But employers are now more willing to consider measures and strategies to prevent and limit sickness absence and its financial impact.

The new legislation gives rise to many conflicts of interest. With regard to professional dilemmas, we observe that the well-being and the autonomy of employees, the financial interests of employers and the professional role and position of occupational health professionals may all be involved.

In this chapter we present three case descriptions.

- *Case 9.1: disability revealed on personal health review*, which deals with a dilemma in which the employee's privacy is weighed against the employer's financial interests.
- *Case 9.2: sickness absence on social grounds at the expense of the employer*, which describes a dilemma in which the principle of justice and the employer's interest are balanced against the health and well-being of the employee and his family.
- *Case 9.3: mandatory referral*, which shows how the employee's autonomy and the occupational health physician's professional responsibility may be threatened by contractual arrangements between occupational health services and subsidiary care providers.

The chapter concludes with a brief final discussion.

Case 9.1: disability revealed on personal health review

In the Netherlands, employers are legally obliged to provide their employees with an opportunity to participate in a periodic occupational health review and to hire a certified occupational health service for this purpose. This obligation is based upon Article 14 of the European Union framework directive (EC 89/391). The participation of employees in any such health review (a kind of general health examination) is voluntary and the contents of the review are derived from assessed health hazards at work. The objective of any such review is to decrease risks as much as possible.

A health review should produce information about workers' health status, especially regarding early health damage from influences attributable to work. What is the balance between workload, on the one hand, and mental and physical health, on the other? With respect to this information, employers and occupational health professionals may intervene by taking either primary or secondary preventive measures. Such interventions may concern either work adjustment or organisational change. But they can only be carried out with employees' consent.

Employers cannot take juridical steps in response to the outcomes of a health review of this kind, since participation in the review is voluntary. They are not allowed to dismiss employees, even if the latter prove not to be qualified for the job, appear not to be fit for the job or fail to meet one or more job requirements.

An employee is being examined by his occupational health professional on the occasion of a regular health review. The employee has to walk a lot (more than six hours) during his working day. He is employed as a city garbage collector. During the physical part of the examination the worker points out that he has a knee injury. It is apparent that the injury will give rise to severe osteoarthritis of the right knee if he continues in his current work. Since it will probably cause permanent damage to his knee joint, it is to be considered as hazardous to his health. In the long term, the situation may have serious consequences not only for the employee (in terms of disability) but also for the employer (in terms of the payment of healthcare expenses). In fact, the employee is to be considered unfit for his current job. The occupational health professional discusses the disadvantages of continuing to work with the garbage collector. The latter says he intends to continue his work 'as usual'. He frequently receives some additional income (tips, etc.), and is unwilling to give up these bonuses.

The occupational health professional faces a dilemma. It is quite likely – although not fully certain – that job continuation will cause health damage to the worker. Two sets of questions arise in his mind.

- Should the employer pay for the consequences of the worker's choice? Should he pay for the worker's right of autonomy?
- Should the occupational health professional consider the health hazard to be covered by medical secrecy? Or is he allowed to inform the employer about the forthcoming disability of this worker? Does he need the worker's informed consent for this? What can he do if the worker refuses to give his consent?

Value premises

In Case 9.1, two main ethical principles or values (of the three commonly employed) have to be discussed – ones that seem to be in conflict with each other. Whatever choice the occupational health professional makes, one of these values will not be complied with.

The two ethical principles are *beneficence* (including *non-maleficence*) and *autonomy*. There is an explicit tension between the two in relation to the garbage collector.

Beneficence means that all people, especially medical doctors, have an obligation to prevent or eliminate the bad, and to promote the good; in particular, they must not harm other people. For the occupational health professional, this implies that he should inform the employer about the need to reduce or eliminate the current workload on the garbage collector.

Autonomy is the principle that all people, again especially medical doctors, have an obligation to respect the wishes, preferences and decisions of people (e.g. their clients), provided that such respect is compatible with the right to self-determination of others (so-called 'third' parties). For the occupational health professional, autonomy implies that the employee's choice is respected and the employer will not be informed, which – in this case – is contrary to the implication of the principle of beneficence.

The ethical value of *equity* (the third principle) is not in danger in this case. All employees are invited to a health review. They are free to participate. If they do, the same approach is adopted – careful examination and personal feedback of results.

Analysis

The stakeholders involved in this dilemma are the occupational health professional and his client (the employee), and also the employer. Although the dilemma as described has been defined in terms of the application of ethical concepts, there are also legislative rules defining the scope for action of the occupational health professional and the employee.

Legally speaking, the extent to which the occupational health professional is allowed to inform the employer depends on the type of health examination. In the case of an obligatory examination the occupational health professional may report results to the employer in terms of 'fit' or 'not fit' for the job. Such a type of examination is not voluntary, but is ordered by a third party (i.e. dictated by law or made mandatory by the employer).

In the particular situation where the employer has convincing grounds for requiring a medical examination, the employer should receive the results or conclusions from any such examination.[1]

Much more common, however, are voluntary health examinations. These are, in some respects, comparable with consultation appointments made with curative physicians. Accordingly, the duty of medical secrecy fully applies, even with regard to any judgement about disability or non-disability.[1] This obligation can only be waived under well-defined conditions.

There are three exceptions to the obligation to maintain medical secrecy.

- An employee or patient can allow his or her physician to waive medical secrecy, but he or she should give this permission in full freedom after having been informed appropriately. In the information accompanying the proposal for adjustment of the Working Conditions Act, the expression 'explicit previous written permission' is used in this respect.[2]
- A physician is obliged to provide medical data in cases where this is prescribed by legislation, for example if certain infectious diseases play a role.
- There is a conflict of duties in the prevailing interest situation. The prevailing interest principle should be applied if a certain interest is judged greater than the interest of the patient in being protected by medical secrecy. Examples of prevailing interest are cases of battered children, and where a physician receives information about a planned crime.

It is the third exception we are most interested in here. Physicians should themselves decide if there is a situation of prevailing interest. Leenen[3] suggests some conditions indicating the criteria that might be helpful in making such decisions:

- the physician has done everything possible to obtain permission for waiving secrecy
- if the physician maintains secrecy, a third person will suffer serious damage
- the physician finds himself in a moral conflict through the maintenance of secrecy
- the physician is not able to solve the problem other than via a breach of secrecy
- it should be almost certain that, in case of breaching secrecy, damage to third parties can be prevented or limited
- the secrecy is violated to as small a degree as possible.

Discussion

First, we discuss some aspects of the ethical principles to be considered by the occupational health professional before he comes to his decision.

May the occupational health professional inform the employer that the employee is not fit for his job? Giving the information is allowed only provided there is a reason for breaching medical secrecy. There is no legal way out; a reason must be supplied. So, there must be either voluntary permission from the employee or a prevailing interest or conflict of duties. Is there a prevailing interest or conflict of duties? This would depend on the nature and seriousness of the damage that arises if the physician maintains his secrecy. On Leenen's criteria, an occupational health professional might indicate, for example, that a truck driver suffering from epilepsy is not fit for his job. This is a situation of prevailing interest where there is a clear danger to third parties. Is this also the case if an employee is damaging his own health by continuing his current job? This is not clear. The occupational health professional should give priority to the health interest of the employee. But, at the same time, he is an adviser to the employer and should try to limit damage to the employer. However, such reasoning does not comply with Leenen's criterion for prevailing interest. In our view, 'damage to own health' or 'financial consequences for the employer' are not usually sufficiently important to justify breaching medical secrecy against an employee's explicit wishes.

A further argument for maintaining secrecy lies in the important societal circumstance that patients should be able to consult their physicians confidentially. Occupational health professionals undermine their own position of trust if they pass information from voluntary health examinations to employers against the wishes of employees. Moreover, occupational health professionals should aim to be transparent in their professional behaviour. If the occupational health professional has stated that the health review is voluntary, such a review cannot have juridical consequences for his client's job. The employee should be able to rely upon this.

Conclusion

What conclusions might we then draw concerning the occupational health professional's 'best' decision?

There are societal and professional arguments for maintaining medical secrecy despite the health damage to be expected. In any case, to avoid misunderstandings, it is important that the occupational health professional discusses the situation with the employee. He should spell out on paper the consequences of continuing working in a comprehensible manner, and pass this on to the employee. Last but not least, both the occupational health professional and the employee should look for solutions for the problems that have emerged. Whatever happens, the occupational health professional should strive to keep the employee's trust, so that he will be able to remain as his work and health consultant.

Case 9.2: sickness absence on social grounds at the expense of the employer

In the Netherlands, employers are legally obliged to continue wage or salary payments to employees in case of sickness absence. A disability judgement ('Is the absence due to medical reasons or not?') is usually carried out within an occupational health service. The occupational health professional in question should act in accordance with the regulations formulated by the government. These regulations include a decree in which a criterion for medical disability is defined.

Sometimes, however, an occupational health professional assessing such a situation faces a dilemma. The case described here concerns the ethical dilemma that arises if an employee takes sick leave, but the real reason for his inability to work lies in social circumstances.

An employee, a sales manager in a large sports warehouse, reports himself sick to his employer. His wife is suffering from a severe schizophrenic psychosis. The couple has a son, two years of age. For the mother, frequent admissions to a psychiatric hospital are necessary.

During consultation with the occupational health professional, it becomes clear that the main reason for the employee's absence is that he has not succeeded in arranging full home care and attention for his wife and child during working hours. He urgently requests the occupational health professional not to inform the employer about his family situation, because he is afraid that such information might have consequences for him. For the same reason, he rejects the option of using the company's care leave regulation, part of which obliges the employee to inform the employer about the reason for care leave (usually for a partner or family member). The employee sees only one way out. He asks the occupational health professional to recommend a 50% disability restriction on his job for the time being. The occupational health professional is being asked to inform the employer that the employee is not able to work more than 50% of his regular working time. From information received from the employee's general practitioner, the occupational health professional is aware that the man's presence at home is genuinely necessary. If there is no care and surveillance at home, the situation might easily deteriorate and become dangerous for mother and child.

Value premises

In this case, all three ethical principles to which we have referred are in conflict.

First, there is the principle of *beneficence* or *non-maleficence*. Doctors have a duty not to harm people. In this case, information from the occupational health professional that the employee is fit for his job might directly cause harm to the employee's family and the employee himself. Care for dependent or vulnerable persons should be designed to provide security against such harm.

Second, however, there is the principle of *justice* (*legal justice* in this case). The law clearly indicates the situations of sickness absence in which there is a right to continuation of salary. It might be said that the principle of justice (which implies equal treatment) would be violated if the occupational health professional acceded to the employee's request. Other employees in similar circumstances might well have asked their employers for help, and not used sick leave to legitimise absence from work. In addition, most company regulations for absence on social grounds are limited in time (weeks) and money (only part of salary), whereas employers on licensed sick leave continue to receive their wages or salaries for at least one year.

Third, there is the principle of *autonomy*. Here, this concerns the professional autonomy of the occupational health professional, who –

within the limitations of his professional competencies – should give well-balanced judgement and advice to the employer.

Analysis

The stakeholders directly involved in this case are the employer, the employee and the occupational health professional. Further, other employees of the company and the population in general are also involved, although in a less direct manner.

Regarding the *employee*, we may assume that there is a major risk of psychological strain if he is forced to resume his job in full. In such case, he has no control over his home situation or the psychiatric crisis of his wife. Further, there is care for his little boy to consider. The employee has been left no choice. It is perfectly understandable that he does not want his employer to be informed about his domestic problems. Psychiatric disease has a bad reputation. How the employer might act in the future, if informed, cannot be predicted. Further, the private situation of the employee's wife should be respected.

The *employer* relies upon the quality of the occupational health professional's advice and the reasons given. He is obliged to continue salary payments in case of illness. His financial capacities are restricted. Long-term sickness absence can lead less profitable companies into financial difficulties and even bankruptcy, especially if they do not have sufficient insurance cover.

The *occupational health professional* is also in a difficult position. He has to opt for one of two primary working strategies. He might follow the principle of non-maleficence, not to cause harm, and tell the employer that the employee is unable to work because of illness. Should an occupational health professional send an employee back to work if the employee's health, and probably also that of his wife and child, will be damaged or at least threatened? Strictly speaking, the occupational health professional is preventing the employee from doing work that will damage his health. From a legal point of view this strategy may not be right, but the aim of occupational healthcare is to protect and promote the health of employees in relation to their work.

The alternative primary strategy is to respect the principle of justice and not to meet the employee's request, despite the tragic family situation. The occupational health professional might take the view that the goal (of caring for the worker) does not justify the means (of writing a false certification). According to professional regulations, the deliberate provision of false medical certification is not allowed. In this case also, this way of acting would be an inappropriate application of regulations concerning unfitness to work. Further, the occupational health professional – if he decides not to fulfil the employee's request – has other ways of offering support and advice. He might try to organise full home care for the employee, preferably in co-operation with the family doctor and social services. The employee might be persuaded to decrease his working hours, for example by a day or two a week. The occupational health professional should realise that he is responsible for the quality of his judgements and the advice he gives to clients, but not for their incomes.

Lastly, the principle of justice applies with regard to other employees in the company and the working population in general. It is not consistent with principles of common justice for an occupational health professional to arrange something for one employee in this particular situation, and not to do so for other employees in the many situations that involve social or family problems. Other employees do not 'medicalise' their private problems, do not present their problems to occupational health services, and would not think it right to claim continuation of payment according to disability regulations under these circumstances.

Discussion

The Dutch legislator has indicated that subjective complaints (which might be the consequences of social circumstances) should not be certified as sickness absence. A circumstance such as 'excessive load in the family situation' is not to be labelled as 'work disability'.

However, people may well develop impairments and handicaps under the pressure of social problems. For that reason, the occupational health professional will act in this case as in any other case, and assess whether there exists a complex of impairments, disabilities and handicaps that give rise to a work disability (according to the legal medical criterion referred to above).

Another consideration in this case is that full continuation of work might cause disability. According to legislation, such an expectation must be very certain in order to be acknowledged as a basis for such a judgement.

The occupational health professional's advice to the employer is medical by nature. Such advice consists of an objective expert judgement about the employee's work capacity. The employer has to be able to rely upon the quality and objectivity of the advice. Other experts must be expected to formulate a similar judgement in similar circumstances. Provision of medical advice that does not correspond with the truth is professionally and legally improper.

The occupational health professional has not only to deal with legal regulations. He should also consider the above-mentioned ethical principles. How can he weight these principles in a correct and justifiable manner?

He might look at the consequences of each of his working strategies. Or he might consider how often such cases actually occur. If they are rare, he might let grace prevail over justice and judge for disability, especially as health damage is likely. Partial absence would prevent a social, and possibly medical, deterioration in the situation. However, if the occupational health professional decides that the employee should not be considered unfit for his job, this has the advantage that a long-term solution might be put in place. In any such solution, support and care for the family need to be organised.

Conclusion

The occupational health professional might consider which ethical values are most important for him, and take this into account in his decision. Written documentation of the arguments is both useful and desirable in case the occupational health professional is asked to defend his decision.

There is no standard approach to cases of this kind. However, practical agreements at company level can contribute to a solution. The employer might leave judgement on care leave to a social worker, especially in sensitive cases. In the case described here, given the private character of the employee's family situation, the latter approach might provide a way out.

Case 9.3: mandatory referral

In the Netherlands, general practitioners have a referral function. In general healthcare, this function makes them the gateway to specialist medical diagnostics and therapeutic procedures, and all curative activities are arranged under their supervision. In contrast, occupational health professionals are not allowed to treat patients. However, since 1994 employers have had to continue wage or salary payments in cases of employee sickness, and there is an increasing demand from employers and employees alike for medical treatment or referral by occupational health professionals.

Case 9.3 deals with occupational health professionals being forced by their own occupational health service to refer employees for treatment. The occupational health service management in question has just signed a contract for employee treatment with two private clinics. 'Fit-At-Work' specialises in the management of musculoskeletal complaints, and the fast-growing clinic 'Master Mind' has developed a successful protocol for the treatment of psychological problems. Employers pay the costs of treatment.

The occupational health service has formulated a number of directives for the referral of employees to these clinics. For employees on sick leave with non-specific low back complaints for more than six weeks, occupational health professionals are *obliged* to advise treatment by Fit-At-Work and to refer the employee to this clinic (also providing the medical data required). If occupational health professionals do not make such a referral, this fact will be noted, and the physician in question will be subject to disciplinary procedures instigated by the medical director of the occupational health service.

In the Fit-At-Work clinic, the patient/employee is examined by an orthopaedic specialist and a physiotherapist, both employed directly by Fit-At-Work. The two draw up a treatment plan. Depending on the complaints and physical symptoms, implementation of such treatment plans usually takes 6–18 weeks, with three sessions a week. The treatment includes exercise therapy, lifting instructions, and in some cases also local interfacetary and/or more superficial paravertebral injections. This so-called 'combined approach' is said to have been tested and found to be very effective in the USA. The treatment is rather cheap, because – it is claimed – no time is lost in ineffective strategies like group discussions and psychological support. The approach is mainly based on the principle of adapting the worker to his work conditions and job demands – 'fitting the worker to the job'. He has to become stronger in a physical sense. This requires muscular exercises, and also learning lifting techniques. This approach reinforces the trend in many occupational health services – that of giving priority to sickness absence management over workplace improvement.

All employees on sick leave with psychological complaints related to work stress but without clear psychiatric symptoms have to be referred to the Master Mind clinic. A psychotherapist at Master Mind will apply a protocol treatment, which includes six counselling sessions. The employer pays for all treatment.

Four out of the 22 professionals employed in this occupational health service do not agree with the mandatory referral procedure. They send their objections to the occupational health service management. The commercial manager of the service replies promptly. He admits that some people might be treated unnecessarily. However, this probability does not counterbalance the fact that everyone who needs treatment will now have it at an early stage, provided their employer is willing to pay for it. The manager makes an urgent request to the four occupational health professionals to co-operate with regard to this new approach. Otherwise, he states, management would consider their resistance as a 'refusal of work'.

Value premises

In this case, all three of the ethical principles we have mentioned have a role to play.

First, we have the patient's *autonomy*. The patient/employee is urged to agree to a given treatment. His employer continues salary payments during his illness, and knows that his employee either has joined the treatment programme or has refused to do so. If the employee does not participate in the programme, his employer might consider this as a refusal to co-operate in the rehabilitation process. So, the patient's autonomy is in genuine danger.

Second, we have the principle of *beneficence* or *non-maleficence*. Some treatment methods applied by Fit-at-Work are not scientifically proven to be effective. They might have harmful effects or prevent the patient from having genuinely effective treatment.

Third, we have the principle of *justice*. The employer pays for the treatment, and he may decide which employees will be treated and which will not. Some employers always pay for treatment, others never do. Of course, these circumstances give rise to differences in the type and quality of treatment programmes applied to employees with similar medical problems. On a macro level there will also be differences between the employed and the unemployed.

Analysis

The stakeholders in this case are the employee, the employer, the occupational health professional, and the occupational health service.

The *employee* is forced to co-operate in a specific treatment. If he prefers a different therapy, he may have problems with his employer. In the Netherlands, freedom of choice of treatment is a right – as regards both type of treatment and its provider. However, if the employee undergoes a different therapy, the employer is likely to conclude that the employee is causing a delay in his rehabilitation. Also, some employees may feel disadvantaged because their employer refuses to pay for the treatment they prefer.

The *employer*, because of his obligation to continue salary payments, may profit from quick and proper treatment of absent workers, especially if the treatment aims to achieve early rehabilitation and the prevention of renewed absence. The employer trusts in the occupational health service. He expects the occupational health service to select a care provider implementing evidence-based treatments. Also, he expects the occupational health service to refer employees to such a care provider only if there is no proper treatment available within the public healthcare system.

The *occupational health professional* should, like all healthcare personnel, act according to professional guidelines. This means acting carefully, taking into account scientific evidence and medical experience, and using means that are reasonable with regard to the objectives of treatment.[4] The concept of professional autonomy means that physicians are responsible for their medical actions. This autonomy is not absolute, but is restricted by legal and corporate rules. Moreover, professional standards and guidelines, and also quality testing, limit the professional autonomy of the individual physician. Physicians are allowed to refuse orders or practices that do not accord with professional standards.[4] And, in accordance with Dutch corporate legislation, they may even be subject to professional disciplinary action if they comply with external requirements that are contradictory to professional legal rules. However, if the occupational health professionals in Case 9.3 refuse to co-operate, they are likely to come into conflict with their employer (the occupational health service management).

The *occupational health service* may have much to gain from a network of good care providers with which it can co-operate. The occupational health service in this case, however, is not operating effectively – from either a medical or commercial point of view. In the short term, the described referral strategy will certainly increase the number of referrals. In the long term, however, the strategy will cause distrust among employers and employees. Employers are unlikely to take kindly to a mandatory referral strategy, especially if the care provider to whom the occupational health service is sending its patients does not apply evidence-based treatment methods, and (for just that reason) does not reach its targets. And the occupational health professional who follows the mandatory referral procedure may eventually arrive at the conclusion that treatment work is not being pursued in a scientific manner.

Discussion

With the referral strategy described, the occupational health professionals concerned are trying to put the employee under pressure to accept the proposed treatment. By doing so, they might act in breach of existing legal rules. In the first instance, the employee has a right to information. This right covers the type and purpose of treatment, its possible consequences and risks, and alternative diagnostic and therapeutic procedures. The physician is obliged to inform his client or patient if the treatment is unlikely to be effective or if there are better methods. The patient should give his free consent, and such freedom is dependent on the type and quality of the information provided. Pressure from an occupational health professional and/or employer can be important in this situation. In this case, we cannot easily assume that patients will always give their free consent. Moreover, the patient has rights to free choice of physician and respect for his or her physical integrity. Given the nature of the referral strategy, these latter rights may well be infringed. The financial interests of the occupational health service and occupational health professionals may persuade patients that they are not objective in their therapeutic advice. This may also apply to employers, who might even choose another occupational health service.

Another related question is the extent to which the employer is allowed to compel the employee to co-operate in this referral-for-treatment procedure. If an employee was really hampering or delaying his or her recovery by refusing to be referred to the contracted provider, the employer might consider stopping salary payments. There is little case law about these issues in the Netherlands. However, the employee is certainly allowed to refuse a medical examination for assessment of the best therapeutic method, provided he or she does *not* intend to delay or hamper recovery.

The Dutch Society for Occupational Medicine needs to indicate the situations in which occupational health professionals are allowed to treat patients themselves, and when they must refer them to other physicians or therapists. Emergency situations in the workplace, and the presence of specific work-related health complaints might provide circumstances of the former kind. In addition, a referral function may be considered for those situations in which waiting times and waiting lists for treatment will cause delay in recovery and rehabilitation. The profession should formulate clear conditions for such referrals. First, the general practitioner should be informed. In most cases, deliberation with curative doctors is also necessary. The occupational health professional should be convinced that the employer is not putting pressure on the employee to undergo any particular treatment. The employee's right to refrain from a proposed treatment should be respected.

The occupational health professional or occupational health service should test the quality of the therapeutic programmes of the provider. Are these evidence based? Is there any quality assurance within the organisation of the care provider?

Test criteria for care providers may be formulated in terms of responses to the following questions.

- Is the care provider applying evidence-based guidelines?
- Is there an opportunity to choose from several evidence-based therapeutic programmes?
- Does the care provider test his own treatments?
- Is there any form of quality assessment?
- Does the care provider measure his clients' satisfaction?
- Does the care provider carry out research into his own therapeutic results?
- How has the care provider performed with regard to outcome, expressed in terms of effectiveness (resumption of work, recovery), quality (satisfaction, multidisciplinarity), and efficiency (time and expense of treatment)?

Conclusion

If occupational health services have business relationships with care providers, they also have to respect professional medical guidelines, and the autonomy of their occupational health professionals, with regard to treatment and referral of employees/patients.

Occupational health professionals are personally responsible for the ways in which they apply their professional guidelines. They are accountable from a juridical point of view, pursuant to both professional regulations and general legislation.

Instructions that do not comply with professional guidelines, or contradict these, may be refused. However, it is important to be aware of the consequences of such refusal.

Up to now, no practical guidelines regarding referral to care providers have been formulated in the Netherlands. Looking at the large scale on which these providers are now working, we request the professional society for occupational health professionals in the Netherlands to prepare such guidelines as soon as possible. With such guidelines, occupational health personnel would have the instruments to resist occupational health services that do not take professional autonomy or patients' freedom of choice seriously.

Final thoughts

In the Netherlands occupational health professionals usually advise about the rehabilitation possibilities of disabled workers. Because of the major interests now involved in rehabilitation, not least financial, ethical dilemmas are almost inevitable for occupational health professionals.

Within the Dutch Society for Occupational Medicine there has been a debate for several years about the ways in which sickness absence consultation should be carried out.

The Professional Charter of occupational health professionals states that the occupational health professional has a consulting or advisory role in the case of sickness absence. Assessment of work disability and advising on return to work are part of that consulting role, but the judgement of claims for continuation of salary payments and absence control are clearly not.

It is a pity that clear definitions of the concepts of 'advice to return to work', 'judgement of claims' and 'absence control' are currently lacking. Should we regard the occupational health professional's advice in Case 9.2, based as it is on social and family circumstances, as a 'judgement of claim' or do we have to describe it as 'advice to return to work'?

From an ethical point of view, Dutch occupational health professionals have to formulate clearly the situations in which they are able to advise the employer and the employee, and when this is not possible.

In this chapter we have presented three cases in which this aspect is relevant. In Case 9.1, our conclusion was more definite than in Case 9.2. In the latter, both parties expected clear and well-balanced advice from the occupational health professional. In Case 9.3, however, the autonomy of both the occupational health professionals and the employee was restricted according to terms defined in a contractual agreement between the occupational health service and a subcontractor. In such a situation, it is difficult to give proper advice to clients (either employer or employee).

Sometimes, situations of this kind may be resolved well in discussions with both the parties concerned. In other cases this is more difficult, especially where there are substantial financial interests involved. In the latter, the occupational health professional has to adopt a balanced stance with regard to which ethical principles should prevail.

It is important that occupational health professionals input experiences from their own practical work, such as those described in this chapter, into professional deliberations with colleagues – so as to test their decision-making processes against the judgements of their colleagues and generally accepted ethical and professional principles.

References

1 Gevers JKM (1996) *De rechtspositie van de werknemer bij sociaal medische begeleiding (The Juridical Position of the Employee in Social Medical Guidance).* University of Amsterdam.

2 Second Chamber of Parliament II (1992–93) 22898, no. 3, p. 26.

3 Leenen HJJ (2000) *Handboek Gezondheidsrecht. Deel 1. Rechten van mensen in de gezondheidszorg. Vierde druk (Handbook of Health Legislation. First Part. Rights of people in healthcare. 4e).* Bohn Stafleu Van Loghum, Houten.

4 Leenen HJJ (2002) *Handboek Gezondheidsrecht. Deel 2. Gezondheidszorg en recht. Vierde druk (Handbook of Health Legislation. Second Part. Health care and law. 4e).* Bohn Stafleu Van Loghum, Houten.

CHAPTER 10

Reducing sick leave: swimming upstream – positioning and multiple loyalties

Stein E Grytten

Background

From 1994 to 2000 sickness absence compensation paid by the Norwegian National Health Insurance Scheme increased by 75%. The Norwegian sickness absence rate is about twice as high as that of most European countries.[1–5] Employees in Norway get full economic compensation for 52 weeks of sick leave. The first 16 days are paid for by the employing organisation, and for the rest of the year via the national insurance scheme.

Occupational health services cover the majority of larger Norwegian companies. Occupational health organisation, the professional qualifications and competence of occupational health personnel, and the level of services vary.

From the perspective of most company leaders, high sickness absence is one of several unacceptable expenses. From the employee's point of view, however, it is often regarded as a result of high job demands and heavy workload. Having colleagues with health problems creates an additional strain, and an increased risk of further negative development. The remaining personnel have to compensate for the productivity losses resulting from reduced effort on the part of unfit personnel or their absence from work. And in the view of occupational health physicians, high absenteeism is a result of a combination of factors. Socio-economic variables, such as unemployment rate and social insurance legislation, are known to be important – while (as described here) internal work and employment conditions also affect the absence rate.

As director of the Health, Security and Environment (HSE) Department in one of 10 factories in a large Norwegian company, with a total of about 4500 employees, I was early confronted by demands for immediate action to counteract sickness absenteeism. The HSE Department was instructed to reduce absence and improve workers' performance, which would result in increased productivity. Here, I provide a personal account of what actually went on.

Swimming upstream

I was originally employed as an occupational health physician in one of the units in the company. During my first year of employment, I accepted the further positions of director of the HSE department at the local factory, and chairman of senior management's Occupational Health Advisory Board.

As director of the HSE department I was part of the company's management team. At the same time, I was an occupational health physician with responsibilities for medical examinations, research and traditional physician–patient relationships. My roles as a manager and as an occupational health physician at a personal level affected both the health of employees and the rate of sickness absenteeism. They therefore have to be described and evaluated separately.

Leading the company's Occupational Health Advisory Board meant co-operating with and counselling the company's senior management on health-related matters. The Board was responsible for developing and ensuring high standards in the occupational health departments of the company's various production units. As discussed later, these tasks increased the potential for ethical role conflicts.

At company management level there was a focus on measures addressing work conditions and personnel management within the company in general. The role of the occupational health physician in this regard was largely 'political', which involved exerting continuous influence on decisions whenever possible. This implied trying to teach engineers and economists to take care of employees in a way that kept them healthy, satisfied and effective – which would reduce sick leave and other losses in production. In-house procedures demanded that all decisions in the company had to include an assessment of health and safety effects. Positioning, participation and influence, whenever a decision was made, was necessary for results, influence and performance. And, at least theoretically, this was feasible.

When writing the company's mission statement, it was easy enough to define personnel as the 'most important resource'. In the 'real world', however, when it came to practical decisions at senior management level, the signals were often for new goals, more demands, cuts in costs, increased effectiveness and reductions in the number of people employed. The local factories continuously had to meets threats of closure if these goals were not reached. When local management moved more slowly than senior management wanted, decisions were shifted from the factories up to company level.

In the factories, this was seen as an infringement of local autonomy and integrity. Decisions made at the 'wrong level' often had negative consequences. Years of experience and local knowledge were over-ruled, which obviously affected the work environment and employees' health. There was a considerable gap between demands and defined responsibilities, and the question of a lack of authority was openly discussed. This made employees frustrated, and resulted in different personal strategies – ranging from resignations to an increase in fighting spirit. Some employees became worn out and consulted the occupational health department for help. Demands for loyalty towards senior management were self-evident, and local leaders had little choice but to show it if they wanted to stay in their jobs.

At person level, work for sickness absence reduction also demanded action in a variety of arenas. Primary preventive action focused on basic environmental factors, and also on local factory culture and employees' attitudes. Secondary prevention consisted of targeting measures at personnel who were absent, or tended to be absent, from work for health reasons.

Appropriate demands, work control (autonomy) and workplace social support are well-documented criteria for a positive work environment and healthy workers.[6] Practical efforts were supposed to start before employment – by recruiting employees with adequate qualities. It then had to continue until retirement – with preventive actions and a focus on work conditions. Taking care of employees and a system for personal follow-up of work-related health problems were established. Implementation took place gradually over a lengthy period – in close collaboration with the principal stakeholders, namely the local plant director, the various trade unions, the personnel department and the occupational health unit.

The main strategies were as follows.

- A procedure for the recruitment of employees with adequate competence.
- Reorganisation into a team-based company. Teams with collective responsibility and authority, reporting directly to the managing director, were established. Team members were chosen on the basis of their own wishes and competence.

- Collegial solidarity was focused upon. Flexibility among colleagues, with temporary reductions in workload caused by health problems, was accepted. This demanded training and habituation. Easy, fast and flexible solutions were found.
- A procedure for close follow-up of sick leave, with personal contact, was established in co-operation with the labour unions. Employees should inform their first-line supervisor or manager on the first day of sickness absence. There was follow-up from the company, based on consideration not control, at least every second week. The employee had no duty to report medical diagnoses. Contacts were made to identify what needed to be done, jointly by the company and the employee, to prepare for return to work. Communication was documented in writing.
- Evaluations, in part statistically based, of developments and differences between departments were performed. Monthly meetings were held in each department, which ended in agreements on necessary actions.
- A rehabilitation panel, comprising trusted employer and employee representatives, was set up. The panel met monthly; employees on long-term sick leave or with health problems related to work environment attended for a discussion of possible solutions. In-house solutions within the company were preferred.
- A scheme for financial support in cases where rehabilitation outside the company became necessary was established.
- The occupational health physician documented personal situations, efforts made and needs for rehabilitation outside the company, and followed up each employee until a satisfactory solution had been reached.
- Extended rights to personal documentation of sick leave were given to employees. The company had to trust employees' own evaluations of ability to manage their work. The old tradition that self-reported short-term 'sick leave', namely the 'right' to take a few days off work when needed, was to be abolished. General practitioners' knowledge of workload and evaluation of ability to manage work were regarded as poor, and deemed unnecessary.
- Support and documentation in cases where early retirement was necessary were given.

The results of all this work were rewarding. Total sickness absence in the factory was reduced from 12.4% to 6.8% between 1996 and 2000, which amounts to 46% over the period in question. Between 1993 and 2001, 95 people (18% of the employees) had a rehabilitation case evaluated, of whom 59 (62%) were still employed after rehabilitation. In particular:

- a dramatic reduction in sick leave with a stable workforce made the work day predictable

- the number of inexperienced substitutes was reduced
- expenses for overtime and hiring extra workers were immensely reduced
- production rate and quality increased with a stable workforce
- pressure from senior management lost part of its focus
- follow-up of employees was documented in a proper manner
- much time was devoted to teach both workers and their supervisors or managers the main goal of 'caring for' employees with health problems; at the beginning, some employees signalled worries concerning increased control, but good experiences of local directors being willing to make necessary investments to adjust workload eventually changed this view
- union leaders, who were sceptical at the beginning, became the most important sellers of the system
- employees made contact with their leader or the occupational health department on their own initiative when they were in need of help
- the financial benefit for the company was much higher than the cost of the occupational health department
- today, systematic work with sick leave is, in Norway, regarded as the 'proper way' of doing things – with benefits for everyone
- the occupational health physician enjoyed increased respect, and was asked to participate in discussions at all levels within the company
- the project and its results were referred to in national news
- other companies asked for help, and lectures were given.

Ethical analysis

Activity at company level and as a member of a management team is one aspect of work, and activity at person level – involving the handling of specific cases – is another. The potential for conflict between different roles is important and ever present. Any ethical analysis will focus on the principles of *beneficence* or *non-maleficence* (doing and promoting good and avoiding harm), *autonomy* (respect for the person) and *justice* (entailing that all have a right to be treated fairly and equally).

Work at company level

At company level most occupational health-related decisions have a direct impact on the work environment and the rate of sick leave. 'Positive' decisions may be a primary preventive, contributing to lowering of sickness absence. By contrast, 'negative' decisions often give opposite results. In the processes described, the key stakeholders were the owners of the company, senior management, local team leaders in the factories, the employees, the occupational health physician and his group, and – to some extent – other companies in the immediate industrial environment.

Beneficence and non-maleficence

In this case, the problem of working consistently for beneficence at company level lay in the differing priorities and goals of the various stakeholders. The main objective of owners and senior management seemed to lie in short-term profit. Increasing global competition and lower prices demanded cuts in expenses and an improved production rate to maintain adequate earnings. For employees in a local factory, long-term improvements and a stable and secure job were most important.

Such goal discrepancy has potential for differences in opinions when consequences of action are evaluated. Senior management's priority was to work for the company's owners (shareholders), and the demand was for a quick return on any potentially profitable investment. Defining personnel as the 'most important resource' when forming a company's ideal goal is always theoretically easy. Pinning personnel-related goals to the wall, displaying them to customers, was perceived as a 'booster' with competitive benefits. But carrying out the mission and waiting for a long-term reduction in production losses and increased profit proved to take too long, and was not a priority for senior management. Short-term results were required. By running factories the 'hard way', at least in their eyes, they succeeded to some extent.

Management in the particular local factory with which I was involved was pressurised by senior company management's desires for efficiency, and by the priority they gave to immediate production. Repeated demands for cutting costs and increasing profits were hard to accomplish in the short term. In the end, this resulted in a decision where senior management defined the plant as a 'marginal unit'. The unit had either to show capacity for fast improvement or be shut down. At the same time, both investment and autonomy at all levels in the factory were reduced. All local decisions had to be accepted by the company's managing director before being implemented.

Decisions were controlled from above in great detail, and a gap between demands and freedom to make decisions developed. Blindly following senior management's decisions would give local management some positive benefits. They would be regarded as loyal leaders, able to fulfil demands, and would be given positive recommendations by senior management when applying for a new job.

It also seemed obvious that reduction in costs would strengthen the unit's ability to survive.

On the other hand, local managers had to face workers who emphasised the risks of negative consequences in the forms of production failure and financial loss. Angry and disappointed workers told the plant director that it was 'expensive to be poor'. Only investment would provide a foundation for financial success. But the director was being forced to reduce the number of personnel at the same time as production should increase.

Cutbacks were driven to a level where local managers met with aggression from employees, which gave rise to a lot of negative feelings among management. On the other hand, the employees also observed the pressure their leaders were under from senior management. In some respects, therefore, they were met with sympathy – which can be regarded as both positive and negative.

The employees' initial reaction was that the company's demands gave them negative signals. They accepted the need for improvement and increased efficiency, but their priority was for long-term improvement that would secure work for the future. Reductions in the workforce and investment, combined with increasing job demands, were creating a really bad situation. Some cutbacks were perhaps necessary, but not to the extent they were experiencing.

On the other hand, this also made them angry, and the organisation developed a strong internal solidarity. The situation was openly discussed, and the 'enemies' were redefined.

The factory team had to become better than competing units, both internally and on a global basis, in terms of efficiency, quality and financial results. It had to fight against senior management's seemingly incorrect 'mental map' of the factory. Rallying together strengthened team spirit. Internal support increased and compensated for the external threats perceived as coming from senior management. The organisation managed the pressure much better, however, than during previous reorganisations. Improvements made production more efficient and profitable. In such a way, senior management's demands could also be regarded as having short-time beneficial effects.

In the long run, however, the increasing demands made it almost impossible for anyone to survive over a full working life. There was continuous heavy work pressure. Employees wanted to prove their ability to manage improvements, worked harder and longer hours, brought work home and were always available. Stress symptoms were observed. Well-qualified staff found other work. This can be regarded as maleficence (negative beneficence).

Working in the management team gave some benefits to the occupational health physician. Being able to influence decisions positively gave him respect and a good reputation in the company, and also among colleagues. Work became challenging and interesting. On the other hand, his position also made it difficult for him to oppose or object when decisions clearly had negative health impacts. Senior management required loyalty, whereas – according to the Norwegian Work Environment Act – occupational health physicians should occupy a 'free and independent position'. One of their main goals is to do good for and not harm people. The stage was set for an ethical conflict.

The situation became increasingly difficult when senior management intensified pressure on the local factory by demanding increased production, quality and profits in an increasingly competitive market. At the same time, costs and the number of employees should be reduced.

I communicated with management, informing them of the situation through the eyes of an occupational health physician. I tried to tell them that leadership based on fear was unlikely to make people work harder. Personnel had to accept work for increased efficiency, but squeezing cost-cutting into economic plans would, in my view, easily increase losses. The trend in the factory had been positive for some time with regard to reduction in sick leave and improved production, but the new regime was raising the risk of a major setback. Senior management had zero acceptance of views of this kind. Having an outspoken occupational health physician not accepting their demands for loyalty developed into a situation of negative beneficence.

The local factory was part of an industrial 'estate' with extensive co-operation between different companies in various sectors. For neighbouring organisations, the position adopted by the company's senior management was a matter of concern. All joint expenses now became a matter of discussion. Earlier agreements were not always followed. The production unit became a problem and co-operation suffered. The factory was no longer trusted by its customers. This was a negative development for everybody.

Autonomy

The issue of autonomy is also relevant when evaluating the process at company level. The owners found senior management to be efficient, in that they had the capacity to make and carry out decisions resulting in increased short-term profits. This was in their view positive. The employees in the company, however, looked at senior management as short-sighted, even brutal. Short-term profits look good but in the long run, the factory and its employees are worn down. In many respects senior management was redefined as the 'enemy', which was clearly negative.

The local directors and middle managers of the company often changed job positions. In a process where senior management had cost-cutting as a priority, local leaders with a capacity to be loyal and obedient were selected. Carrying out what had been decided at the company's top level gave them respect. On the other hand, local leaders had to face employees and their reactions. The staff observed the enormous pressure put on local directors to implement decisions from above, which in many ways made them regard the local managers as 'errand boys'. Such a situation gives little respect! However, pressure from employees did sometimes result in flexible solutions. The local leader then had to face senior management's reactions. After all, the factory was also dependent on its director as the reporter of results to senior management. He was the one fighting for the plant's survival at board meetings, and success over time would also earn him the respect of employees.

The autonomy of the occupational health physician regarding work at company level depended on what I like to call 'positioning'. Senior management seemed to have great respect for the competencies in occupational health medicine, and accepted argumentation for and implementation of various projects, at least as long as they did not have to be involved themselves. The result of internal work in the factory was very good, and was applauded. The result of the work of the occupational health department was systematically reported in order to document achievements and the company's need for occupational health competence. The positive side seemed to be forgotten, however, when disagreement and 'opposition' from the occupational health department developed.

Suggestions that could threaten senior management's main goals were set aside; opposition was never responded to, and was silenced to 'death'. For the occupational health physician, lack of response, opinion and discussion was much more difficult to cope with than disagreement. The situation was negative, and developed into a very difficult one. Locally, within the factory, the occupational health physician enjoyed significant respect. Commitment to work for improvement for everyone in the factory and taking care of employees' interests gave him a good reputation. The occupational health service became an arena where frustrations could be discussed and handled.

The autonomy of the surrounding companies on the industrial estate was challenged. They perceived a lack of interest and difficulties in decision making whenever subjects of common interest came up. An endless discussion of essential costs and their distribution usually ensued, which was a negative development. As time went by, staff became increasingly resigned to the situation.

Justice

The effects of management's decisions with regard to justice must be assessed on the basis of the position one chooses to adopt. Senior management would consider their decisions as positive, and implementation of them as necessary for survival and continuous profit. The local director had accepted his job, and regarded turbulence as part of it. He would, at times, consider the opposition of employees as unjust, for he was working for their future. The employees certainly found the process unjust. They saw the need for improvement, but often regarded decisions taken at top level as unwise. Given their operational knowledge, they thought that the long-term results would have been much better if only they had been listened to. For the occupational health physician, assessing the situation with regard to justice became difficult. Active work based on new ideas was appreciated. And title, position and salary were part of the rewards. But senior management seemingly avoided discussions and decisions threatening their main short-term goals. To the occupational health physician, this showed a lack of professional knowledge, and was regarded as unreasonable and unfair.

Work at personal level

In working for sick leave reduction at a personal level, the key stakeholders were the local management team in the factory, the employees, and the occupational health physician and members of his unit. Senior management of the company, which demanded results, was also a stakeholder, but took no active part in the practical work. The social security system in Norway is state controlled. Co-operation within and financial support from this system were often an element in sick leave reduction activities. In this respect the system was also a stakeholder.

Beneficence and non-maleficence

Stakeholders' evaluations of benefits at personal level changed over the period. The organisational change effort was extensive and took time. Senior management at company level wanted results fast, and were impatient and sceptical for a long time. When major improvements were demonstrated during the final couple of years of the period referred to, they applauded and wanted the new system (described above) spread to the rest of the company. For the local management team reduced sick leave was an important element in work to reduce unnecessary costs. At the beginning, its members had to act as defenders of the occupational health service against senior management's demands for results. When results were finally achieved, they became part of a 'winning team'.

For the employees, the introduction of a system with close contact and communication during sick leave was seen as a threat from the very beginning, with the potential of being perceived as negative. 'Even when we are sick, the factory wants to check up on us!' The occupational health physician introduced most of the new ideas involved in this work, and took the risk and responsibility involved in implementation. Succeeding was a positive incentive and perceived as a benefit. Although the activities were largely secondarily preventive by nature, they were considered good occupational health practice both in the company and among colleagues. But, at the same time, work at both personal and managerial level represented a challenge – posing a great risk of negative consequences.

High ethical standards are important when balancing on a 'knife's edge' between various professional roles. Loss of trust can easily be a consequence of unprofessional management of a rehabilitation case. That would have been a really bad negative outcome, and a complication, but it never became a problem. At the beginning, scepticism on the part of all the other stakeholders had been a burden for the occupational health physician. If results had been perceived as a failure, it would not have been easily forgotten.

For the local social security agency, participation in work of this kind demanded flexibility. We could not wait for bureaucratic decisions later; we needed action now. Traditionally, the agency had a fairly bureaucratic system, and we had to find and practise an easier way of communicating and promoting acceptance. Members of the agency had to believe in us, and also defend us against their own superiors' questioning about what we were really doing. Suspicion about the efforts of another industrial enterprise to get rid of workers with health problems was communicated to us. Our ideas and focus were new, progressive and often not described in regulations. They needed to be explained, and – by doing so – we managed to convert their concern into enthusiasm.

Autonomy

At a personal level, autonomy also changed dramatically and positively for all stakeholders. In the local factory, the system and the communication surrounding it represented what could even be called a 'cultural revolution'. Open discussions became commonplace in order to find solutions from which everybody could benefit, creating a 'win–win' situation. Employees could be trusted and were allowed to increase self-reporting of sick leave.

Local leaders built up trust. There was no risk attached to telling them about health problems. Flexibility and investments in good solutions were provided.

Justice

Part of the discussion concerning work for the reduction of sick leave involved considerations of justice. A few of the senior managers wanted the system to be implemented for production workers only. They perceived 'interference' with their own sickness absences as unnecessary and a nuisance. That was the area that presented the greatest challenges. But, building up a system for just one part of the workforce was impossible, and the discussion soon faded out. The first rehabilitation cases for managers required some customising. Having leaders meeting a rehabilitation group to discuss their own health problems was a new setting, but became a natural part of the work. Discussions of fairness and justice were no longer a theme.

Positioning and multiple loyalties

Background

In large companies, having influence on decision makers in order to achieve occupational health improvements demands 'positioning' on the part of occupational health professionals. Members of occupational health staff have to 'change hats', which has many ethical aspects. The process described above shows the ethical dilemmas that occupational health physicians may encounter.

I was originally employed just as an occupational health physician. During my first year I was offered the position of local HSE manager and head of senior management's Occupational Health Advisory Board. This was a career promotion, and in many ways I was proud and satisfied. However, I also recognised the possibility of conflicts of loyalty. I took some time before accepting the position, discussing the option with various trusted individuals in management, the trade unions and in my own professional organisation. I was also a member of the Norwegian Medical Association's Board for Occupational Health Physicians, and discussed the implications of the change in my position with other members.

Description

The stakeholders involved were the employers and the company, the collective workforce of the company, individual staff members, the occupational health service organisation and myself as an occupational health professional.

The company's senior management wanted a respected occupational health professional as leader and co-ordinator of the company's occupational health team, and took the initiative to appoint one. From their point of view, this was looked upon as beneficence and gave them respect – internally in the company, and in relation to customers and external alliances. At the beginning they accepted, and even positively acknowledged, processes in the company in order to improve quality on a range of occupational health issues. They saw the potential for financial savings. But as the international market became more difficult, demands for savings from a short-term perspective increased. Occupational health improvements usually take time, have initial costs and are not prioritised. An occupational health physician with opinions, and without fear, started to be perceived negatively by senior management, on the grounds that he was showing too little respect and loyalty.

The collective workforce and the individual staff members soon came to realise that having an occupational health physician in senior company management was a positive factor. I had close contact with the union. Initiation of the changes they had wanted for a long time was looked upon as a positive development. They perceived me as a spokesman for the 'soft values' of the company. Actions resulted in improvements that increased their autonomy and improved justice for all parties. When senior management intensified pressure for savings and staff cutbacks, I employed my professional knowledge to reveal inherent dangers for the workforce, and also for the company's long-term personnel and their health status. Staff looked upon me as fighting for the good, and never regarded me or the position I was in as a threat.

Our multidisciplinary occupational health service developed close co-operation in a team. The various health professionals worked closely together, and – in ethical discussion – we could look upon the team as a united group. For the occupational health physician, the new role initially gave great benefit and autonomy at all levels.

The Norwegian Work Environment Act defines the position of an occupational health professional as 'free and independent'. In my case, there was a compromise in that my revised job specification clarified and specified my 'free and independent role', which was important. Having direct communication with senior management had been one of my demands when I was first employed, and – in many ways – I already had such a position. But the new roles could and did significantly improve the basis for professional independent acting, and the possibility of exerting influence on decisions increased considerably.

I was looked upon with respect and given new and interesting tasks. Establishing an occupational health service at 'company quality level' in a new factory in China was one example. Working with sick leave and introducing systems for follow-up in the other plants was another. These were actions that promoted justice from an occupational point of view. Systematic procedures resulted in predictable actions and outcomes when problems arose.

When demands for savings and personnel cutbacks increased, however, senior management seemed to lose focus on occupational health matters. The need for change was, at least to some extent, evident – even from an occupational health physician's point of view. Advice from the occupational health physician on the way the processes should be carried out in a proper and humane manner was initially accepted, but the pressures increased as time passed – resulting in demands from senior management that were increasingly difficult to accept. The management demanded loyalty from local managers. This action had, from an occupational health physician's point of view, many negative effects on staff's health at all levels. It also affected negatively the future of the particular factory in which I was involved for longer than just a few months.

It became impossible for me to participate in a process where 'soft values' came across as irrelevant – a point of view that I clearly demonstrated to all the parties involved, both in writing and in other forms of communication. I genuinely believed that better results would be achieved – both economically and for the company's and employees' health – through co-operation and long-term improvements. The self-evident choice of position, that is, supporting local points of view and openly opposing senior management decisions, gave increased opportunities for beneficial action and professional autonomy on the part of the occupational health physician in the plant. Senior management obviously disliked such disloyalty, avoided all discussions and even 'went silent'. And silence is more difficult to handle than open disagreement. The occupational health physician perceived a marginalisation of occupational health issues.

Occupational health projects at company level more or less stopped. Even decisions without considerable costs but with considerable potential for negative consequences, both personally for the employees and economically for the company, were not taken. One simple but important example was the withdrawal of a high-quality system for healthcare developed for employees who are injured or sick when travelling in countries with low-quality healthcare systems.

As head of the Occupational Health Advisory Board and HSE director for senior management, I was being compelled to make decisions with negative occupational health, safety and environmental consequences. This was extremely frustrating and a heavy strain.

Years of activity had made me well known in the Norwegian local community, branch of industry, and various professional networks. I felt like a hostage, trapped in a situation contrary to my ethical standards. The negative health effects locally in the plant, in terms of lack of autonomy and justice, were overwhelming compared with the positive results achieved.

Discussion

The situation described above, connected as it was with what I have called 'positioning', demands closer discussion of possible role conflicts faced by occupational health physicians. As leader of an occupational health team working closely together, I often had to act as spokesman and had access to meetings and discussions at top company level.

Close connection to decision making did significantly improve the basis for professional, independent action. As a member of the Norwegian Medical Association's Board for Occupational Health Physicians, one of my major projects had been clarification of the occupational health physician's various roles. This was performed in close co-operation with legal experts. I knew more about these matters than most of my colleagues. When there was no conflict involved, my opinions and suggestions were usually easily accepted. The management group needed my competence. In many respects, its members were not negative to health and safety projects and evaluations in decision making. Lack of action was often based on a lack of knowledge. And in such a situation the occupational health physician provides a lot of beneficence through influence on the development of projects and decisions.

Being close to management resulted in information and discussions about future plans that would be clearly negative for employees. I could be part of the discussion, but also had to accept some decisions I did not like or approve. Acceptance of maleficence was part of the price to pay for the opportunity to exert positive influence. But when the financial results became unsatisfactory in management's eyes and 'immediate action' was demanded, the difficulties escalated. The situation had become impossible, and I had to make a choice.

I could continue fully to occupy the role of occupational health director, with the loyalties to management that this entailed, or I could affirm my professional independence, with a loss of influence and impact on management decision making.

I pondered over the issue for quite some time. Being close to management gave a lot of beneficence, and I did not want to lose this. As the saying goes, 'If you can't beat them, join them'. However, as time went by, the frustration level rose. I slept badly and people close to me clearly recognised I had changed for the worse. The priority of professional independence was never doubted, either by myself or by people in my immediate surroundings. In many respects, this was of benefit to all groups within the company. The staff recognised and appreciated my efforts. Senior management also seemed to respect my work in many regards. They used me and the results we had achieved locally as an example to follow. But, when it came to difficult discussions and decisions, they over-ruled occupational health arguments and made important decisions over our heads. I regarded such ruling 'by threat' as devastating and impossible to accept. Locally, however, we could work freely within a limited frame.

My autonomy largely increased during this process. I had a job specification specifically stipulating my 'free and independent' position. I could always ask 'difficult' questions and argue professionally without risk of 'punishment'. This was not always easy for other personnel. Staff reductions and reorganisations were a continuous threat.

A situation where multiple loyalties have to be managed is always difficult. Being a participant in 'negative decisions' by a managerial group might be perceived as inequitable or unjust by some personnel. On the other hand, the company had to make some changes even to survive. Not making decisions could, in the long run, have greater negative consequences. There was a choice between 'pest and cholera'.

As an occupational health physician in a situation where I was 'frozen out' by senior management, I felt I had been unjustly treated. First, I was presented as the initiator of a successful occupational health system that had given documented financial results; then, I was not listened to at all. This was an impossible situation. My goal had been to develop an organisation with healthy employees, working together in order to increase profit for the company. The impatience and demands for immediate 'improvements' of senior management resulted in decisions that clearly were unjust for the local plant and its employees, and had negative consequences for them and the company in the long run. This clearly affected my positions as HSE director and leader of the occupational health department.

Continuous evaluation and discussion of changes in working life and the health impacts related to increasing demands are essential. Well-defined and high ethical standards must be an important basis when working at the interface between demands for financial achievements while managing real and potential health problems. This is a fundamental basis in setting the objective of achieving a 'win–win' situation for all groups involved.

'Positioning' is important for an occupational health physician. You have to be present when decisions are taken and use your competence constructively. Maintaining high ethical standards is an important element in balancing on the 'knife edge' between various professional roles, sustaining the trust given you by the parties involved. Role conflicts can put you into a situation where you have to evaluate your own position and the consequences of different choices. And this is a position where guidance would be very much appreciated.

Very little has been written about the dilemmas involved in trying to satisfy several key stakeholders with different demands at the same time. Nevertheless, in the introduction to the *International Code of Ethics for Occupational Health Professionals* of the International Commission on Occupational Health (ICOH), reference is made to the need to pay 'special attention to ethical dilemmas which may arise from pursuing simultaneously objectives which may be competing, such as the protection of employment and the protection of health, the right to information and confidentiality and the conflicts between individual and collective interests'.[7] In many articles of the Code, there are repeated references to the obligations of occupational health professionals with regard to integrity and impartiality in professional conduct. In the Faculty of Occupational Medicine *Guidance on Ethics for Occupational Physicians*, it is stated that 'conflicts of interest between the physician's obligations to an individual and those to the managers can usually be resolved by discussion'.[8] In a *Good Practice* document issued by the World Health Organization's Regional Office for Europe in 2002, reference is made to the extent and scope of the occupational health professional's duty of care, taking into account the multiple loyalties involved.[9] It is, however, obvious that the balancing and resolving of the various interests, opinions and values of the major stakeholders and players in a company or a workplace remains a most difficult challenge for occupational health professionals.

There is no law of nature, or law of man, to do the job. A close association between professionalism and autonomy is inescapable. Professionalism involves acting on autonomous judgements, and management involves getting other people to do what one wants.[10] The situation has to be resolved by individual occupational health physicians or professionals, based on their personal and professional values.

A last thought

I have described my positions and dilemmas. In the end, I felt like a 'hostage' – as leader and representative of an occupational health service in a company making decisions with visibly negative health impacts. All of this ended in my writing and distributing an open letter of resignation to the company's senior management and the occupational health departments in its various plants. The letter stressed the ethical reasons for my decision. It was, and still is, a relief to me to have given priority to professional ethical standards over title and position.

References

1   Odelsproposisjon nr 29 (2001–2) *Om endringer i folketrygdloven – tiltak for å redusere sykefravær mv (Norwegian Government proposal to the Parliament of Norway for amendments of Norwegian Law on the National Social Insurance System – Measures to reduce sickness absenteeism, etc.')*.

2   NOU 2000–27 *Et inkluderende arbeidsliv.* (Norwegian Public Investigation. *Sickness Absence and Disability Pensioning – an inclusive working life*).

3   Pedersen AW (1997) *Fravær i arbeid – utvikling i sykefraværet på 90-tallet (Sickness Absence from Work – developments in sickness absenteeism during the 90s)*. Fafo-rapport 218.

4   Eide HG (1999) *Sykelønnsordninger i Europa (Arrangements for Sickness Benefits at Work in Europe)*. Sintef Unimed, Oslo, Norway.

5   Kolstad A (2000) *Effects of Changing Government Policies on Sickness Absence Behavior*. NOVA-report, Oslo, Norway.

6   Karasek R and Theorell T (1990) *Healthy Work. Stress, productivity and the reconstruction of working life*. Basic books Inc., New York.

7   International Commission on Occupational Health (1992) *International Code of Ethics for Occupational Health Professionals 1992* (www.icoh.org. Updated 2002).

8   Royal College of Physicians (1999) *Guidance on Ethics for Occupational Physicians* (5e). Royal College of Physicians, London.

9   World Health Organization (2002) *Good Practice in Occupational Health Services: a contribution to workplace health*. WHO Regional Office for Europe, Copenhagen.

10 Harrison S and Pollitt C (1994) *Controlling Health Professionals – the future of work and organization in the National Health Service*. Open University Press, Buckingham.

CHAPTER 11

A case of workplace drug and alcohol testing in a UK transport company

Olivia Carlton

Introduction

A railway company in a large city in the north of England requires all people who undertake tasks defined as 'safety critical' to be subject to its drug and alcohol policy. This includes the requirement for unannounced (so-called 'random') drug and alcohol testing. The external regulator of the industry is aware of requirements and managerial issues that allow the testing regime to form part of the health and safety arrangements of the company.

Alcohol testing is done by breath test. Drug testing is performed by collecting a sample of urine and having it analysed for a specific list of drugs by a laboratory contracted to do so. An external testing firm undertakes the collection of urine samples and unannounced breath testing. A positive result for alcohol leads to disciplinary action, usually resulting in loss of job. A positive result for any drug test leads to initial medical review by a physician in the occupational health team, who is specifically trained in medical review for drug testing. If the occupational health physician decides that there is no medical reason for the person taking the drug(s) in question, the physician advises the manager that the test is positive. This leads to disciplinary action, usually resulting in loss of job.

Case 11.1: a case of wrong identity?

Mrs A is a 41-year-old station manager for the railway company. Some of the tasks of a station manager are classified as safety critical, and she was subjected to unannounced drug and alcohol testing. One day, without prior warning (as is the procedure), she was tested along with nine of her colleagues. Her urine test was found to be positive for cocaine, and a physician in the occupational health department, acting in capacity as Medical Review Officer, saw her to review the result. Mrs A expressed astonishment at this result, finding it impossible to explain. She did not make any comments about the testing procedure that she had undergone. The Medical Review Officer advised Mrs A's manager that she had tested positive and provided Mrs A with a copy of her result, confirming that the drug in question was cocaine. This followed agreed procedures.

The manager and personnel manager were surprised that Mrs A had a positive result. Mrs A showed them the report so they knew she had tested positive for cocaine. She had worked for the company for 16 years, had an exemplary record, and was known to be a mature and sensible person.

The manager arranged a disciplinary hearing, during which Mrs A gave a description of the process on the day of testing. She stated that other people had come into the room while the nurse was completing the labelling of her urine sample. She thought that it was possible for her urine sample to have been wrongly labelled. This description led the manager to believe that the test had not been undertaken according to all prescribed procedures. He therefore adjourned the hearing and made further investigations. He interviewed all the other employees who had been tested on that day. The interviews with other employees confirmed Mrs A's account. The manager then asked the testing firm to give their account of what had happened. He also asked the occupational health department to review their records to advise if they had any information that would help the investigation.

The testing firm agreed that full procedures had not been properly implemented, but stated that they were absolutely certain that the sample that tested positive was that of Mrs A. The manager at the railway company felt he could not be absolutely certain that this was the case.

Mrs A was assessed by the railway company's drug and alcohol adviser, but he was unable to give any definitive opinion as to whether she had or had not taken cocaine. This was in the context of a major increase in the use of cocaine as a recreational drug that year throughout English major cities.

The railway company was left with the knowledge that Mrs A may have taken cocaine, but there was sufficient doubt about the procedure for drug and alcohol testing for it to be inappropriate for her to be subject to disciplinary action that might lead to dismissal. If the sample had been wrongly labelled, then they knew that one of the other nine people tested was positive for cocaine.

The action the company decided to take was to stand Mrs A down from her safety-related duties for a period of six months, subject to her taking regular but unannounced drug tests during that time. Her pay was protected. They also subjected all the other employees who had been tested on the same day to two further unannounced tests over the six months following the initial incident. They consulted extensively with their occupational health advisers in deciding on these actions. The company considered offering an 'amnesty' – just testing everyone who might be involved on one single occasion. However, in view of the certainty of the testing firm that the result was of Mrs A's urine sample, they decided that this would not be appropriate.

Ethical analysis

Autonomy and integrity

Integrity can be described as behaviour and decisions that are consistently in line with a person's principles and which are honest. Words used to describe the concept include *principled*, *honest*, *scrupulous*, *truthful*, *fair*, *consistent*, *faithful*, *whole* and *trustworthy*.

In this context, autonomy and integrity are usually maintained through clear communication of the drug and alcohol policy to all employees of the railway company, and through the application of strict procedures during testing. Employees working for the railway company understand the behaviour that is expected of them in relation to drugs and alcohol use, and also understand the consequences of a positive drug test. Because the procedures had not been strictly adhered to, it was not possible to be sure that Mrs A had autonomy over her own behaviour. It also made it difficult for her manager and the advising occupational health physician to be absolutely sure that they were behaving with integrity. Their autonomy and integrity were impaired because the procedures had not been followed properly. They considered that they had to find a 'best compromise'.

The occupational health physician was also well aware that his department was liable to potential criticism. Its assurance to the railway company that the drug and alcohol testing company was working to required standards had been demonstrated not to be sufficiently robust, and its ability to be seen as acting with integrity was also subject to question. For an occupational health department, where integrity is so important for maintaining the trust of both employees and managers, this is a very serious situation.

Beneficence and non-maleficence: doing good and not causing harm

The breach in application of procedures proved harmful to all concerned. The testing firm admitted a breach in procedure but denied that it was substantive. Its reputation for reliability was harmed, creating the possibility of losing future business from the railway company, and even the business of other customers. The occupational health department had to take a measure of responsibility for the harm caused, and suffered damage to its own reputation by assuring the railway company of good service from an external provider. The management solution certainly harmed Mrs A if the positive cocaine result was not hers. On the other hand, if it was her result, then she got away with not losing her job. All Mrs A's colleagues who were tested for drugs and alcohol on the same day were harmed, since they came under suspicion of having taken cocaine, and were subjected to further tests. On the other hand, if the positive result for cocaine was actually from one of these employees and not from Mrs A, then that individual obtained the 'benefit' of not being identified. The travelling public were harmed in that they did not have as absolute an assurance of their safety as they would normally have from the railway company. The railway company was harmed, at least potentially, in terms of loss of reputation.

The compromise solution showed reasonable beneficence and minimised the harm to all concerned, in particular to the travelling public. The travelling public could maintain a reasonable degree of confidence in its safety. The presence of a positive cocaine test in someone undertaking safety-critical duties resulted in some level of ongoing monitoring, even though it was not absolutely sure to whom the result belonged. At the same time, all the employees involved were subject to a degree of monitoring, but none of them lost their jobs.

Fairness and justice

A so-called 'chain of custody' arrangement was used in order to ensure that the result of the drug test could be indisputably linked to the person who produced the sample that was tested. Chain of custody arrangements are crucially important because the consequence of a positive drug test is likely to be loss of employment. In this case, the chain of custody arrangement had not been adhered to strictly enough for the railway company to be absolutely sure that the positive result came from the urine sample of

Mrs A. What they were sure of was that the positive result came from one of the employees tested that day.

If a chain of custody arrangement is sufficiently stringent, the person who has a positive drug test loses his or her job. As it was, the action the company took was not really fair to anyone, but the company considered it was the best compromise. If the test result was that of Mrs A then she could be described as lucky because she kept her job. Her colleagues were, however, subjected to two further drug and alcohol tests, and were all under a degree of suspicion.

If the test result was not that of Mrs A, however, then she was very unfairly treated. She was subjected to six months' monitoring, and was thereby under the continued suspicion of her employer. In such a case, one of her colleagues could also be considered as lucky; not only did he or she keep the job, but was also subject to just two further tests and only to minimal suspicion. The travelling public was reasonably well protected, but did not have the absolute protection it would have had if the chain of custody arrangements had gone to plan.

If all this had been subject to the rules that apply in legal cases, no action would have been taken against the people subjected to the drug and alcohol tests. This is because, when it became clear that the procedures were not adhered to, the case would automatically have been dropped. The railway company did not adopt this approach, because it considered that it had to act in some way on the basis of its knowledge of a positive test for cocaine on the part of one of its safety-critical employees. This meant that the price for the breach of procedures was not paid entirely by those responsible for it. The price, at least in the main part, was paid by the employees who had no responsibility for the offence – rather than by the testing firm, its client (the railway company) or the occupational health department responsible for ensuring that the testing firm provided the railway company with adequate assurance of good practice.

In this case, there is also the question of whether the response of the railway company to the situation reflected prejudice. If the person whose test was positive for cocaine had been a 25-year-old man from an ethnic minority background, with or without an exemplary record, would the railway company have investigated the alleged breach of chain of custody so rigorously and then acted as it did on its findings? It is impossible to answer this question, but there is room for suspicion that the behaviour of the railway company might have been different. This emphasises the need for a clear and agreed line of action if procedures have not been followed, so that there is no possibility for prejudice to have an impact, or be perceived as having an impact, on behaviour.

Ethical analysis of other alternatives

Comparisons between the ethical analysis of the option chosen by the railway company (Option 1) with two other options are given in Table 11.1. The other options were for the railway company to have taken no action at all because the procedure was flawed (Option 2), and for the railway company to have kept all involved employees in their safety-critical roles and tested them once or twice more (Option 3).

Table 11.1 Three principles of practical ethics for the railway company in relation to the options available

	Option 1 (adopted)	Option 2 (cancel process)	Option 3 (re-test 'safety-critical' employees)
Autonomy and integrity			
Employees	Does not support Mrs A's or other employees' autonomy and integrity	Supports employees' autonomy and integrity	Does not support employees' autonomy and integrity
Railway company management	Supports autonomy; integrity threatened	Supports integrity, but takes away ability to deal with a positive cocaine result	
The railway company's occupational health department	Supports autonomy; integrity threatened	Supports integrity	
The testing firm	Supports the testing firm's autonomy and integrity; the testing firm's conviction that the test was that of Mrs A is acknowledged in this scenario		
The travelling public	Minimal effect	Minimal effect	Minimal effect
Beneficence and non-maleficence			
Employees	Harmful to all, but no one lost their job	Beneficent	Harmful to all, but no one had to change duties and no one lost their job

Continued

Table 11.1 Continued

	Option 1 (adopted)	Option 2 (cancel process)	Option 3 (re-test 'safety-critical' employees)
Railway company management	Some harm – all management arrangements to be made throughout the six months – but some reassurance may be offered to the travelling public	Maleficent – cannot demonstrate that it has acted on knowledge of a positive test for cocaine	Some harm – can only offer limited assurance to travelling public
The railway company's occupational health department			
The testing firm	Potentially beneficent, although redress through other means was sought by the railway company	Maleficent; its failure to follow procedures is clearly illustrated	Beneficent; their failure to follow procedures is not highlighted (although the testing firm has other forms of redress to turn to)
The travelling public	Minimal harm – reasonable confidence in safety is maintained	Harmful – loss of confidence in safe travel	
Fairness and justice			
Employees	Unfair to all; very unfair to Mrs A if the positive sample was not hers	Fair and just	Unfair to all
Railway company management			
The railway company occupational health department			
The testing firm		Fair and just	
The travelling public	Moderately fair and just – provides reasonable assurance of safety	Not fair and just; does not support their perception of safety – a known positive for cocaine in a safety-critical position and 'nothing done'	Not very fair and just; does not support their perception of safety

On such an analysis, the option adopted by the railway company was the best for the travelling public. This is based on the assumption that the travelling public does not feel safe if it knows that someone who has tested positive in a drug test continues to work in a safety-critical position. It is also based on the assumption actually made by the railway company, and serves to illustrate why the railway company considered that the action taken was the best compromise under the circumstances.

Ethics of workplace drug and alcohol testing

Drug and alcohol testing by an employer may well be an invasion of privacy. The action that the employer takes as a result of a positive test can range from offering personal help to sacking the individual in question. A company needs to be able to justify its actions from an ethical point of view. If the argument is that a testing programme is necessary on the grounds of safety to employees, customers, the public or the physical assets of the company, then it follows that the level of risk posed by employees inappropriately using drugs or alcohol and the effectiveness of a testing programme in reducing this risk should be assessed. Such risk assessments are difficult to perform; there is little hard evidence available and the pressures of government bodies, industry organisations of various kinds and wider society may be very strong.

In the UK there is little current societal objection to the widespread practice in safety-critical environments of making it a criterion of continued employment that a person can produce a negative urine test for a range of drugs – despite the fact that any such risk assessment is not based on the same level of evidence as a similar risk assessment for alcohol. The decision to use a breath test for alcohol can be easily justified. There is clear evidence of diminishing performance with increasing level of alcohol. For drugs tested in urine the effects of a particular level of drug cannot usually be related to performance, because there is no direct relationship between level in the urine and active level of the drug in the blood. This is an area where considerable research is being undertaken, looking at other methods of testing – such as that of saliva or sweat – to see if an accurate proxy for blood levels of drugs can be related to specific changes in performance. In the meantime, two approaches can be adopted. One is not to test for drugs at all; the other is to state that the finding of any drug in urine (from the group of drugs that cause concern) is not acceptable. The latter approach has been adopted in the UK.

In Western Europe the most frequently used argument for workplace drug and alcohol testing is safety, and – in the UK at least – it is widely accepted that it is reasonable to insist that employees who undertake safety-critical tasks have to undergo drug and alcohol testing at work. In the railway industry there is a legal definition of safety-critical tasks provided by regulation. Each employer has to decide which of its employees undertake the tasks that meet the legal definition. Employers can also determine, for the purposes of running their business, that other tasks should be defined as 'safety critical'. Some employers insist that all their personnel should be subjected to drug and alcohol testing so that everyone is treated equally or because they believe that this contributes to enhanced performance. There is a suspicion, especially in Scandinavian countries, that drug and alcohol testing is introduced at work ostensibly for safety purposes, but is actually for reasons of productivity. The prevalent attitude in the UK is one of risk aversion, as displayed by industry, regulators and society at large.

Where mitigation of a risk includes employees being sacked if they are found to be in breach of procedures, it is not part of any risk assessment to consider the effects on them. However, that might form a part of a wider societal risk assessment, which is currently not taken into account.

Background information to Case 11.1

Attitudes to risk in railway companies

A very high level of safety is demanded of railway travel, in both the UK and elsewhere. The levels of injury and death tolerated for road travel are much higher than those tolerated on the railway. This continues to engender an attitude to risk that is extremely negative in managers of railway companies, as well as in their regulators. A risk assessment is therefore often likely to focus on potential loss of reputation – because of the nature of the media coverage if an event were to take place even when the actual risk of an accident or injury ensuing from that event is very low.

In the UK, legislation requires railway companies to be able to demonstrate due diligence in their approach to preventing people undertaking safety-critical tasks being affected by drugs or alcohol. Railway companies have taken the view that their approach must include drug and alcohol testing in order to demonstrate due diligence.

Procedures used by the railway company

The railway company in question had carefully thought through the procedures for drug and alcohol testing. This is because the consequences of a positive test are very serious – both to the employee concerned, who is likely to lose his or her job, and also to the travelling public, since it indicates that someone has been undertaking safety-critical tasks when they may have been under the influence of drugs or alcohol. The assurance that the testing procedures give the travelling public is that when individuals do test positive, they are appropriately dealt with and usually lose their employment. The travelling public also gains reassurance from the very fact that testing takes place within the framework of a clear policy. To ensure beneficence, autonomy and integrity, and also fairness and justice, procedures have been carefully developed – some of which apply to good practice in any industry and some of which are specific to a railway company. An account of some of these practices is now given as background to the ethical discussion above.

Unannounced testing

Unannounced testing is undertaken only for those personnel whose job is classified as safety critical. The arrangements for unannounced testing are such that only one senior manager knows that it will be undertaken, and ensures that appropriate facilities are available. An external firm does the testing. The testing firm liaises with the senior manager of the railway company. Testing firm personnel arrive and secure an appropriate area for testing. The senior manager identifies the people to be tested using a computer program, which identifies all the people working at that location and lists randomly the names of employees in each grade. The testing firm is required to test a proportion of people at each grade. They use the computer list provided to them by the senior manager. Where someone is on holiday or absent for some other reason, they move to the next name on the list randomly generated by the computer. The people who have been chosen are asked to stay in a waiting area (which they cannot leave) and are then taken into the testing area one by one to produce their urine sample for laboratory analysis for drugs, complete the relevant paperwork and undergo the breath test for alcohol. The alcohol result is immediately available.

Chain of custody

The arrangements used for all types of drug testing to ensure that a result can indisputably be connected with the person who produced a urine sample are called 'chain of custody'. They include arrangements to check the person's identity and to check his or her signature. The person is asked to empty his or her pockets as a reasonable precaution to prevent substitution of the sample or contamination with a masking agent. The person is alone when passing urine. All sources of water are sealed off or coloured with a dye to prevent substitution with water or dilution of the sample. The people go back into a room where they are alone with a person called the 'collecting agent'. The collecting agent checks and notes the temperature of the urine. The sample is poured into two bottles and sealed in front of the person; the person signs the seals and checks the name on the accompanying paperwork before signing it. All of the steps are checked and signed by the person and by the collecting agent (who is often a nurse). When the samples reach the laboratory, similar precautions are followed to ensure that the samples and paperwork can be tracked throughout laboratory procedures and matched with the results.

Urine test showing presence of a drug

At the railway company, where the laboratory has found a drug in someone's urine above the agreed threshold limit, the occupational health department is informed. The occupational health department contacts the manager and advises that the individual should be temporarily stood down from all safety-critical duties and attend an urgent medical review appointment. This is undertaken by one of the physicians of the railway company's occupational health service. Occupational health physicians are trained to do this. This role of the Medical Review Officer is not primarily related to the occupational health of the individual. It is related to ensuring fairness in the drug-testing programme. Having said that, if the Medical Review Officer concludes that the positive drug test is for acceptable medical reasons, then the case is considered a medical case and will be dealt with according to the usual occupational health procedures of the railway company.

Where the outcome of the medical review appointment is that the result is considered to be positive, the manager is informed that there is a positive test. At the railway company the occupational health team does not inform the manager of the actual drug where there is a positive test. A positive test will always lead to a disciplinary hearing. Employees can show their managers the result if they consider that this will help their case, but there is no obligation to do so.

Other arrangements at the railway company include a clear drug and alcohol policy that is explained to all new employees when they start, inclusion in the employment contract of requirements for drug and alcohol testing, a full explanation to employees of exactly what is expected of them in terms of their behaviour in relation to drugs and alcohol, training for managers in how to implement the policy, comprehensive guidelines for managers to help them to arrange for testing and how to manage a positive result in one of their employees, and training for the occupational health team.

Another option

In Case 11.1, on a purely practical level, it would have been possible to arrange DNA testing to identify whose urine was positive for cocaine, if the employees had agreed to this. This has only become apparent in subsequent discussions about the case, and was not considered by any of the stakeholders at the time. It would, however, have involved use of the second samples that are stored on behalf of the employees. It would have been an *ad hoc* solution, and there was no prior agreement with employees about the use of such a method. If Mrs A had requested this herself, she would have had a strong case for insisting that it was performed, since the second sample is considered to be, in a sense, the 'employee's sample'. The employee is not allowed direct access to it, but can demand that it is transferred to a laboratory of his or her choice (providing the laboratory can demonstrate that it meets satisfactory standards for drug and alcohol testing) to repeat the drug and alcohol test.

Role of the occupational health team

It is hotly debated across Europe whether or not occupational health teams should be involved in drug and alcohol testing in the workplace. There is a school of thought that it is inappropriate for them to be involved because they are acting in a policing capacity, and – as a result – employees will lose trust in the team. On the other hand, there is a contrasting school of thought that an occupational health team is well placed to ensure that the process is undertaken in a fair way and to acceptable professional standards.

At the railway company, the occupational health team in question is involved in:

- reviewing the effective working of the drugs and alcohol policy
- providing support to those employees who declare problems with drugs and alcohol
- managing the contract with the testing firm and the laboratory that undertakes the analysis
- providing the railway company with assurance that the testing firm and the laboratory are using good practice
- receiving the results of drug testing

- providing medical reviews for those whose drug test is found to be 'positive' by the laboratory
- communicating positive and negative results to the senior managers of the railway company.

Roles of the occupational health physician and other occupational health personnel

Medical review

In Case 11.1 the first involvement of the occupational health physician was at the point of medical review.[1] At that time Mrs A made no criticism of the procedure of unannounced testing, and the occupational health physician did not question the validity of the result. During the disciplinary hearing it became apparent that there may have been irregularities with the procedure during the unannounced testing. The disciplinary hearing was suspended, and the manager asked the occupational health physician whether he had further information. This involved a review of the medical review notes and required the written consent of the employee. No additional information was obtained from these notes.

Using specialist drug and alcohol adviser resources

The occupational health physician was then asked for advice on how to manage the case. The physician suggested that a drug and alcohol adviser assessed Mrs A to advise on the likelihood of her having taken cocaine.

Assurance of quality of work of external supplier

The occupational health department had provided the railway company with assurance of the standard of the work undertaken by the analysing laboratory, and by the company that performs unannounced testing. The assurance was made by means of regular review of the work of the collecting company and by audit of this work, undertaken on an annual basis. The most recent audit had identified some minor problems, but these had been rectified. The occupational health department was aware of some recent complaints about procedures, and had been intending to perform another audit, but had not yet made the necessary arrangements to do this.

Provision of case management advice

The occupational health physician and other members of the occupational health team were closely involved in discussions about how to manage the case, which involved managers, and human resources and legal advisers. During these discussions they remained aware that their own performance was liable to criticism in view of their role in assuring the quality of the work of the testing firm. The final compromise was reached in discussion with Mrs A herself and with her employee representative.

Concluding remarks

The case illustrates the importance of following procedures consistently at all times when the consequences of not doing so can be so serious. The nub of what happened here was that there could not be total confidence about who had produced a particular urine sample, and there was no acceptable way of finding out whose sample it was later on. This was combined with the fact that a positive test results in loss of job, and also implies a safety problem for the railway company.

In such a situation there is a clear ethical duty for all parties involved in the process of workplace drug and alcohol testing to assure themselves that they are carrying out their role properly, and to have clear agreements in place as to what happens if procedures are not properly complied with.[2,3]

The ethical discussion has also highlighted some of the underlying issues of fairness and justice in the implementation of a workplace drug and alcohol testing programme. From an ethical point of view, such a programme should be justified by evidence that it actually mitigates the risks that it was introduced to mitigate, and that in doing so, the ethical principles of autonomy and integrity, beneficence, and fairness and justice are properly adhered to.

References

1 Faculty of Occupational Medicine of the Royal College of Physicians (1999) *Guidance on Ethics for Occupational Physicians* (5e). Royal College of Physicians, London.

2 Shahandeh B and Caborn J (2003) *Ethical Issues in Workplace Drug Testing in Europe*. International Labour Organisation. Prepared for the seminar on 'Ethics, Professional Standards and Drug Addiction'. Strasbourg, 6–7 February 2003.

3 Faculty of Occupational Medicine of the Royal College of Physicians (1994) *Guidelines on Testing for Drugs of Abuse in the Workplace*. Royal College of Physicians, London.

CHAPTER 12

Alcohol abuse in the workplace: some ethical considerations

Tommy Alklint

Alice went timidly up to the door, and knocked.
'There's no sort of use in knocking' said the Footman, 'and that for two reasons. First, because I'm on the same side of the door as you are: secondly, because they're making such noise inside, no one could possibly hear you.' And certainly there was a most extraordinary noise going on within – a constant howling and sneezing, and every now and then a great crash, as if a dish or a kettle had been broken to pieces. 'Please, then' said Alice, 'how am I to get in?'
'Are you to get in at all?' said the Footman. 'That's the first question, you know.'

Alice's Adventures in Wonderland (Lewis Carroll, 1832–98)

Background

Alcohol consumption and alcohol-related health problems have increased in most European countries over the last decades. Problems of heavy drinking are generally regarded as the cause of a number of severe health difficulties. In the International Labour Organisation (ILO) programme for the management of alcohol- and drug-related issues in the workplace it is stated:

> that problems relating to alcohol and drugs may arise as a consequence of personal, family or social factors, or from certain work situations, or from a combination of those elements. Such problems not only have an adverse effect on the health and well-being of workers, but may also cause many work-related problems including a deterioration in job performance. Given that there are multiple causes of alcohol- and drug-related problems, there are consequently multiple approaches to prevention, assistance, treatment and rehabilitation.[1]

Alcohol consumption among women has increased during the last decades, and the prevalence of severe alcohol dependence in women has been reported to be around 2%, compared with men at around 6%.[2–4] Therefore, in most workplaces there will be some cases of alcohol abuse among employees.

In a health service workplace, as in others, the acute effects of alcohol may cause accidents and might in this way be hazardous not only for problem drinkers but also for their fellow employees, customers, and patients or passengers.

Absenteeism is another workplace problem associated with problem drinking, and constitutes a major stress for fellow employees, employer and the enterprise. Frequent episodes of absence tend to put an extra strain on interpersonal relationships. In this way, social support in the workplace is endangered, and the risk of acquiring stress-related diseases is increased.

The cost for the business relates to lost production and poorer quality of goods or services. There are also costs in administering sick leave and rehabilitation, and for higher personnel turnover.

For these reasons, and even more so on ethical and humanitarian grounds, it is considered worthwhile for businesses to take alcohol-related problems seriously. In many workplaces there are well-functioning programmes for the detection of, early intervention in and rehabilitation of alcohol-related problems. The ethics behind programmes of this kind are thoroughly outlined in the ILO *Code of Practice*,[1] which states that 'A balanced program should include prevention, identification, treatment and rehabilitation components'.

The ultimate goal of such programmes is to diminish accidents leading to injury or disease, reduce absenteeism and the risk of bad health and alcohol-related disease, and to enhance the possibilities of creating a safe and healthy work environment. In this way, they constitute a part of both proactive and reactive actions in the workplace, and therefore, represent an important part of the daily work of an occupational health unit.

Here, I concentrate upon the ethics of a single case of alcohol abuse in the workplace. Such a case will consume much time and effort on the part of occupational health personnel – to inform the employer and fellow employees, and to offer therapy to the suspected abuser. It will mean a lot of rehabilitation work, and resources and effort will need to be requisitioned. It is well known that such work is of great importance and value for the individual, the workforce and the employer,[5,6] but various ethical problems arise during the process. Two major phases of the problem are focused upon here: Phase 1 – if and how to get involved; Phase 2 – how to inform the workforce and the employer in order to improve rehabilitation efforts and prospects.

Alcohol and drug abuse among employees can provoke conflict in the workplace, and become hazardous for personnel as well as production. In some environments there are more dimensions to the problem than in others. In hospitals, for example, there are concerns for patient safety, and opportunities to acquire narcotics or sedatives. In Case 12.1 I have concentrated on alcohol misuse because it is the most common form of substance abuse in Sweden, but the possibilities of concomitant use of sedatives and tranquillisers should always be borne in mind.

Case 12.1: Signals of an alcohol problem

Anne is a nurse, 42 years of age. She is single and has no children. She is considered to be a competent nurse, and there have never been any complaints about her work performance. Lately she has been doing a lot of overtime work due to a shortage of staff. She has never refused to do extra shifts when called upon, except for three or four times in the previous few weeks on the grounds that she had to visit her ageing parents the following day. One day another, newly employed, nurse tells the head nurse that she has detected a faint smell of alcohol on Anne's breath, but no action is taken. A few weeks later there is a new report of a scent of alcohol, and the head nurse becomes involved. She chooses to call the occupational health unit, and asks if someone can give advice or come to the ward to confirm the suspected alcohol abuse.

Phase 1

As an occupational health professional, when the request arrives, you basically have two options – to intervene or not to intervene. There is usually a demand for rapid action, and postponement is scarcely an alternative.

Ethical issues

From an ethical point of view, you can identify at least five stakeholders: Anne; her fellow employees; the employer; patients in the ward as representatives of the community; and yourself as a representative of occupational health services.

The non-intervention option

This is almost never an option because it would allow the problem in the workplace to drift, and might end up in a situation with manifest and severe problem behaviours. Nevertheless, sometimes it can be necessary to give the non-intervention option a thorough sounding. You can then identify ethical aspects, strengthening your eventual intervention. This sort of 'reverse-angle thinking' may often be very helpful.

When you get the telephone call Anne is not your patient. This should be borne in mind, and must be made clear in your discussions with the employer.

Beneficence

A non-intervention attitude towards Anne is not beneficial to her. Alcohol problems are serious; they almost never cease by themselves, and the longer they last, the worse they get. So, if Anne has an alcohol problem, it will benefit her if you intervene. Non-intervention will probably diminish her chances of dealing with her problem, and the situation can be harmful to her. Remember that the purpose of intervention is not policing; rather, it is meant to open ways for rehabilitation of the individual.

If, on the other hand, Anne really has no alcohol problems at all, a non-intervention approach will be of no benefit to her and perhaps even harmful, since gossip and speculation in the workplace are likely to continue as long as nothing is done.

For fellow employees, non-intervention may, at least for the moment, feel like 'the easiest way'. It might give them a way to blame the employer or the occupational health unit. If nothing happens, they can assume the problem does not exist and detach themselves from it. This attitude is not of advantage for the future psychosocial environment in the ward, but it can be seen as a survival route for fellow employees. In the long run, such an attitude will create suspicion, gossip and emotional strain in the workplace, and staff will be tempted to leave the ward. This situation is of benefit to no one, and may be harmful to some.

The head nurse and management must act in accordance with safety regulations, but they might be tempted to pass responsibility on to the occupational health unit. No intervention at all is not an option for them, but they might think that they have done enough by calling upon you. However, such an attitude can seriously delay handling of the work environment problem, and chances to resolve the problem may be diminished or completely lost.

So here you are in the midst of the turmoil. And you and your credibility are at stake. A non-intervention approach is not expected from you – for this is one of the situations in which an occupational health service is needed and requested. It is of benefit to you if you intervene in a way in which your integrity is not questioned. Your actions are carefully watched and discussed. You are not Anne's doctor. If you were you could confront her with the situation, and thereby maybe pave the way for an intervention including the employer and the workplace.

If you choose not to intervene you cannot do anything wrong, but you can harm your personal reputation badly, and also that of your occupational health unit. This can severely diminish your chances of acting on other important occupational health matters. It can render the unit powerless – in that nobody will call you, even when needed. A non-intervention approach is therefore not only of no benefit to you, but might even be harmful. Nevertheless, you can and must thoroughly discuss the question of 'how to intervene'.

For patients in the ward a non-intervention stance creates a possible danger. It might be harmful, and lacks beneficence.

Autonomy

Anne's autonomy is also at stake, but the possibility of her acting wrongfully towards the patients in the ward in a medical sense is of greater importance at this point. The legal and moral consequences of maltreatment are far more harmful to patients, the employer and society than her loss of autonomy, and could in the long term be a total disaster for her.

For the employer non-intervention can cause serious harm in the long run. Staff may leave the workplace, and the quality and performance of the ward will require a lot of resources to be rebuilt. And respect for the employer as a just, considerate and active agent is most certainly at stake.

The autonomy of an occupational health unit is not preserved by a non-intervention attitude. It is best maintained by acting in a professional way. (*See* 'How to intervene', p. 172.)

Intervention

Beneficence

If Anne has a drinking problem, she will benefit from intervention.[7] You will do her good in the long run because your intervention will give her a chance to tackle her drinking habits. Alcohol abuse is a fatal and serious illness. In the short term it can cause her harm, since she probably does not want her problem to be revealed. Therefore, you must act in a careful manner, so as not to cause her harm by doing her good. It is important to adopt an ethically correct way of confronting her.

Fellow employees will, as a whole, be satisfied with your intervention if they feel that you are acting in a professional manner, but there may always be someone who feels shame for not having taken action earlier. The intervention can give them a chance to act as caring colleagues, and it will most certainly put a halt to some of the gossip and speculation in the workplace, and also the drain on energy resulting from that.

The employer will most certainly benefit from your taking action, but there may be some hesitation. He or she may try to disregard the problem, because if Anne is sent on sick leave and for rehabilitation it might mean a further shortage of staff. That can cause problems, since Anne is a competent nurse. In the long run an intervention will do good, but in the short run it will just cause problems. And what is immediate is always more visible than what may happen in the future!

Patients will also benefit in the long run from your taking action, but in the short term there may be problems for them because of the shortage of staff. But the long-term risks of maltreatment and medication theft from patients will diminish.

The community as a whole cannot accept the risk of maltreatment, and therefore will benefit from your actions. Even a suspicion of drug abuse among hospital workers will certainly damage the reputation of the hospital.

How to intervene

Your second duty as an occupational health professional is to act in a manner that does not cause any harm to the stakeholders involved. To achieve this you must act with discretion and carefully regard your duty of secrecy as an occupational health practitioner not to reveal more details than necessary. You must rely upon a programme for dealing with abusers. Such programmes are always of benefit, and it is well known that they should be established and tailored to the individual in advance.[4] It is also well known that if they are followed by repeated educational measures targeted at the workplace, they can serve you well as ethical 'guardians'.

The first and most important thing to consider is your own occupational health resources. You must always bear in mind that occupational health work is teamwork, not a 'one man show'. This gives you the opportunity to discuss the problem with colleagues and other members of your unit. Inside the unit there is room for this type of discussion, and it does not violate the principle of confidentiality. You can distribute various tasks within the unit, and thereby obtain social support and back-up from team members. Your actions at this stage create the setting for the management of the entire case.

You should consider the option of making first contact with the workforce yourself, and letting someone else be the contact person for Anne. In this way, Anne can feel more confident that her case is being handled with the utmost secrecy and consideration. You cannot take on all the roles in the drama yourself. That might create confusion among the other stakeholders. By discussing the problem in advance you enhance the possibility of a favourable outcome.

If your intervention approach is wrong, there is no beneficence to anyone, and harm may be done to some (especially the occupational health unit). In such circumstances, Anne will probably not accept a treatment pro-gramme, and that will cause harm to her. Nor is the employer likely to rely upon you, either in this particular case or with regard to future occupational health assignments. And the employer needs you as a well-functioning unit. So, you have a narrow path to follow if you are not to cause harm to the employer or your occupational health unit. And your unit is only of benefit to the employer if he or she, and also employees, have confidence in your unit's skills and ethics.

Autonomy

It is mandatory for you to maintain a stance of great integrity. Otherwise, you compromise your own autonomy and respect for your unit. Your role as an occupational health practitioner in a hospital service is to help personnel and patients in the workplace. You can only accomplish this by acting in such a way that your integrity and professionalism are never doubted.

It is also of value to have a discussion with the employer, in this case represented by the head nurse, about the ethical values and rules of occupational health services and the workplace.

Such a discussion can most easily be pursued on the basis of a drug and alcohol abuse programme already in operation in the workplace. In this discussion you must outline the different roles of the employer, the employee and yourself as a neutral party. You must state clearly that you are not supposed to act either as a police officer or as a surrogate manager.

During the intervention phase Anne is not yet your patient, and this should be borne in mind. But she still has the right to secrecy and respect. This phase is critical for the final outcome of the rehabilitation process. As stated in the ILO *Code of Practice* referred to above,[1] each individual has the right to choose his or her own doctor.

Phase 2

Anne enters an alcohol rehabilitation programme consisting of cognitive and supportive therapy, and also aversion therapy and repeated laboratory tests. She responds well to the treatment, and in due course there is a call for a rehabilitation meeting in the workplace to discuss when and under what circumstances Anne is to return to work.

The treatment mentioned above can be handled inside or outside the occupational health unit, but it is usually most successful if it takes place outside. Alcohol and drug therapy consumes a lot of resources, and there is a great risk that by taking on treatment within the occupational health service, you will diminish your opportunities to work on other important tasks (such as risk assessment and other preventive measures). So, by taking on the assignment and doing good to Anne, you may well reduce the good you are doing towards other employees and the employer.

Ethical issues

Now that Anne is about to return to work, you have to consider the various stakeholders, and your possibilities of acting in an ethically appropriate manner. The stakeholders will usually be the same as those at Phase 1.

Beneficence, harm and equity

For Anne it would be good to come back to work. But if she is not yet ready to return, you can harm her by forcing her back too soon or under the wrong circumstances. This is a fundamental question that you have to discuss thoroughly with her. You cannot do her any good, and might actually harm her, by keeping her on sick leave for too long. She has lost her identity as a nurse, and if she cannot come back it will harm her both financially and socially. However, letting her face an 'impossible' situation in the work-place will harm her even more. And her autonomy will be put at stake.

Fellow workers will probably benefit from her coming back if they can feel 'sure' that she will not start drinking again. But if they have obtained a competent substitute nurse in the ward, they may be more reluctant to let her back. The question of doing good is not easily answered, but in the long term it is always of value to maintain a good human resource policy in the workplace. Such policies have been shown to help people who have been ill to return to work. If fellow employees feel that they cannot rely upon Anne, their psychosocial situation at work may become unbearable, and they might feel a need to supervise and control her in a way that diverts resources from other important tasks in the ward.

The employer will benefit from Anne's return if there is a shortage of nurses, and may also be credited for good management of rehabilitation (although this can entail a lot of effort needed for other tasks). So, even if you consider your action as good for the employer, he or she might consider it a burden or a nuisance. Swedish and common European legislation states that you cannot be dismissed from work because of alcohol or drug problems if these are handled and treated in a correct manner. Justice is done by helping her back, but justice is not free. It costs money and effort.

For patients, the risk of maltreatment might mean that, if rumours of a substance-abusing nurse remain, they will feel insecure – with harm and lack of safety as a result. From the patients' point of view, there is no room for even the suspicion of possible maltreatment. Justice to them means total safety.

For the community it is of the utmost importance to get people back to work. In this sense you will be doing good by helping Anne back. But the community also has the right to be absolutely sure that patients' safety in hospitals is not endangered. Justice to the community requires opportunities to exercise control by means of drug tests and repeated check-ups. Under current legislation, representatives of the community have the right to ask for control measures and relevant information.

Outcome

Following discussion with Anne, her employer and her fellow employees, and with due regard to the safety of the patients, it was decided that Anne should return to work in accordance with a specific rehabilitation programme. Her return started in another workplace with better supervision and support facilities, and she had no direct or crucial patient caring responsibilities. It was also agreed that she was not allowed to work with the administration of medications during her rehabilitation. For a period of at least one year, she was called for random drug tests at the occupational health unit.

Three years later, Anne is back in her regular workplace, but she still keeps in contact with the occupational health unit – now entirely of her own free will.

References

1 International Labour Organisation (1996) *An ILO Code of Practice: management of alcohol- and drug-related issues in the workplace.* ILO, Geneva.

2 Lidfelt J (2003) *Health in Middle-aged Women.* Department of Community Medicine, Malmö University Hospital, Lund University, Sweden. Blom Printing, Lund.

3 Jenkins R (1986) Sex differences in alcohol consumption and its associated morbidity in young civil servants. *British Journal of Addiction.* **81**: 525–35.

4 Österling A, Nilsson L-H, Berglund M, Moberg A-L and Kristensson H (1992) Sex differences in problem drinking among 42-year-old residents of Malmö, Sweden. *Acta Psychiatrica Scandinavica.* **85**: 435–9.

5 Hermansson U (2002) *Risky Alcohol Consumption in the Workplace.* Department of Clinical Neuroscience, Karolinska Institutet, Stockholm, Sweden.

6 Mangione T, Howland J and Lee M (1998) *New Perspectives for Worksite Alcohol Strategies: result from a corporate drinking study.* JSI Research and Training Institute, Boston, USA.

7 Hermansson U, Knutsson A, Rönnberg S and Brandt L (1998) Feasibility of brief intervention in the workplace for the detection and treatment of excessive alcohol consumption. *International Journal of Occupational and Environmental Health.* **4**: 71–8.

CHAPTER 13

Blood-borne viruses as workplace hazards

Ian S Symington

Introduction

Occupational health physicians and nurses who provide occupational health services for healthcare workers are faced with a range of ethical issues arising from problems involving blood-borne viruses. These viruses create interactive risks, which can lead to transmission of infection between healthcare workers and patients. 'Needlestick' or so-called 'sharps' injuries provide the usual mechanism through which healthcare workers can become infected by blood from patients that contains a blood-borne virus. In turn, patients can become infected by healthcare workers during surgical procedures if an incident occurs when, for example, a surgeon is cut by a scalpel blade while operating, and his or her blood is then transmitted directly into the patient's wound.

A wide range of micro-organisms have been recorded as being transmitted via these routes, but currently most attention is focused on human immunodeficiency virus (HIV), hepatitis B virus (HBV) and hepatitis C virus (HCV). Each of these viruses is capable of producing life-threatening illness and has a high hazard rating. Incidents affecting healthcare workers and patients do therefore generate considerable concern, although the risk of transmission of infection to a healthcare worker from a single needle-stick injury, or to a patient from a single surgical operation, is relatively low. Overall, healthcare workers are more at risk of being infected by their patients than vice versa. If the blood involved in a significant needlestick injury is confirmed as containing a blood-borne virus, it is estimated that approximately 30% of high-infectivity HBV incidents, 3% of HCV incidents and 0.3% of HIV incidents will lead to infection in healthcare workers who are not immune to these viruses.[1]

Preventing the transmission of these infections and the management of incidents that do arise can lead to a range of ethical issues covering the clinical care and clinical governance of patients, and the health and safety at work and employment rights of healthcare workers. Although these affect occupational health professionals, other clinical personnel involved, and also hospital managers and those responsible for public health, will also have to examine their ethical standpoint. Even patients themselves may have to be asked to consider their own ethical stance.

Case 13.1: injury to a healthcare worker, involving blood from a patient

An experienced phlebotomist had been taking a blood sample from a patient in an infectious diseases unit, using a standard technique with a needle and syringe. Just after she had taken the sample but before filling the container, the patient suffered a vasovagal episode and fell against her. During this event, the needle she was holding, still attached to the syringe containing the patient's blood, penetrated the skin of her left thumb. The phlebotomist applied appropriate first aid measures, reported the incident to her supervisor and then visited the occupational health department to obtain further advice. She was seen by the occupational health nurse, and was clearly concerned that the patient might be a carrier of a blood-borne virus. The phlebotomist asked for the blood taken from the patient to be tested so that she could be advised about the risk of infection. Does the phlebotomist have a right to insist that this is done so that she obtains the reassurance she seeks? What action should occupational health personnel take to fulfil their duty of care?

Ethical analysis

In most simple injuries involving patients, basic first aid is all that is required. In this example, however, we are faced with a number of additional problems. Healthcare workers will usually have some awareness of the risks of blood-borne viruses, and their main concern is the likelihood of becoming infected at a future date. Here, we are dealing with two key stakeholders – the phlebotomist and the patient. In order to allay the anxieties of one, however, we may indirectly increase the concerns of the other. The rights and responsibilities of both parties must be considered.

Needlestick injuries of this kind are among the most commonly encountered in healthcare work, and they can cause much concern to those who have been injured. The occupational health personnel providing treatment and advice to the injured person are in a 'patient relation' – a relation between a doctor or a nurse and the patient. They have a duty to ensure that the best possible care is given. This would, first of all, involve a detailed risk assessment, followed by appropriate management to prevent transmission of infection and also to prevent the anxiety which is often a feature of such injuries.

Discussion

In Case 13.1, a risk assessment of the actual injury confirmed the involvement of a hollow bore needle, the presence of blood within the needle and penetration of the needle into the subcutaneous tissues. These are all factors known to increase the risk of transmitting infection if blood in the syringe is infected with a blood-borne virus (BBV). It is therefore necessary to proceed further and extend the risk assessment process to find out more about the patient whose blood has been involved in the incident (the source patient). This can reveal additional problems, since the source patient will not usually be under the clinical care of occupational health personnel. Therefore, some liaison with the clinician who has responsibility for the care of the source patient is needed in order to identify whether the patient is an infectious risk. But the injured healthcare worker may not be perceived by either patient or clinician as someone to whom they owe a duty of care – 'This is not my problem!'. The challenge might then be to ask what consideration they would expect for themselves in the same circumstances. Sometimes co-operation is more likely to be forthcoming when the injured healthcare worker is recognised as a member of the same clinical team. Clearly, effective systems need to be in place to facilitate an even-handed approach to this issue.

Information from the case notes of the source patient may already be capable of identifying a previously diagnosed HIV or HBV infection, but this occurs only in a minority of cases. Occasionally, there will be evidence of a risk factor that will point to a higher risk of transmission, but most frequently there is no evidence of such factors in the case records. The absence of risk factors has often been used to reassure those with needle-stick injuries that the risk is low, but reassurance that infection has not been transmitted can only be fully confirmed after the injured person has had a final serology check six months later. For many, this is a long time to wait when they know that reassurance could be obtained without delay by testing the source patient's blood at the time of the injury. In this case, there is no established information from the patient's case record to indicate current infection with a BBV, but a past history of having experimented with intravenous drugs has been noted and this increases the level of concern.

So, what do we do now to provide appropriate clinical management for the injured worker? She has been injured in the course of her work, and is at risk of acquiring a serious viral infection. A sense of justice would suggest that there should be access to the information needed to manage her case effectively, and every effort should be made to test the blood of the source patient. After all, she still has the blood sample ready to go to the laboratory. A further venesection would not even be required. But what would the source patient think of this?

Respect for the autonomy of patients is a strong ethical principle that has to be considered. On the one hand, they may be quite relaxed about having blood tested for evidence of HBV, HCV or HIV. Alternatively, they may be totally averse to the prospect and would rather not know if they were carrying a serious virus. Patients may react adversely to a positive test result by developing a clinical depression or even attempting suicide. In these circumstances it seems prudent, with hindsight, to seek properly informed consent from the source patient before testing. It is also important to consider who should seek that consent – for it might be argued that the injured healthcare worker is too close to the situation to ensure a fair and balanced approach, and may be less likely to respect the patient's wishes. Recent guidance from the Department of Health[2] has advocated, in the interests of equity, that a universal approach to source patient testing is introduced to avoid selecting for testing those who may be subjectively judged as being at higher risk because of lifestyle factors or appearance. In this context, it is worth noting the maxim: 'Carriers [of blood-borne viruses] look like ordinary people!'. A universal approach, it is argued, would normalise the process – and presumably result in fewer refusals.

But what happens if consent is refused? Under these circumstances, the occupational health physician or nurse must manage the case using information available. Prophylactic treatment employing specific hepatitis B immunoglobulin can be given if there is significant risk of HBV infection – but, as most clinical healthcare workers are now effectively vaccinated against hepatitis B, it is unusual to find work-related transmission of this virus. Prophylactic treatment using combinations of anti-HIV medication can effectively reduce the risk of transmission of HIV, but the occupational health physician has to consider the overall balance of advantage, since there is a substantial incidence of side effects. Consequently, treatment tends to be confined to the minority of cases where there is confirmed or highly suspicious evidence to suggest HIV transmission. In the case of HCV infection, there is no vaccine or prophylaxis available – but recent evidence suggests that if seroconversion is detected early, through regular surveillance, treatment with interferon may be effective.

The reality is that when consent is sought by an experienced clinician and the situation is explained to the source patient, it is seldom that permission is refused. After all, patients themselves, as fellow citizens, have ethical standards and their sense of fair play generally extends to those who are trying to assist with their own care. Concerns about being tested for HIV are also not as intense as they were a decade ago. The situation, however, is more complex if the source patient is unconscious or, indeed, has died. How should these situations be handled? The General Medical Council has published guidance for doctors on serious communicable disease.[3] This advocates a cautious approach when consent cannot be obtained directly from an unconscious patient, and advises that testing without consent should only occur when there is a strong suspicion of a serious infectious condition. If the patient is deceased, this guidance does advocate testing if there is thought to be a significant risk, but advises that the agreement of a relative should normally be obtained before testing.

One further aspect of the occupational health physician's duty of care that deserves attention is responsibility for the whole working population in the organisation covered, including the requirement to develop policies and procedures that will help prevent needlestick injuries occurring. In this case, for example, it could be argued that the role of safer devices has not been fully explored. If a suitable retractable needle had been made available, the injury may not have taken place. There is also scope to ensure that systems are in place so that each injured person and each source patient are dealt with equitably, and that all those involved in the process know precisely what their responsibilities are. A question that might reasonably be asked is whether or not an occupational health professional has failed in his or her duty of care if satisfactory policies to protect the workforce as a whole are not in place. This challenge draws attention beyond the purely clinical aspects of care, which cover mainly treatment and management of disease rather than its prevention. It should be recognised, however, that the provision of professional advice on such matters does not always equate with its implementation, and that liaison with managers who have executive authority to establish policy can enable the occupational health professionals to achieve more effective care for the total workforce.

Conclusions

In Case 13.1, respect for the autonomy of the source patient, in relation to consent for blood to be tested, is the predominant ethical issue that has potential to interfere with the injured person's need to receive effective assessment and management of a potentially serious risk of infection, and – for some individuals – to prevent significant anxiety. In practice, when informed consent is sought and the reasons fully explained, it is relatively seldom that permission to test is declined. It is thought that routine rather than selective testing arrangements should provide a more equitable approach and may help to normalise the process.

Case 13.2: employing a surgeon who is a carrier of a blood-borne virus

Two patients have presented with illnesses identified as hepatitis B, and both were found to have had a surgical operation performed in the same unit by the same surgeon within the previous five months. Tests on the surgeon confirm that she is a previously undiagnosed hepatitis B carrier with a serotype identical to the infected patients. She has asked to see the occupational health physician to discuss the situation and, in particular, the implications for her future employment. She is most concerned that she might have to consider giving up surgery and feels that this would be a most unfair outcome. Now that she knows of her infectious status, she feels that she can take appropriate measures to limit further harm to patients, allowing herself to continue with the expert work she has been trained to do over many years. Is the occupational health physician justified, in the interests of protecting patients, to recommend that the surgeon stops working? Would withdrawing the surgeon's skilled services do more harm than good to the wider population she serves? How can employment decisions in this case be managed with fairness and equity?

Ethical analysis

Surgeons who discover that they are carrying a blood-borne virus have an ethical dilemma quite literally 'on hand'. They know that there is a possibility that they could infect patients, but they are generally not aware of ever having harmed a patient in this way. They also realise that volunteering this information may have major consequences, affecting their ability to maintain their professional practice, status and income. They may decide – because of these pressures – to 'carry on regardless', but what would be the outcome if they were found to have transmitted infection at a future date? They could then be accused of having disseminated infection with the knowledge that they were infectious, and – within the ethical codes of many countries – could be found guilty of serious professional misconduct, with loss of practising privileges. In some countries, criminal charges could also be brought. So, faced with this dilemma, there is an ethical duty for surgeons to consult with appropriate medical advisers. Occupational health physicians in the healthcare sector are well placed to provide advice.

In Case 13.2, the surgeon who previously had no knowledge of her infectivity has been found to be the source of an outbreak, and this has been investigated by a public health team. In a sense, the decision to seek advice from the occupational health physician has already been thrust upon her. In giving advice, the occupational health physician will have a duty of care to the surgeon to ensure the case is dealt with fairly. Usually, however, it will also be necessary to give advice to a hospital manager about the surgeon's capacity for work so as to ensure that the welfare of patients is protected. In other words, the occupational health professional must 'wear more than one hat'.

Discussion

Let us first consider what the risks to patients are. The literature confirms that blood-borne viruses can be transmitted from healthcare workers to patients,[4] and definite evidence of this is reported for HBV, HCV and HIV – all of which have the capacity to cause significant ill-health (including cancers and liver disease, which may be life threatening). For HIV, over the past 20 years, reports of transmission throughout the world literature have confirmed only one definite case involving a surgeon, and just one suspected case involving a dentist. The chances of an HIV-positive surgeon transmitting infection in this way must therefore be infinitesimal. Nevertheless, the general interest in and fear of AIDS have led many countries to withdraw infected medical personnel from surgical work. There is an increasing body of literature describing HCV transmission during surgery, and HBV is now very well recognised in many reports as the most easily transmitted virus of the three. Consequently, many countries are moving towards the withdrawal of surgeons infected with these viruses.

But do these harmful risks outweigh the positive life-saving benefits that surgeons can achieve in the course of their work? Let us take an HIV-positive surgeon as an example. As a group, surgeons are generally a scarce resource – expensively trained over many years and difficult to replace. In a surgical specialty with a shortage of replacement personnel and a growing waiting list of patients who require 'life-saving' surgery, the balance – in terms of lives saved – is likely to favour the option of keeping the HIV-infected surgeon at work. Perceptions of risk, however, will vary from country to country, and some patients may choose not to take the risk of being operated on by an infected surgeon (if, of course, they are offered the choice). Moreover, many organisations that employ doctors may not wish to expose themselves to the risk of causing any possible harm to patients even if that risk is very low. Other factors may also have an influence, such as the supply of surgeons in different countries. Some developing countries, for example, which experience a high prevalence of blood-borne virus infection in the general population and a shortage of doctors, may take a more relaxed attitude to detecting and restricting surgeons who are carriers of blood-borne viruses than some developed countries, which adopt a more stringent approach.

In this case, what advice should be given to our surgeon about her future employment? The occupational health professional has checked all the clinical data available, and it is clear that the surgeon is a confirmed carrier with serological markers that indicate definite infectivity (including the presence of the high-infectivity marker hepatitis B 'e' antigen). There is a prospect of treatment that provides a limited chance of clearing carrier status, but the outcome of such treatment will not be known for at least a year. Taking into account the national guidelines[5] that have been agreed (in this case in the UK), the occupational health professional advises the surgeon that she is not fit to undertake her full range of duties, some of which involve participating in exposure-prone procedures. These are defined as those invasive procedures where there is a risk that injury to the worker may result in the exposure of the patient's open tissues to the blood of the worker. Clearly, this definition applies to the work she does as a gastrointestinal surgeon and – although she is upset by the advice – she understands that it is based on the agreed guidance applied to all healthcare workers in the country. Indeed, it is recognised as an ethical standard by the General Medical Council (the body in the UK that determines the right to practise) and by medical insurance organisations.[3] This hierarchy of consensus, with national guidelines supported by medical and governmental bodies, strengthens the authority of the advice given. It does not give much flexibility to either the occupational health physician or the surgeon to interpret freely, but each case is considered on its own merits and decisions can be applied equitably and fairly to all those affected.

Having made the recommendation on fitness for work, the occupational health professional's duty of care needs to be extended to consider other employment possibilities. Although not 'disabled' within the usual definitions employed in disability discrimination legislation, the surgeon has a health-related condition – possibly acquired through her work – which is preventing her from undertaking the full duties of her post. She is otherwise well, has extensive experience of clinical practice, and a reputation as an effective teacher. In the interests of fairness and justice, it would seem appropriate for her employer to consider the hospital's duty of care as an employer and explore what reasonable adjustments could be made to allow to her to continue in paid employment.

Is it possible to adjust a job so as to avoid its 'exposure-prone' component altogether? Some surgical specialties, such as ophthalmology and ear surgery, use operating techniques that can be performed with the hands outside the operating site, and restricting work to such duties might be feasible. Other examples include creating a focus on endoscopy, and shifting the scope of duties closer to those of a physician rather than a surgeon (which was considered in this instance). In some cases, retraining in another specialty or moving to a research-based post can be considered and effected.

Other possibilities to consider might include making 'reasonable adjustments' in relation to contact with patients, but these may raise further ethical issues. In the case of hepatitis B, there is a highly effective vaccine available that would protect patients from a surgeon with such an infection. How would patients react to being offered immunisation to hepatitis B as a precondition for surgery? Clearly, patients' views would be paramount before embarking on the route of retaining infected surgeons in employment. Nevertheless, faced with the choice between a waiting list delay and more immediate treatment, the immunisation option may be attractive to some patients. Although this approach may not yet have been implemented, it serves to demonstrate the need for innovative attitudes to work adjustment.

A further cause for concern arises for the surgeon who has infected a patient, when the question is asked if it is necessary to engage in a 'look back' exercise to identify any other patients who have been operated on and who may have acquired an infection. The decision to embark on such an exercise is made on public health grounds in a spirit of transparency, and the process aims to identify any infected patients so that early support and possible treatment can be given. The cohort of patients is identified, and if addresses are known, contact is made by post explaining the situation and inviting contact by telephone for further discussion and the offer of a blood test.

All healthcare workers are bound by medical confidentiality not to divulge the details of any patient, and the correspondence to each patient will not identify the name of the surgeon. However, once the letters are received by patients, they are likely to remember the name of the surgeon who performed their operation and discuss the issue with friends. In this situation, if a large number of letters are sent out, it will just be a matter of time before press interest is aroused. Examples of newspaper headlines 'naming and shaming' the surgeon involved, such as 'DOCTOR TRANSMITS KILLER VIRUS', can be most distressing for both the doctor involved and patients alike.

Benefits of the exercise include early detection of disease and possibly access to treatment, but the procedure can also add to the burdens of the 'worried well' – by raising anxiety levels in the population contacted. When a 'look back' exercise is regarded as justifiable, employing authorities can make special arrangements to support the healthcare worker involved – if necessary by imposing a legal injunction on the press to protect confidentiality. Any decision to embark upon such an exercise, however, must be based on expected benefits for patients; the effect on the healthcare worker must take second place behind sound clinical governance of patients.

As discussed in Case 13.1, occupational health professionals have a duty of care not only to the individual but also to the entire working population for which they are responsible. They are required to ensure that the organisation they work in has arrangements in place to prevent problems arising. In the context of preventing harm to patients from infected healthcare workers, this means that effective policies must be in place to ensure that all new applicants for posts considered to involve exposure-prone procedures are immunised against hepatitis B and free from infection with any blood-borne virus.

Many medical and nursing schools in the UK and elsewhere are already implementing these arrangements for applicants to medicine and dentistry before the start of their courses. Thus, the likelihood of problems at time of entering employment should be less. Some medical schools, however, deny access to applicants who are known to be carriers of a blood-borne virus – on the grounds that medical students might be involved in exposure-prone procedures during some parts of their course. These schools run the risk of legal claims against them of discriminatory practice if it were shown that the medical curriculum could be completed satisfactorily without taking part in exposure-prone procedures. Arrangements for both students and healthcare employees will be more effective if they can be agreed by consensus at national or international level. Applied equitably to all employees, they will protect the health and safety of healthcare workers and contribute to sound clinical governance of patients.

Conclusions

Beneficence in relation to patient care is the predominant ethical issue of concern when a decision is being made to withdraw surgeons infected with a blood-borne virus from their duties, but the balance between doing good and doing harm through such action is not always clear-cut. Indeed, in a global sense, it may well depend on the supply of skilled surgeons in a particular area. Fair and equitable employment decisions can more readily be reached through consensus-based guidance.

References

1 Department of Health (1998) *Guidance for Clinical Health Care Workers: protection against infection with blood-borne viruses.* DoH, London.

2 Department of Health (2000) *HIV Post-exposure Prophylaxis: guidance from the UK Chief Medical Officers' Expert Advisory Group on AIDS.* DoH, London.

3 General Medical Council (1997) *Serious Communicable Diseases.* GMC, London.

4 Hasselhorn H-M (1999) The hepatitis B, hepatitis C or HIV infectious healthcare worker. In: H-M Hasselhorn, A Toomingas and M Lagerstrom (eds) *Occupational Health for Health Care Workers – a practical guide.* Elsevier Science, Edinburgh.

5 Department of Health (1993) *Protecting Health Care Workers and Patients from Hepatitis B: recommendations of the Advisory Group on Hepatitis.* HMSO, London.

CHAPTER 14

Workplace rehabilitation

Knut Erik Andersen

The halt can manage a horse,
the handless a flock,
The deaf be a doughty fighter,
To be blind is better than to burn on a pyre:
There is nothing the dead can do.
It is always better to be alive.

From: *Håvamål*, Verse 71 (1222, Snorri Sturlason, Iceland)

Background

The topic of workplace rehabilitation is of interest and importance for society as a whole, and – in particular – for the present and future workforce. Accordingly, rehabilitation is about much more than regaining the ability to work and getting results. Work is linked to social and work-related networks. It gives each of us dignity and identity as a unique individual and as a member of a group. Work is important for fulfilling ourselves and for safeguarding our families.

The International Labour Organisation (ILO) estimates that there are about 60 million young people between the ages of 15 and 24 who are in search of work.[1] In this arena, disabled workers have to compete with the workforce as a whole. Rehabilitation programmes have more than medical aspects, either physical or psychological; they also encompass skills development, coping, training and retraining.

Workplace rehabilitation should be borne in mind as a fundamental health objective of occupational health services and clinical occupational health departments. But back-to-work schemes can give rise to various ethical dilemmas and considerations. Some of these will be exemplified and discussed in Case 14.1 below.

Various sets of ethical guidelines have been published for occupational health physicians and services. The Faculty of Occupational Medicine of the Royal College of Physicians of London states in its *Guidance on Ethics for Occupational Physicians* that:

> the need for special consideration of ethical standards in occupational medicine arises because the occupational physician plays different roles from those of other specialists and general practitioners. It also arises because employers and other employees may well be unaware of the ethical constraints under which the occupational physician operates.[2]

Johnston and colleagues make a similar point.[3]

Case 14.1: a worker with a problem

John is a 43-year-old male in the production industry. Over a period of 25 years, he has increased his alcohol consumption. It started during his time as a seaman, but he left sea and started onshore. He hid his problems and denied the consequences, which became more and more obvious. As time passed, he developed typical signs of alcohol-related problems, such as increased sickness absence without communicating with the workplace. Eventually, John developed neuropathy in his legs, with sensory nerve damage and reduced muscular activity from foot to knee. Blood samples showed reduced liver function, and he had an increased liver size. He started to drink methylated spirit in an amount of about 1–2 litres a day, alongside other kinds of 'normal alcohol'. He was referred to a variety of medical professionals, such as a neurologist, a drug abuse specialist, and – in co-operation with them – specialists in a psychiatric institution. He developed depression, and was periodically suicidal. During his stay in the institution, he drank in secret and was eventually discharged. John was regarded more or less as a 'hopeless case' by external specialists, and told that his physical health would gradually deteriorate, and his psychological and emotional dysfunction increase, if he continued to drink. He had a poor social network, and was divorced because of the problems that had arisen during his years of drinking. One of his children had also started to abuse alcohol and narcotic substances. His focus and wish was, as usual in such cases, to keep his job.

John showed insight and a kind of understanding, but also fear of not having a personal future. He was well aware of the consequences of his way of living, with impending poor health and job loss, and the subsequent destruction of the entire social and financial foundation on which he depended.

Employee assistance programmes

Through an earlier internal process, the employer and the company's trade unions had worked out an agreement in accordance with Norwegian national recommendations for how to handle abuse problems in enterprises. Many so-called employee assistance programmes aim to help the problem drinker, but have only a reduced focus on prevention. Accordingly, the basis for setting up a programme usually lies in job-related indexes, such as those measuring reduction in absenteeism, accident rates or work performance, violation of company regulations, and – ultimately – a wish for job retention. The objective of an employee assistance programme is usually to reduce the negative effects that have led to the establishment of the programme itself. Application of the employee assistance programme concept and the treatments to which it gives rise vary from country to country and from company to company.

In Norway, such a programme has been given the acronym 'AKAN'.[4] This derives from the Norwegian Tripartite Committee for the Prevention of Alcohol and Drug Problems in the Workplace, which was founded in 1963 by representatives of the Norwegian Confederation of Trade Unions (LO) and the Confederation of Norwegian Business and Industry (NHO). Today, the national AKAN Committee (the organisation's board of directors) consists of two representatives from LO, two from NHO, and one from Norway's Ministry of Social Affairs. These parties also pay for AKAN's operations. The aims are to prevent alcohol and drug problems in Norwegian enterprises and to provide help and assistance for employees already with a substance use problem.

Each client has to agree to the same baseline contract, but follow-up and advised therapy are worked out individually to the greatest extent possible. During the time of contract clients remain in employment, keeping their salary. The contract represents a commitment by both the employer and the client. Commonly, the trade union is consulted on the content of an employee assistance programme contract.

In Case 14.1, the client admitted that he needed help and support to deal with his drinking problem. The rehabilitation programme started with the signing of a contract. At time of signing John had been a heavy drinker for about 25 years. An occupational health professional was made responsible for medical supervision and follow-up, as defined in the employee assistance programme contract. Accordingly, the occupational health professional also became an important co-ordinator between the stakeholders – the client, the employer, middle management, trade unions, co-workers, the social security agency involved and the occupational health service. The procedure was cleared with the employee. The contract stipulated strict follow-up through both external and internal consultations. Follow-up through the occupational health service was designed to give the client good personal contact so that he felt secure. As a part of the internal rehabilitation programme, the occupational health physician – in co-operation with the general practitioner – referred the client to specialists in psychiatry and neurology. During the rehabilitation period, and as agreed in the employee assistance programme contract, a great deal of attention was paid to work adjustment and the structural adjustment of work organisation. Also, conversational therapy was provided to support coping with drinking and psychosocial problems, and also follow-up of the physically harmful effects of alcohol abuse.

Ethical issues

How can employee assistance programming[5] give rise to ethical problems in the three key aspects of beneficence, autonomy and justice?

Note that the reader can generalise the particular issue of alcohol abuse, and discussion of it, to other types of problems, alcohol related or not. These include problems related to physically or mentally ill employees, and management strategies aimed at rehabilitation.[6]

Beneficence

In Case 14.1, an employee assistance programme was seen to be beneficial to the client, which provided the basis for the decision taken at the outset of the programme. The benefits of an employee assistance programme are taken on faith, implying that uncertainties as to the client's development over time will remain. The client obtains the benefits of keeping his job and of sustaining and improving his social network. He is given an opportunity to change his existing way of life, and learns to deal with problems without abusing alcohol. An important benefit lies in support in building up self-respect.

An employee assistance programme is also seen *a priori* as basically sound and beneficial to company or employer, who may get back a qualified, healthy and productive staff member following treatment. This also applies to work colleagues and the other stakeholders involved. The employee assistance programme formalises an approach to abuse problems, which can be of benefit to both the employer and co-workers. If the programme turns out to be successful a 'win–win' situation arises for all involved. However, it should be borne in mind that this assessment is made prior to programme implementation.

Occupational health professionals carry out tasks that are expected from any professional when acting within a structured programme. Accordingly, there seems to be no specific benefit to them.

A contract is usually signed for one year, with the option of prolonging the contract period. During the initial period there is regular follow-up from the employer, the union and the occupational health service. If time has elapsed without effect or the employee assistance programme has been shown to fail, a new scenario arises. The beneficial effects of the employee assistance programme are no longer certain. They are, in fact, doubtful. The client may, however, still benefit from the programme because it may take time (more than a year) to change lifestyle. The expectations of the employer and work colleagues are not met, and it cannot be assumed that they will accept contract prolongation if a subject is blocking resources over time without any signs of positive effects. Resources could also have been used for other personnel with problems, and co-workers may be unwilling to accept work overload arising from poor performance or even non-performance of a colleague and team member. This is understandably non-beneficial to them.

Successful rehabilitation will be beneficial to society. Even if rehabilitation takes time, there will still be a benefit to society in that a citizen will have returned to work. The employee assistance programme will have relieved the burden on society by supporting a troubled client.

Autonomy

When a client signs an employee assistance programme contract, all the stakeholders involved must accept its formal content and rules. The contract can be very strict in form, and both the client and employer may perceive it as a 'straitjacket'. Clearly, the client can choose between accepting and rejecting the offer of a contract. But is his autonomy harmed? An employee assistance programme imposes limitations on autonomy, but this is balanced by gains in terms of beneficence. The limitations depend on the individual case. Examples include the client's acceptance of home visits when absent from work, consent to his general practitioner being informed about the employee assistance programme contract, and approval of a change in work tasks for a defined period (related to the development of the abuse).

The employer experiences an infringement of autonomy. This applies, in particular, to the managerial prerogative; that is, the right to manage an enterprise within the framework of accepted laws, regulations and agreements. One implication of such a contract is an imposed restraint to discharge an employee who is incapable of carrying out his work task.

And how might an employee assistance programme affect the autonomy of the occupational health professional? Employee assistance programme regulations also need to be consistent with the ethics of occupational health professionals to be accepted by them.

Colleagues in the work unit involved are stakeholders who should not be disregarded. An employee assistance programme contract commonly entails that the client's colleagues are expected to carry out his tasks when he is absent. This may be perceived as an infringement of their autonomy even if the programme has been approved by the trade union. If there is no change in behaviour over time on the part of the client concerned, this is likely to be perceived as a burden by the other staff members.

Justice

Employee assistance programmes seem to be a good and fair company policy. The client may encounter mistrust from other stakeholders until he shows a different attitude to his own problems. But an employee assistance programme policy gives all employees a fair chance, and the programme will be perceived as just. The employer and/or co-workers can conceal a worker's abuse for many years. The offer of an employee assistance programme contract often comes when employer or colleagues have lost patience with the employee. In terms of time taken for rehabilitation, the period before the contract is signed is often added to the rehabilitation period by some stakeholders because they feel that demands for their solidarity with the person concerned have already been overstretched.

At time of signing an employee assistance programme contract the client is vulnerable and de-privileged, and his self-respect is usually low. If, at this time, a non-action strategy is chosen by the occupational health professional, implying that no active measures are taken to rehabilitate the client, this may certainly be regarded as non-compliance with the principle of justice and, thus, unethical.

In our type of society it seems difficult to argue that there is societal concern over how much time is consumed within an enterprise on any particular rehabilitation project. The stakeholders may therefore have different conceptions of how the client improves. The occupational health professional will usually compare current status with the starting point for rehabilitation. The professional registers an improvement, whereas other stakeholders may focus on the time consumed for treatment and other out-of-work activities. The hard question concerns the point in time when continued efforts and prolongation of an employee assistance programme can be assessed to carry only low probability of achieving their objective. Obviously, futile efforts may be perceived as questionable from an ethical point of view. Thus, an ethical dilemma may develop when time is regarded as the main factor in making a decision in a particular case. The occupational health professional may consider referral to the 'time factor' as unjust because of its simplicity in a complicated case involving a vulnerable person. Nevertheless, it is difficult to evaluate how much time and improvement should elapse before applying the argument of justice or injustice. In Case 14.1, the professional based his opinion on the employee assistance programme and used that as an objective. The occupational health professional should not, however, hide behind employee assistance programme regulations and forget that every case is an individual one.

It is always important to bear in mind that the commitment in an employee assistance programme is voluntary. This applies to all parties to the agreement: the individual staff member concerned, the employer and the occupational health professional involved. The underlying assumption is determined motivation on part of the subject to undergo rehabilitation. If convincing motivation cannot be ascertained, or if there are serious doubts about it, the prospects of a programme achieving the objective of rehabilitation are, in common experience, bleak. In such a situation an entirely different scenario for ethical considerations emerges. The likelihood of reaping benefits decreases. The regime imposed according to contract may be perceived as an infringement on autonomy by the subject concerned. On the bottom line, there is the question of available resources, which may be more effectively deployed on other employees needing rehabilitation. In the absence of motivation, this may actually be seen as a squandering of resources in contravention of the ethical principle of justice or equity.

Discussion

Occupational health professionals must work within the confines of their free and independent role in rehabilitation. It is important that all the stakeholders involved occupy this role – to some extent or another – because acceptance of this may beneficially affect the framing of ethical dilemmas. When professionals become involved in the process at an early stage, strong 'ownership' of a particular case may develop – especially if they feel that other stakeholders are insecure and shunning responsibility. From the professional's point of view, this is not the case. In the longer term, it can lead to reduced autonomy – for both the employer and the client.

Politicians, employers' organisations and unions in Norway seem to have reached virtual consensus in sharpening focus on management accountability for the physical and psychological work environment. Increased efforts are also being made to reduce days of sickness and to prioritise rehabilitation programmes. This gives rise to an ethical paradox in real life when companies are signalling the priorities of high efficiency (including downsizing), increased productivity and a stable workforce. All these factors can give rise to difficult ethical dilemmas for the employer, unions and occupational health professionals. Working with rehabilitation finance[7] can sooner or later lead stakeholders into troublesome ethical situations. To what lengths should rehabilitation programmes be pursued in the face of an assessment of diminishing returns? Although it is important that the various stakeholders have individual considerations with regard to ethical assessments, the decisions involved can be perceived as troublesome.

Words such as *impairment*, *disability*, *efficiency*, *inefficiency* and *competence* come up much more frequently in dialogue about a client than used to be the case. The occupational health professional should not try to 'medicalise' any disability; rather, the client must be an active part of the entire process. He must seek to understand how he functions at work with his changed capacity. It seems that many companies have a wish to achieve objectives as quickly as possible. A long-term rehabilitation programme is much more difficult to operate today than it was some years ago.[8–10] The client can easily be branded as an inefficient resource, and positioned on the debit side in a team setting. Use of time and resources cannot be formally weighted when beneficence, autonomy and justice are handled in a proper manner. It is a challenge for the occupational health professionals to take individual considerations into account when operating on an ethical basis.

John is now 59 years old, and he has stayed sober for more than 13 years. His neurological condition is almost normal. His liver function is quite normal. He has, however, developed asthma and grave rheumatism. John is now working part time in a well-adjusted but normal job situation, and carrying out his tasks to the satisfaction of management and colleagues. Also, nine months ago, he quit smoking.

Concluding remarks

The objective for all involved may be the same, but understandings of how to obtain it will differ, thereby giving rise to ethical dilemmas.

Occupational health professionals always have to capture the complexity in a case. The facts of the case provide the basis for the health professional's contribution to the challenge of adapting conditions at work to the capabilities of the client, taking into account medical and psychosocial considerations. This is the prima facie ethical obligation of occupational health professionals. It is usually, however, difficult to say anything about an employee's future ability and coping position. They are not only dependent on medical factors, but also on a person's willingness to make internal adjustments, and also the attitudes of the employer and co-workers.

At the early, unsettled stage of a rehabilitation programme, occupational health professionals should not be used to seek medical reasons for an early retirement or disability pension. Some companies argue for disability benefit even when the prognosis is unsettled. They may even 'buy out' the client if they feel the situation to be troublesome. In this way, autonomy is infringed – because the employer places the client on an edge where he has little opportunity to defend himself against paid exclusion. The client's autonomy and sense of justice can be impaired if an occupational health professional supports any such argument or solution. In addition, one fundamental difficulty to confront is the fact that occupational health professionals working under contract with an employer commonly have no accountability or responsibility extending beyond that of their employers.

Rehabilitation is a process that, for the client, should develop better life quality, vigour, knowledge, capacity for coping with disease and recognition of opportunities and limitations. Not least, rehabilitation should lead to the feeling of not being rejected. Occupational health professionals have an important function in the rehabilitation process – not least because there is a need to focus on the ethics of any operational rehabilitation programme.

References

1 International Labour Organisation (1998–99) *World Employment Report*. ILO, Geneva.

2 Faculty of Occupational Medicine of the Royal College of Physicians (1999) *Guidance on Ethics for Occupational Physicians* (5e). Royal College of Physicians, London.

3 Johnston MV, Keith RA and Hinderer SR (1992) Measurement standards for interdisciplinary medical rehabilitation. *Archives of Physical Medicine and Rehabilitation*. 73(12–S): S3–23.

4 AKAN (1993) (www.akan.no/info/english.html).

5 Walker K and Shain M (1983) Employee assistance programming. In search of effective interventions for the problem-drinking employee. *British Journal of Addiction* 78(3): 291–303.

6 Ament WW (1986) Legal and ethical considerations in managing the troubled employee. *Occupational Medicine State of the Art Reviews.* **1**(4): 673–82.

7 Aronsson T and Malmquist C (2002) *Rehabiliteringens ekonomi (Economy of Rehabilitation).* Bilda førlag, Stockholm, Sweden.

8 Imrie R (1997) Review: rethinking the relationships between disability, rehabilitation and society. *Disability and Rehabilitation.* **19**: 263–71.

9 Scheer SJ and Weinstein SM (1992) Industrial rehabilitation medicine. 1. An overview. *Archives of Physical Medicine and Rehabilitation.* **73**(5–S): S356–9.

10 Causey J and Mcfarren T (2000) In search of a method: permanent disability revisited. *New Solutions.* **10**: 207–15.

CHAPTER 15

Insurance medicine and work-related diseases: some ethical and legal aspects

Juhani Juntunen

Introduction

Insurance medicine practices differ greatly between countries due to variable legislation.[1–5] It is an area of social medicine that often gives rise to suspicions of the partiality of an insurance physician or a physician seeking a third-party funder for patient procedures.[6] Occupational health professionals in particular are subject to many conflicting pressures.[7] In Finland, insurance medicine has developed into a medical specialty, and the impartiality of insurance physicians has been strongly emphasised. This chapter considers ethical issues in recognition of work-related diseases within the insurance medicine system (scheme) in Finland. The issues are probably similar in every country.

Insurance medicine

For the purposes of determining benefit entitlement, insurance medicine breaks down into four major areas of competence: risk assessment; establishment of any causal relationships; assessment of working capacity; and assessment of any impairment. In this setting, medical examiners and legal experts have a duty practically to ensure the fair and equitable treatment of individuals in respect of benefit entitlement. In addition to legal and medical aspects, this also involves many ethical considerations – which are common to all experts and their competencies.

Although insurance medicine consultants are rarely directly involved in deciding whether to grant or refuse a benefit application, their expertise still carries exceptional weight. In Finland, the financial significance of decisions requiring the contribution of a medical examiner represents more than six billion euros annually, which underscores the importance of this area of competence. Notwithstanding this, the extensive literature on ethics and moral philosophy does not expressly address the issue of the ethics of expertise, of which insurance medicine is a good example.[8,9]

- **PRINCIPLE OF THE OBJECTIVE ORIGINS OF EXPERTISE**
- Statutory qualifications for certain expert assignments
- True expertise is born out of external recognition and demand

- **REQUIREMENT OF TRUTH AND JUSTICE AS THE ULTIMATE AIM**
- Truth should be the aim, although absolute truth is an abstraction
- A just and fair decision is often the product of many different truths
- Truth and justice are culture-specific notions

- **INTEGRITY TO DEFEND ONE'S JUDGEMENT IF CHALLENGED**
- Ignoring irrelevant influences
- Bringing strongly forward the significance of the considerations relevant in the expert's own area of competence

- **REQUIREMENT OF INDEPENDENCE**
- It is morally right for an expert to disqualify himself if he finds that he is dependent on external influences
- The credibility of an expert arises out of his independence
- Confidence in the independence of an expert is decisive for his credibility

- **IN-DEPTH UNDERSTANDING OF THE RELATIONSHIP BETWEEN THE RIGHTS OF AN INDIVIDUAL AND THE INTERESTS OF SOCIETY**
- Recognising different viewpoints
- Considering the interests of the insured person

- **CRITICAL APPROACH TO ONE'S OWN COMPETENCE**
- Keeping up with developments in one's own area of expertise
- Keeping back the feeling of omnipotence
- Avoiding excessive identification with the expert role
- Declining an offer to act as an expert, when necessary

Figure 15.1 Cornerstones of ethics in insurance medicine.

Accordingly, here the issue of recognition of compensible work-related traumatic stress disorder is approached in the context of general ethics and insurance medicine.

There are six cornerstones for the ethics of expertise in the practice of insurance medicine (Figure 15.1) which are argued to be relevant in any social system.[10]

The Finnish compensation system for work-related diseases

In Finland compensation for occupational diseases and work-related accidents is payable by insurance companies under the Finnish Accident Insurance Act. Compensation under the statutory earnings-related scheme is higher than that provided for periods of sick leave or disability pension. The Accident Insurance Act and the acts on statutory earnings-related pension set out the disability criteria, among them the requirement that – to be eligible for benefit – the applicant must suffer from an illness, defect or injury that reduces his or her capacity to earn a living from gainful employment. The most important determinant of compensation is the strength of causality between illness and any work-related factor(s). This is a non-fault system, with no requirement to prove negligence on part of the employer. The law also includes flexible provisions, giving adjudicators some power of discretion in individual cases – provided that the applicant satisfies certain conditions concerning, for example, working career and overall life situation.

The medical examiners in the service of authorised insurance companies make an assessment of an applicant's health situation and its relationship to work on the basis of available medical evidence, and express an opinion accordingly. All evidence submitted to the insurance company serves as a basis for adjudication. In the event of a refusal (in Finland the refusal rate is less than 10%), the applicant may lodge an appeal with the Accident Appeal Board (about 5000 cases reviewed per year), with final appeal to the Insurance Court. Insurance medicine consultants serve on all appellate bodies. They are often medical examiners of long-standing experience, and they must not, of course, simultaneously be employed by an insurance company. That is, they are regarded as completely impartial.

Traumatic stress disorder

The concept of traumatic, or post-traumatic, stress disorder is highly problematic from the point of view of insurance medicine. Psychological reactions after considerable traumatic experience are obviously quite normal. The diagnosis of traumatic stress disorder requires the presence of a typical set of symptoms (*see* Table 15.1) after a traumatic event that is outside the range of normal human experience (war, environmental catastrophe, mass murder, torture, etc.). There is controversy as to whether or not these symptoms can appear months or years after the traumatic experience. Diagnostic criteria vary somewhat between different diagnostic manuals, which adds to the complexity of the issue. The benefits of psychological debriefing in the prevention of traumatic stress disorder have been questioned.[11] It is even the case that the disorder has been defined as an entity constructed as much from sociopolitical ideas as from psychiatric ones.[12]

Table 15.1   Diagnostic criteria for post-traumatic stress disorder[13]

A   The person has been exposed to a traumatic event in which both the following were present:

- the person experienced, witnessed or was confronted with an event or events that involved actual or threatened death or serious injury or a threat to the physical integrity of self or others
- the person's response involved intense fear, helplessness or horror

B   The traumatic event is persistently re-experienced in one (or more) of the following ways:

- recurrent and intrusive distressing recollections of the event, including images, thoughts or perceptions
- recurrent distressing dreams of the event
- acting or feeling as if the traumatic event was recurring (includes a sense of reliving the experience, illusions, hallucinations, and dissociative flashback episodes, including those that occur on awakening or when intoxicated)
- intense psychosocial distress at exposure to internal or external cues that symbolise or resemble an aspect of traumatic event
- physiological reactivity on exposure to internal or external cues that symbolise or resemble an aspect of the traumatic event

Continued

Table 15.1 Continued

C **Persistent avoidance of stimuli associated with the trauma and numbing of general responsiveness (not present before trauma), as indicated by three (or more) of the following:**

- efforts to avoid thoughts, feelings or conversations associated with the trauma
- efforts to avoid activities, places or people that arouse recollections of the trauma
- inability to recall an important aspect of the trauma
- markedly diminished interest or participation in significant activities
- feeling of detachment or estrangement from others
- restricted range of affects (e.g. unable to have loving feelings)
- sense of a foreshortened future (e.g. does not expect to have a career, marriage, children or a normal life span)

D **Persistent symptoms of increased arousal (not present before trauma), as indicated by two (or more) of the following:**

- difficulty falling or staying asleep
- irritability or outbursts of anger
- difficulty concentrating
- hypervigilance
- exaggerated startle response

E **Duration of the disturbance (symptoms in criteria B, C and D) is more than one month**

F **The disturbance causes clinically significant distress or impairment in social, occupational or other important areas of functioning**

The following examples highlight the problem from the point of view of insurance medicine, and also demonstrate the multifaceted background and variability of cases. All the patients discussed below had suffered from post-traumatic symptoms in the various combinations listed in Table 15.1. They had all undergone psychiatric and psychological evaluation, and been diagnosed as suffering from traumatic stress disorder. Their claims were denied by the insurance company, and all were submitted for review to appellate bodies in Finland. Consequently, causality between trauma and symptom(s) was very thoroughly assessed during the process by a number of experts.

Case 15.1: robbery at work

A previously healthy bank clerk had been threatened with a sawn-off shotgun in a hold-up at his place of work. He had been given two days of sick leave because of post-traumatic shock resulting from the event. Approximately six months later he had gone to see a doctor for ailments in the upper extremities – the neck and shoulder region, and the back. He also reported that he had been suffering from sleep disorders, nightmares, conditions of fear, depression and anxiety. He was diagnosed with traumatic stress disorder by his attending psychiatrist. His claim for compensation was refused by the insurance company, and subsequent appeals were also refused by the Accident Appeal Board and the Insurance Court – on the grounds that the stress reaction to the accident had not warranted any longer sick leave. No probable causality was shown between the mental symptoms later developed by the applicant and the accident.

Case 15.2: accident while driving

A bus driver had run over a woman and her child, who both died of their injuries. On the day of the accident the driver had seen a doctor, complaining of exhaustion. He also said that he suffered from sleep disorders, anxiety and nervousness, and he was consequently found to be incapacitated for work as a bus driver. He later had nightmares about the accident, and was diagnosed as suffering from fear neurosis. In the absence of any indication of prior severe psychopathology, his attending psychiatrist diagnosed traumatic stress disorder. The insurance company refused the claim for compensation on the grounds that the diagnosed stress was not a consequence of the accident. The insurance company's decision was reversed by the Accident Appeal Board, which ordered the company to pay compensation for temporary disability caused by traumatic stress disorder for a total of six months.

Case 15.3: fell asleep while driving

A man was driving a car on his way to work with his seven-year-old son when he fell asleep at the wheel and had a frontal collision with a lorry. The car was totally demolished and the boy was immediately killed, with the father suffering severe injuries. The father had to spend about two hours in the wrecked car with his dead son before the emergency service arrived. The father was taken to the central university hospital, where he underwent several major operations. As a complication of the operations, he contracted an infection and was in a bad state for a very long time. For some of this period he was unconscious and connected to a respirator. After his physical recovery from the accident, which took approximately one year, he developed severe depression, sleep disorders and conditions of fear, which rendered him incapacitated for work. He had displayed an inclination to depression even before the accident. The insurance company refused the claim for compensation for mental symptoms on ground of the presence of pre-traumatic mental disorder. The Accident Appeal Board, however, found in favour of traumatic stress disorder, and ordered the insurance company to pay compensation.

Case 15.4: stress at work?

A man with a long employment history as a charger had started to develop fear of his work, pain in the chest, sleeplessness, tremors, nightmares and tension. During psychiatric consultations he was diagnosed with severe depression and work-related symptoms consistent with traumatic stress disorder. The insurance company refused his claim for compensation on the ground that the symptoms were consistent with mental rather than occupational disease. The Accident Appeal Board also refused the appeal on the ground that no probable causality could be shown between the symptoms and the work.

Case 15.5: hurt at work

A youngish construction worker was hit on the head by the hook of a tower crane in his workplace. He suffered an impression fracture of the skull, and was unconscious for approximately one hour. The fracture was operated upon, and the patient made a good recovery. Nevertheless, he started to develop mental symptoms, such as depression, conditions of fear, sleeplessness and nightmares, which added several months to his period of disability. Anamnestically speaking, he had had difficulties at school, and also drug and alcohol problems before the accident. He was diagnosed with traumatic stress disorder by his attending psychiatrist. The insurance company, however, refused the claim for compensation on the ground that probable causality between the symptoms of the patient and the accident could not be demonstrated. Appeals were also refused by the appellate bodies on the ground that the trauma was not severe enough to account for the symptoms.

The key ethical issue in assessing causal relationships in the above cases concerns application of rules regarding individual susceptibility to the development of psychological symptoms and the pre-traumatic psychiatric constitution of the patient. Pre-existing psychiatric disease by no means rules out the possibility of developing traumatic stress disorder. The individual symptoms listed in the most recent diagnostic criteria of traumatic stress disorder (Table 15.1) are quite common and non-specific. They may present themselves in various combinations. Since the concept of traumatic stress disorder has been widely discussed in the media, attending doctors very often tend to make such a diagnosis even in cases where the evidence of causality is rather poor. Estimation of the severity of trauma is therefore very important. Does the traumatic event fulfil the criteria of traumatic stress disorder? That is, is the trauma severe enough to evoke significant symptoms of distress in almost everyone? The escalation of benefit applications after relatively minor trauma is a challenge to insurance medicine consultants, who try to identify 'the real cases' that qualify for compensation.

What, then, are the consequences of misclassification of compensable traumatic stress disorder? In 'false-positive' cases expenses are paid within the private insurance company, and eventually by the employer. In 'false-negative' cases the patient obtains compensation within the general social security system, that is, from taxpayers. The decision of the impartial appellate body is always based on evidence 'beyond reasonable doubt' (as in the courts in general). In this process, the cornerstones of ethics provide valuable guidelines for taking final decisions.

Cornerstones of the ethics of expertise

Definition of expertise

Commonly, people are referred to as experts if they clearly have more profound and extensive knowledge in a particular field than the average person. The value of expertise is highly specific to environment and culture. In terms of consequential ethics, the value of expertise also varies greatly (e.g. expert in nuclear weapons or expert in etymology). The greater the asymmetry of information in a society in a particular field (i.e. the fewer experts exist), the greater are the power and responsibility of the experts (i.e. the less chance there is for a second opinion).

The law sets out qualifications for certain professions requiring expertise, which include the professions of judge, medical doctor and university lecturer. However, those experts that are not defined by law, particularly the top-level experts, pose the biggest problem in terms of ethics. It is not easy to be recognised as an expert. You do not gain the status of an expert merely by appearing in the media or criticising the current state of affairs! Nor can you declare yourself to be an expert. Who, then, is the expert in assessment of traumatic stress disorder? Is it the attending physician or a psychiatrist with considerable experience? Or is it a medical adviser in an insurance company or a member of an appellate body?

An insurance medicine consultant in Finland must be a medical doctor by profession, and generally have built up experience in his or her area of competence over many years – *inter alia*, through medical practice, clinical work with patients, scientific research and studies in the field. As a rule, insurance medicine consultants are consulting physicians with considerable clinical experience. They have received a thorough scientific education, and have thus developed critical thinking skills and learnt to understand that causal relationships apply to varying degrees. Therefore, they are required to have very good expertise in decision making even in cases outside their own specialty. True expertise is born out of external evaluations, recognition and demand. The *principle of requiring recognised and solid competence and professional expertise* is the first cornerstone of ethics.

Expertise, truth and justice

When assessing the significance of expertise, consideration must be paid to the fact that the world is becoming increasingly complex and more reliant on expertise. Consequently, the power and responsibility of experts are growing all the time. For example, society needs insurance medicine consultants to ensure the just and fair provision of social security benefits according to health status.

Expertise must thus be recognised as a value in itself, which according to the ancient philosophers represents 'truth' (from among the so-called Platonic values of beauty, truth and virtue). The Common Law system is still based on these values (truth, justice, mercy).

In theoretical terms, truth is an abstraction for which experts should strive – well aware as they are of the absence of absolute truth. Tolerance of ignorance and acceptance of truths contrary to one's own convictions are also part of the essence of the value of truth. It has been argued that the requirement of truth has developed out of practical necessity. Untruths often given rise to troublesome situations!

Insurance medicine consultants have to consider different truths in their work, and observe the requirement of fairness in their judgements. Are the symptoms presented by the cases of traumatic stress disorder true? What is the probability of causality in an individual case? Insurance physicians should present culture-specific objective information, and strive for justice and the absolute truth, unaffected by priorities or value judgements. This is, however, a practical abstraction. For example, the value judgements of presiding judges determine the range of punishments they apply. In the field of insurance medicine, assessments of causality and work capacity go beyond medical expertise. A medical examiner acting in line with an ethical code should, however, avoid making far-reaching interpretations of the flexible provisions of social insurance legislation in situations where an illness, defect or injury cannot be accurately measured in precise quantitative terms. This holds particularly true in the cases of traumatic stress disorder. The medical examiner must make the rationale for his adjudication as clear as possible, both to himself and to others. It is the prime interest of benefit providers to make fair and equitable decisions within their power of discretion; otherwise, their activities are not solidly based. The *requirement that experts must strive for truth and justice* constitutes the second important cornerstone of ethics in the practice of insurance medicine.

Expertise and morality

Morals refer to the general norms, customs and habits applied in the interest of the right and good as understood within a particular culture. Every person is obliged to do the morally right thing.[8] Experts should be aware that the combined effect of expertise and decision-making power may have far-reaching consequences. This is especially true in assessing work-related psychiatric disorders. The practice of insurance medicine is therefore characterised by a certain degree of conservatism. In handling claims, medical examiners must not go beyond the terms and conditions of the applicable insurance contract or accept forms of treatment other than those generally recognised, although new and as yet non-established forms of treatment may in some individual cases provide subjective benefit to a patient. The critical interpretation of scientific findings constitutes an essential element of expertise.

Professional ethics may sometimes clash with rules and regulations, and the conflicts that thereby arise may be difficult to handle. Is it ethically correct for a medical examiner to change his adjudication policy because he is told that the costs are too high? Can he find medical grounds for an award even when the flexible provisions involving the human element do not support it? The third cornerstone of the ethics of expertise lies in the *integrity to defend one's judgement within one's own area of competence.*

Independence of experts

Finland's adjudication practice in the context of compensation for occupational diseases has recently come in for strong criticism in the Finnish media. The impartiality of medical examiners in particular has been challenged. In accordance with statements made by the Council of Europe,[14] attention has been drawn to the fact that the parties involved in the adjudication process must not only be impartial, but also must be perceived to be impartial.[15–17] This discussion should be interpreted in light of understanding how deeply rooted the practice of insurance medicine is in the cornerstones of the ethics of expertise.

Independence from outside and improper influences constitutes a key prerequisite for the work of insurance medicine consultants. Medical examiners must not let their own interests, or the interests of their immediate circle, influence their decisions. Such decisions must be based solely on the facts of the case and the standards applicable, and be consistent with legal practice and uniform adjudication practice. The circumstances under which an adjudicator is to be found formally incompetent to participate in the adjudication process are laid down in legal provisions and emerge from legal practice. Independence and integrity are, however, ultimately questions of ethics, which the medical examiner must be able to determine himself.

The practice of insurance medicine aims at decisions that are just and fair. When laws are enacted, flexible provisions are generally introduced to allow adjudicators some power of discretion. On the borderline, there are no right or wrong decisions – only ones that are just and fair in relation to other equivalent cases. It is therefore just as wrong to award compensation on false grounds as it is to deny one on false grounds. There is, however, one difference. An adverse decision delivered on false grounds is open to appeal, whereas appeal is seldom lodged against an award. The primary duty of insurance medicine consultants is to apply social security law independently, and thereby ensure that all insured people receive equitable treatment. For the sake of credibility alone, medical examiners in the service of insurance companies should be as independent as possible. Considering that the notion of independence is still being given somewhat varying interpretations in legal practice, the medical examiner's own interpretation, which is based on his own very strict ethical principles, is highlighted. The *requirement of independence* is the fourth cornerstone of the ethics of expertise.

The expert, the individual and society

Experts often have to consider a conflict of interests between the individual and society. This is a key issue, particularly in medical law. At what point do the interests of society take precedence over the interests of the individual? To what extent is value relativism acceptable? Whereas environmental expertise holds that prevention of the establishment of a factory that pollutes the environment is good, those who are planning to build the factory, together with the unemployed and the employment authorities, may regard it as bad.

The expert may have to play a dual role, which is difficult to manage. For example, the ethical code of medical doctors highlights the importance of recognising the universal nature of human dignity. When treating a patient, the doctor's main concerns are the well-being of his patient and treatment of the patient consistent with the ethical code of doctors. He may even think of himself as the patient's legal counsellor. This seems to happen quite often in cases of traumatic stress disorder, where initiation of psychiatric symptoms coincides with the trauma. It should be remembered that association is not the same as causal relationship. The role of the medical examiner is that of an impartial expert on social insurance charged with making a decision that is just and fair. In reviewing a case, representatives of the insurance scheme must be concerned with the effectiveness of the legal system, the rights of other applicants to the same benefit, and the rights of the current applicant. They must be able to put themselves in the position of the applicant when considering the claim and the evidence submitted in support of it. This imposes high demands on the morals of experts. Accordingly, the fifth cornerstone of ethics of the practice of insurance medicine consists of *in-depth understanding of the relationship between the rights of an individual and the interests of society.*

Maintenance of expertise and the dangers of omnipotence

An expert is recognised as an expert only for so long as his or her knowledge and skills are generally held valid and there is asymmetry of information in the community. This is determined by those in authority who call on the services of an expert. The only way any expert will be able to maintain his position is to keep in the forefront of knowledge in his or her own area of expertise. Considering that scientific truths are constantly changing, for example in the field of natural science, insurance medicine consultants must keep abreast of developments in the fields of medicine and social insurance legislation. Studies of traumatic stress disorder are constantly reported in scientific publications, and sources of exceptional traumatic stress in this world seem to persist. Regular review of the scientific literature is therefore essential for maintaining expertise in the field.

One common problem related to expertise is the potential sense of omnipotence to which it gives rise. Sometimes we believe that we understand something better than others simply because we are already recognised experts in a particular field. An expert may also entertain the belief that he will always remain an expert in his own field. Someone who has held an expert position within the same area of competence for a lengthy period of time may begin to identify himself too much with his job. Those calling on the services of the expert may not have the requisite skills to take these considerations into account, and might end up receiving distorted information as a basis for their decisions (by trusting a false expert).

An expert should be humble and wise enough to decline an assignment for which he feels he does not have the necessary competence. The requirement that *an expert should be critical of his own competence* constitutes the sixth cornerstone of the ethics of expertise, and often leaves him or her with considerable discretionary power.

Attending doctors and medical examiners with possibly different ethical codes

In the practice of insurance medicine, one key problem relates to the occasional differences of opinion between the attending doctor and the medical examiner with regard to the disability of the patient, the aetiology of the illness in question, and the resulting impairment. This issue has also raised public concern in Finland.[18] It has, for example, been asked how a medical examiner representing an insurance company can decide against a benefit solely on the basis of written evidence, without meeting and examining the patient. Is the medical examiner ethically correct in recommending refusal of a benefit application contrary to the opinion of the attending doctor?[19] For example, a diagnosis of traumatic stress disorder requires considerable in-depth psychiatric evaluation by an attending physician, who certainly knows the patient better than anybody else. His or her prime concern is to attend to the health and well-being of the patient in the best possible way. The medical opinion of the attending doctor is of prime importance for assessment of work-related diseases. The attending doctor and the medical examiner generally agree on the patient's level of incapacity owing to occupational disease if they have access to the same medical evidence. Assessing the causal relationship between work-related factors and the disease is, however, a much more complex issue, requiring considerable expertise in the fields of epidemiology and occupational health.

Nevertheless, the role of the medical examiner is different from that of the attending doctor.[20,21] The medical examiner must review each individual case in the context of the broader picture, paying attention to general adjudication and legal practice. Unlike the attending doctor, he or she does not have to take on another role when drafting a medical opinion, and – what is more important – also possesses adequate expertise in insurance medicine. Adverse decisions are never made on the basis of insufficient evidence, but the insurance company or appellate bodies will obtain additional information whenever necessary.

It is regarded as understandable, indeed acceptable, that the attending doctor is biased towards his or her patient. In the adjudication practice applied in the insurance business, due consideration is given to the medical opinion of the attending doctor, and any decision is based on considerations of insurance medicine. Indeed, one great misconception is that this approach is always contrary to the interests of the insured person. This is, of course, not the case. Award practices within personal insurance schemes are geared towards the provision of benefits to all those who are entitled. Such a demarcation policy, of course, always leaves those who are refused a benefit dissatisfied, but changing the policy does not remove the problem.[22,23]

A statutory accident insurance scheme is part of the Finnish social insurance system. This holds true despite the fact that the scheme's implementation is largely delegated by legislation to private accident insurance companies. It is employers who are obliged to pay the insurance premiums, and employees do not pay anything. The insurance companies perform a statutory public duty, and an insurance physician is subject to the same kind of administrative regulation as a civil servant. Accordingly, within the social insurance scheme, the function of appellate instances is not to force any liable party who is unwilling to co-operate into legal proceedings or to pay damages resulting from appropriate evidence submitted. Instead, their duty is to re-examine the claim and rule on the correctness of the decision of the benefit provider and the adequacy of the evidence. The alternatives to such a demarcation policy, that is, consistently to grant or refuse all applications, would not be realistic.

Medical examiners in Finland are subject to very strict monitoring, *inter alia* by actors in the social insurance field, the Ministry of Social Affairs and Health, and appellate bodies. The doctor–patient relationship implies that the attending doctor does not have to draft a medical opinion in capacity as an objective expert on insurance medicine, but as an expert on the health of his or her patient. Indeed, for purposes of determining causality and

disability, the attending doctor should only describe the patient's functional capacity – which can then be assessed on the basis of medical
expertise, and a detailed history of work-related factors and work conditions. Generally speaking, the attending physician primarily acts in accordance with the ethical code of medical doctors, whereas the insurance
physician (medical examiner) has to observe the ethical code applied in
his or her own field of expertise (*see* Table 15.2). Adjudication in the field of
social insurance therefore requires the contribution of medical examiners.

Table 15.2 Attending and insurance physicians – ethical dilemmas

Attending physician	Insurance physician
Expert on health of the patient	Expert on insurance medicine and social security legislation
Follows the ethics of a medical doctor	Follows the ethics of medicine and the ethics of expertise in insurance medicine
Patient–doctor relationship	No patient–doctor relationship Impartial
Seeks solution most beneficial to patient	Seeks fair and equitable solution in light of available scientific evidence and prevailing compensation practice
Under pressure from relatives and employer	No outside pressure
Paid by the patient	Paid by the insurance company or by the appellate body, no financial interest
Stakeholders: patient, doctor	Stakeholders: employers, taxpayers

Concluding remarks

In their everyday practice, experts on occupational health, insurance
medicine and insurance law have to pay close attention to the above-
mentioned ethical considerations. Strict adherence to these considerations
is fundamentally important to the existence of the professional doctrine of
insurance medicine. Notwithstanding this, public attention is constantly
drawn – through the press and television – to alleged violations of people's
civil rights, especially in the practice of insurance medicine. Such suspicions and misunderstandings put the entire insurance scheme in a bad light
in the eyes of the public, whereas in fact insurance companies and appellate
bodies are working hard to ensure consistent decision-making practices in

line with applicable provisions. These efforts necessarily require the contribution of insurance medicine consultants. If available expertise is of low standard, practices will show increasing inconsistencies in decisions taken, deeper dissatisfaction, and possibly even the loss of public trust. Compensation for traumatic stress disorder provides a good example of this. One approach to restoring public confidence would be the clear statement of the grounds of decision, although this would not make those who are denied a benefit any less dissatisfied with the decision. Another approach to strengthening public confidence would be to disseminate information about the practice of insurance medicine and the process of diagnosing work-related disease. For this reason, the key ethical principles of insurance medicine addressed above should be discussed not only among insurance medicine consultants themselves, but also in public – irrespective of the sociopolitical system prevailing in any particular society.

References

1 Marpet MI and Primeaux P (2001) Using decision science to gain insight into ethical issues: an example involving thresholds in workers compensation. *Journal of Forensic Science.* **4**: 969–77.

2 Kronick R (2001) Valuing charity. *Journal of Health Politics, Policy and Law.* **5**: 993–1001.

3 Barnighausen T and Sauerborn R (2002) One hundred and eighteen years of the German health insurance system: are there any lessons for middle- and low-income countries? *Social Science Medicine.* **10**: 1559–87.

4 Brown LD (2003) Comparing health systems in four countries: lessons from the United States. *American Journal of Public Health.* **1**: 52–6.

5 Light DW (2003) Universal health care: lessons from the British experience. *American Journal of Public Health.* **1**: 25–30.

6 Freeman VG, Rathore SS, Weinfurt KP, Schulman KA and Sulmasy DP (1999) Lying for patients: physician deception of third-party payers. *Archives of Internal Medicine.* **19**: 2263–70.

7 Higgins P and Orris P (2002) Providing employer-arranged occupational medical care: conflicting interests. *Occupational Medicine.* **4**: 601–6.

8 Airaksinen T (1987) *Moraalifilosofia (Moral Philosophy).* W Söderström Oy, Finland.

9 Juntunen J (1999) Työkyvyttömyyseläkeasian käsittely eläkevakuutuslaitoksessa (The disability pension determination process of authorized pension providers). *Suomen Lääkärilehti (Finnish Medical Journal)* **13**: 1593–6.

10   Juntunen J (1999) Vakuutuslääketieteen asiantuntijuuden eettinen näkökulma (The ethical aspects of the practice of insurance medicine). In: T Aro, A Huunan-Seppälä, J Kivekäs, S Tola and I Torstila (eds) *Vakuutuslääketiede (Insurance Medicine)*. Kustannus Oy Duodecim, Helsinki: 46–51.

11   Kenardy J (2000) The current status of psychological debriefing. *British Medical Journal.* **321**: 1032–3.

12   Summerfield D (2001) The invention of post-traumatic stress disorder and the social usefulness of a psychiatric category. *British Medical Journal.* **322**: 95–8.

13   American Psychiatric Association (2000) *Diagnostic and Statistical Manual of Mental Disorders* 4e (rev.) APA, Washington DC.

14   Council of Europe (1998) *Human Rights and Fundamental Freedoms.* The European Convention on Human Rights, Rome. 4 November 1950; Protocol No. 11.

15   Lehtimaja L (1998) Tuomioistuin tarvitsee yleisön luottamuksen (Courts need public trust). *Lakimies (Journal of the Finnish Lawyers' Association).* **1**: 79–81.

16   Portin G (1998) Miltä oikeuden pitää näyttää? (What should justice look like?). *Lakimies (Journal of the Finnish Lawyers' Association).* **8**: 1355–61.

17   Rintala E (1996) Tuomarin roolista ja riippumattoman aseman takeista euro-oppaoikeuden mukaan (On the role of judges and the guarantees of impartiality under European Law). *Defensor Legis.* **5**: 562–70.

18   Juntunen J and Havu T (2000) Onko vakuutuslääkäri viisaampi kuin hoitava lääkäri? (Is the insurance physician wiser than the attending physician?) *Duodecim.* **22**: 2453–5.

19   Juntunen J and Havu T (2001) Vakuutuslääketieteen eettisiä ja juridisia näkökohtia (Some ethical and legal aspects of insurance medicine). *Sosoiaalilääketieteellinen aikakausilehti (Journal of Social Medicine).* **37**: 72–9.

20   Havu T (1999) Vakuutuslääkäri on henkilövakuutuksen asiantuntija (Medical examiners are experts on personal insurance). *Suomen lääkärilehti (Finnish Medical Journal).* **7**: 855–8.

21   Havu T (1999) Vakuutuslääkärin asema ja juridinen vastuu (Position and juridical responsibility of medical examiners). In: T Aro, A Huunan-Seppälä, J Kivekäs, S Tola and I Torstila (eds) *Vakuutuslääketiede (Insurance Medicine)*. Kustannus Oy Duodecim, Helsinki: 28–31.

22   Havu T (1999) Vakuutetun oikeusturva (Legal protection of the insured). In: T Aro, A Huunan-Seppälä, J Kivekäs, S Tola and I Torstila (eds) *Vakuutuslääketiede (Insurance Medicine)*. Kustannus Oy Duodecim, Helsinki: 32–41.

23   Havu T and Juntunen J (2002) Lääkäri tuomarina-lääkärijäsenen roolista toimeentuloturvan muutoksenhakuelimissä (Physician as a judge – on the role of physician members in the review of social insurance appeals). *Lakimies (Journal of the Finnish Lawyers' Association).* **100**: 594–617.

CHAPTER 16

Recognition of work-related diseases

Bengt Järvholm

Case 16.1: chemical exposure

A man of 57 with acute non-lymphocytic leukaemia (ANLL) is working in a small firm for the finishing of metals (electroplating, painting, etc.). He has worked in the firm since he was around 25 years of age. The work environment is rather complex, and has varied over the years. He has been exposed to strong acids and some solvents, such as xylene and trichloroethylene, but there is no current obvious heavy exposure to benzene. Although benzene might have been present in the workplace in small amounts several years ago, the information is uncertain. He has been treated successfully, and his disease is now in remission. He is now back at work and is consulting occupational health services to discuss his job. He is tired, and the employer would like to be sure he is not exposed to anything that may further impair his health.

He has been, and still is, intermittently exposed to low concentrations of alkaline cleaning agents, but such exposure is not considered to give rise to any increased health risk. However, did his previous exposure to chemicals have any importance for his disease, and can that disease be recognised as work related?

Exposure to benzene and ionising radiation is a well-accepted cause of ANLL.[1] Also, exposures to some solvents have been discussed as possible causes of ANLL.[2] Although the evidence is much weaker in the latter case, a clever lawyer and some 'luck' may give him a chance of compensation (at least in some countries).

Thus, if he reports the case to his insurance company (or some governmental agency), there is a chance that it will be accepted as an occupational disease and compensated for accordingly. The outcome of any such reporting is not known when the worker comes to the occupational health service for advice. Should the occupational health personnel concerned, for example the physician, the safety engineer or the nurse, tell the patient that he should report a possible occupational disease? This chapter focuses on the ethical dilemmas surrounding this question.

Stakeholders

There are several stakeholders involved, and they have different interests:

- the patient
- the employer
- the insurance company
- society
- other workers associated with the occupational health service
- the occupational health service.

The patient

It may seem obvious that the patient's primary interest would be to have the case presented to his insurance company if there is any chance of compensation.

However, if the case is not accepted as an occupational disease, the patient will be disappointed. He might be able to appeal to a higher court (legal procedures for appealing differ between countries). In the worst case, the patient will spend most of his time and money on legal proceedings, and then eventually lose. Thus, advising the patient to embark on an appeal might do him harm (in the forms of losing money, getting too preoccupied with the appeal, etc.). Even patients who accept a negative decision from an insurance company will have some adverse experience of reporting the disease (certainly in terms of loss of time and money).

The paternalistic view would be for you, as an occupational health professional, to decide for him, but the principle of autonomy (of the worker) requires that he himself decides after being fully informed. However, how do you inform him so that he understands the uncertainty and, at the same time, has the courage to report and fight his case? It might seem simple in theory to advise him, but anyone who has faced a case like this recognises the difficulties involved.

The employer

The employer would probably prefer the case not to be reported, especially if there is a low chance of compensation. Just the possibility of an association might cause concern in other workers and some feeling of guilt, since the employer has not been able to protect the worker from exposure. Further, reporting is likely to give rise to a lot of paperwork.

Also, the relation of the occupational health service to the employer may be impaired if several cases that are not accepted are reported. In many cases, occupational health personnel do not have the opportunity to inform the employer in the same way as the patient. Thus, in deciding how to inform the patient, you – as an occupational health professional – must also consider the possible maleficence you may do to the employer.

The insurance company

For an insurance company, receiving a report is a cost under all circumstances. The company has to investigate the case, which costs money. If it is not accepted, it has been a waste of money for the company (or for taxpayers if a governmental compensation system is involved). On the other hand, any compensation system must be prepared to handle uncertain cases. Since you do not know the exact chance of compensation in a case like this, you have to consider whether raising it is a waste of money or a matter of justifiable uncertainty. If you recommend reporting of every case of illness to the insurance system, it would collapse under the cost of investigations!

Society

A compensation system for occupational diseases is not just a system for compensating patients, but also an information system for recognising work hazards. Based on the statistics derived, preventive measures are implemented. If possible cases are not reported, preventive opportunities are hampered. Thus, for society, the interest might be to report many 'possible' cases and detect environments where preventive measures should be implemented. New hazards will rarely be detected if no one reports a possible risk, but only very well-known risk factors. On the other hand, the costs of investigations may also be of concern to society.

Other workers associated with the occupational health service

Justice requires that you treat all workers in the same way. Thus, other workers with a similar chance of compensation should be treated just like this patient. This is likely to mean more work and costs for you as an occupational health professional, since the principle of autonomy requires that you inform all patients (so they are able to make their own decisions).

If other workers with similar exposures hear that the case is reported to the insurance system, they may be anxious about having an increased risk of disease (cancer in this case). They will not have a chance of compensation if they remain healthy, but will always have to deal with the stress of being reminded of a potential risk exposure.

The occupational health service

For the occupational health service, recognising an occupational disease is usually largely a cost. Only when an insurance company asks for help may some financial compensation be provided to the occupational health service. Further, a negative attitude on the part of the employer may mean a less favourable contract, or even no contract at all, the next time it is negotiated.

Since there may have been some exposures way back in time in this case, the patient would be helped by a careful exposure assessment by the occupational health safety engineer. This would take a workday or even more time. The chances of compensation will heavily depend on the quality of the exposure assessment. Thus, a good exposure assessment may be of benefit to the patient, but it will certainly be a cost for the occupational health service.

Discussion

There are several interests that give rise to a general ethical dilemma for you as an occupational health professional – that of deciding how you should inform a patient about the possibilities of compensation in a case like this. Obviously, powerful stakeholders, such as the employer and the insurance company, think they benefit from cases not being reported. Thus, their interest is that occupational health services do not recommend uncertain cases for compensation.

In the Netherlands, there is no special compensation for occupational diseases, but such cases are still reported by occupational health physicians to a central registry for use in statistics, prevention, etc. However, although there is no financial cost to the employer, few cases are reported compared with some other countries. In 2001 there were 5593 cases of occupational disease reported in the Netherlands, which compares with 26 496 in Sweden (with a much smaller population). Lumbago, a well-known disorder caused by whole-body vibration, is reported to be much lower in the Netherlands ($n = 10$) than in Belgium or France.[3] The reason for the low frequency of reporting in the Netherlands has not been investigated, but it is possible that occupational health physicians, who are paid by employers, feel that it is easier not to report cases of the disorder.

One resolution of the dilemma would be to inform the patient carefully about the possibilities of compensation, which would mean that the autonomy of the patient is given priority over maleficence to the employer, the occupational health service and the insurance company. There are cases where the chance of compensation is low and the possibilities of the patient understanding the legal requirements of compensation are small (e.g. because of a mental handicap). Under such circumstances, attaining a balance between possible maleficence to and autonomy of the patient in any decision is even more difficult for the occupational health professionals.

In Case 16.1, the patient was informed about the compensation system and his chances of obtaining compensation. He decided not to report his disease to the insurance company. A contributing factor may have been that the disease was in remission, and he felt well. If he had had a relapse his decision may well have been different.

References

1   Zeeb H and Blettner M (1998) Adult leukaemia: what is the role of currently known risk factors? *Radiation and Environmental Biophysics.* **36**: 217–28.

2   Lynge E, Anttila A and Hemminki K (1997) Organic solvents and cancer. *Cancer Causes and Control.* **8**: 406–19.

3   Hulshof CTF, van der Laan G, Braam ITJ and Verbeek JHAM (2002) The fate of Mrs Robinson: criteria for recognition of whole-body vibration injury as an occupational disease. *Journal of Sound and Vibration.* **253**: 185–94.

CHAPTER 17

Workplace genetic screening

Lisbeth Ehlert Knudsen

Introduction

Workplace genetic screening is a sensitive area within occupational health owing to a history of misuses, and potential future misuses, with regard to workforce selection. The matter is discussed, for example, on websites such as www.genetic-testing-and-work.be and www.nuffield.org.uk (from the Nuffield Council on Bioethics). However, the issue is not 'black and white', since sensitive people may benefit from protection against harmful exposures. A distinction should be made between, on the one hand, the biological monitoring of genotoxic exposures and testing for heritable susceptibility to exposure to genotoxicants and, on the other, disease predisposition. Validity of tests and the predictive capacity of a positive or a negative test result are also very important issues.

Ethical concerns arise in the following areas.

- *Autonomy*. Pre-employment testing and screening programmes very often lack a voluntary element in terms of participation; also, the right to know or not to know results may be irrelevant since future employment will depend on the outcome of the test.
- *Beneficence*. A person may avoid an unnecessary risk when a test shows vulnerability, which may allow him or her not to work in a risky workplace; both the employer and society will benefit from diminishing the costly treatment of disease through the selection of best-fitted workers.
- *Non-maleficence*. Stress may be imposed on a family by the delivery of information about heritable characteristics.
- *Justice*. Societal context is important; in some countries, like Denmark, special rules prohibit unjustified pre-employment testing or the denial of insurance in cases of non-beneficial genetic test results.

McCunney,[1] in his review of the ethical implications of genetic testing in the workplace, raises a number of important questions.

- Should genetic testing results be afforded special treatment, in comparison with other medical and health-related information?
- How should genetic information be defined? Is family information included? Should symptomatic conditions be differentiated from asymptomatic risks?
- How predictive should a genetic test be to be considered as representing an increased risk?
- Should access to genetic information be restricted? Should legislation address discrimination due to inappropriate use of genetic testing?
- What restrictions are necessary on the use, access, disclosure and retention of genetic information?
- What is the physician's role and liability related to genetic tests?

This chapter will address only some of these questions. The author's experiences are within genetic testing as part of biomonitoring research programmes, the preparation of Danish regulation on the use of health information in relation to job application, and the maintenance and preparation of European terminology and guidelines for use of genetic testing in the clinical testing of medicines.

History

The term 'ecogenetics' was introduced in the 1930s following increasing evidence of individual differences in drug sensitivity, and also in sensitivity to exogenous exposures in the environment and in the workplace.[2] US job applicants with glucose-6-P dehydrogenase deficiency were excluded from employment in occupations with exposures to aromatic amines in the 1970s, and applicants in Denmark with atopy were excluded from employment in occupations with a high allergen load, for example enzyme production. In a later follow-up study, however, atopic predisposition at time of engagement was not found to be a significant risk factor for enzyme allergy.[3]

Applications of genetic polymorphisms (defined as mutations present with a frequency of >1%) in risk assessment were not made on an individual basis in the 1980s – a period when most limit values were set sufficiently low to allow susceptible people to be exposed. But in recent years, increasing analytical opportunities and capacities have enabled the use of genetic polymorphisms in individual risk assessment and drug treatment. Thus, the discipline of pharmacogenetics takes differences in metabolic capacity and differences in drug–target response into account, enabling individualised drug treatment. Similarly, toxicogenetics now has a role to play in environmental and occupational toxicology.

Genetic testing in the workplace may take the form of screening for heritable susceptibility to exposures or disease predisposition or of monitoring the effects of exposures on genetic material. Both kinds of testing are practised today, with monitoring often forming a part of surveillance programmes. Recently, the Human Genome Project has led to very impressive advances in understanding the genetic basis of the individual's risk of disease, which opens new challenges even in the arena of occupational health. However, the validated number of genetic characteristics relevant to workplace genetic screening is not very high. There are great expectations, and it has even been predicted that everyone will carry a gene map, showing all relevant characteristics, in future. The occupational scenario has been set up – for a gene map would offer a preview with regard to skills, susceptibilities, risks of diseases and so on. Fortunately, however, such genetic determinism does not apply to most human characteristics (indeed, to virtually none at all), which are regulated by a number of genes in combination.

For disease predisposition with a largely monogenic origin, high-penetrance genes, such as those associated with Huntington's disease and breast cancer, have been reported in relation to the selection of (discrimination against) workers and the denial of insurance. The rationale is that a person is prone to develop the disease, and is thus more 'costly' for the employer or insurer.

Genes of low penetrance (susceptibility genes), usually active in association with the metabolism of foreign compounds, often interact with other genes. This makes any risk association less significant, and there is as yet no report of discriminatory action due to an unfavourable genotype in the scientific literature. However, stories are often told about discrimination against job applicants with a monogenic disease trait in their family. Also, the so-called 'healthy worker effect' (which keeps healthy people at work) seems to be associated with an over-representation of people with favourable genotypes in certain exposed occupations.[4]

Biomonitoring of occupational exposure to genotoxic substances

Occupational exposure to genotoxic substances implies an increased risk of cancer, reproductive failure and, in some cases, damage to the immune defence system, as shown by epidemiological evidence.

The most effective preventive measure is to eliminate the exposure. However, this is not always possible, since genotoxic and carcinogenic substances have unique uses where replacement is not possible. Examples of the personnel involved are nurses and healthcare personnel handling cytostatics, laboratory workers handling carcinogenic substances as part of analytical and research work, workers handling pesticides, and workers processing material that releases carcinogenic substances, for example polyaromatic hydrocarbons (PAHs) via combustion. Processing of asphalt and stainless steel welding entail exposure to toxic fumes containing carcinogenic substances, and the production of reinforced plastics gives exposure to styrene (which, in humans, is metabolised into styrene oxide with carcinogenic activity).

Occupational exposure assessment by environmental monitoring has been a traditional and legal requirement for decades. The results of environmental monitoring are compared with occupational exposure limits to estimate whether exposures are acceptable. Safety improvements may also be evaluated on the basis of comparative measurements. The specific analytic methods used to detect individuals' exposure through breathing air require detailed knowledge of kinds of exposures. Very often, the detection limit is too high for exposures to be detected in Danish or other European workplaces. Procedures to ensure the sampling of peak exposures are not always technically feasible. Also, exposure through the skin or gastrointestinal tract is not quantifiable via environmental monitoring.

Over the last decade, attention has been drawn to biological markers as indicators of events in biological systems and samples, which take individual factors such as uptake, metabolism and excretion into account. Biomarkers also have the potential to indicate minute interactions between xenobiotics and critical macromolecules, and identify changes that occur at an early and, hopefully, reversible step in the progression of occupational disease. Biological markers may be classified as markers of exposure, effect and susceptibility.

A biological marker of exposure is an endogenous substance, or its metabolite(s), or the product of an interaction between a xenobiotic agent and some target molecule or cell that is measured in a compartment within an organism. A biological marker of effect is a measurable biochemical, physiological or other alteration within the organism that, depending on magnitude, can be recognised as an established or potential health impairment or disease. A biological marker of susceptibility is defined as an indicator of the sensitivity of a person towards exposure to a xenobiotic compound. The measurement of biological markers is performed by biological monitoring. If the monitoring activity covers genetic endpoints or material the term 'genetic monitoring' is used.

Monitoring of selected parameters in single samples from selected groups or individuals is most common, and usually performed in smaller studies. Such monitoring activity provides a cross-sectional description of an actual occupational exposure and may give rise to interventions. The results of a monitoring activity may also satisfy scientific research purposes by describing the exposure of the people tested and by giving data for validation of the methods used. Repeated testing of genotoxic exposures by biological monitoring is, however, practised in some instances, for example in the surveillance of people exposed to radioactivity. Also, the repeated monitoring of blood lead concentrations is common as part of surveillance or control programmes. Ethical questions raised in such programmes are concerned with beneficence. This is normally small for the participant, but increased knowledge is expected to be beneficial to the future workforce (provided that it is used for later interventions). Further, the autonomy of study subjects is a matter of concern regarding appropriate information, proper consent to participation, and future use of data. Lastly, there is the question of data protection to prevent harm to subjects from the misuse of available information.

The use of biological monitoring in occupational hygiene has been a matter of debate in Denmark for several years. Currently, regulation only covers the routine monitoring of blood lead concentrations in selected exposed groups. The debate has been about the risk of substituting selection of staff for preventive occupational work.

Experimental methods determining individual susceptibility are available. At present, approximately 50 human genetic diseases have been identified as having the potential to enhance an individual's susceptibility to toxic or carcinogenic effects of environmental agents.[5] A few examples are shown in Table 17.1.

Table 17.1 Examples of genetic factors affecting susceptibility to environmental and occupational conditions

High-risk group	Estimated occurrence	Genetic characteristic	Testing methods	Health impact
Sickle cell traits	7–13% American blacks are heterozygotes	Change of basepair in beta-globin gene	Haemoglobin or DNA testing	Haemolytic anaemia, infarcts, increased susceptibility to lead poisoning
Thalassaemias	Alpha 4–5% Beta 2–3%	Several variants	Haemoglobin or DNA testing	Anaemia, increased susceptibility to lead poisoning
Glucose-6-P dehydrogenase deficiency	1–8% Mediterranean 16% American blacks	X-linked, recessive	Enzyme or DNA testing	Acute haemolysis from exposure to certain chemicals
Serum alpha-1 antitrypsin deficiency	4–9% Northern European	Basepair substitution	Protein or DNA testing	Predisposition to emphysema from exposure to irritants
Aryl hydrocarbon hydroxylase induction	Several variants	Mutations and deletions	Protein or DNA testing	Risk of lung cancer
Acetylation geno/phenotype	50% fast and 50% slow metabolisers	Slow, recessive	Protein or DNA testing	Risk of arylamine-induced bladder cancer
Low superoxide dismutase activity	<0.1%	Recessive	Enzyme activity or DNA testing	Decrease in cellular resistance to oxidative stress
Catalase variants	2%	Recessive	Enzyme activity or DNA testing	Susceptibility to ozone, radiation
DNA repair and chromosome instability	1%	Several variants	Enzyme activity or DNA testing	Risk of cancer, immune suppression, etc.
Activated proto-oncogenes	Unknown	Several variants	Enzyme activity or DNA testing	Risk of cancer, immune suppression, etc.

Ethical aspects of biological monitoring

The use of human biological samples gives rise to special considerations with regard to information, consent, confidentiality and follow-up (as stated in the second Helsinki Declaration). In Denmark the collection of personal information about health status used for research or surveillance must be preceded by a notification of the project in question to a county-based ethical committee. Such notification must contain a protocol describing, *inter alia*, risk to the persons participating, information (oral or written) given to persons participating, and a way of obtaining informed consent. If a register (data set) with personal information is to be created, rules for running the register must be approved by the Data Inspection Service. The rules must state who should have access to and how to obtain the information. Information about exposure and susceptibility gained by biological monitoring is personal, and may predict health impairments. Such information may therefore be discriminatory, and thus sensitive, in relation to future work opportunities and health insurance. It is therefore of utmost importance to keep the information confidential, with precise guidelines on who is allowed to use it.[6] On the other hand, it is also of importance to make sure that information about test results showing a health impairment that might be treated or prevented is given in time. This may be a problem if data and sample banks keep information anonymously.

The concept of validation

Before a test is used to monitor a certain working population it has to be validated. Validity has a variety of definitions. From a scientific point of view, a valid test must have acceptable sensitivity, specificity, predictive value and reliability. In this context, it is relevant to consider laboratory validity and population validity. Laboratory validity depends on the characteristics of the test (feasibility, reliability, accuracy and precision) and on the biological characteristics of the marker. Laboratory validity implies studies of sensitivity, traditionally considered as the minimum level of an analyte that an assay can detect (i.e. the smallest single value that can be distinguished from zero with 95% confidence limits). For an analyte value above this minimum, the assay is positive; for lower levels, the assay is negative. In genetic monitoring, background levels are almost always present, and the values measured are distributed over a range – caused by, among other things, inter-individual variation. Thus, the statistical test used to distinguish between levels to be tested and background levels requires knowledge of the expected distribution of values (normal, lognormal, Poisson, etc.).

Specificity traditionally indicates the ability to detect a unique analyte from a group of closely related structures. In genetic monitoring, this implies identification and statistical analysis of the test outcome with due respect to confounding factors, such as sex, age, smoking, medication and X-ray examinations, to mention the most common ones.

Reproducibility under conditions of routine use must be demonstrated as a prerequisite for the comparability of test results. This implies repeatability. That is, tests of the same specimen must repeatedly give the same result whether performed by several different laboratories (inter-laboratory) or by the same laboratory on several occasions (intra-laboratory). This requires the strict following of standardised protocols for the processing of material, analysing, scoring and data processing. Along with standardisation of techniques, laboratory quality assurance and quality control are essential.[7]

The feasibility of the test is another prerequisite that is provided by scientific and technical skill, housing, technical equipment and data management.

Population validity refers to how well the markers depict an event in a population. The sensitivity of a test is a measure of how accurately the test identifies those people with a disease or abnormality who will correctly test positive. Those who have the disease or abnormality and are correctly identified by a positive test are classified as true positives. Specificity is a measure of how accurately the test identifies people who do not have the disease or abnormality. Those persons correctly identified by a negative test are classified as true negatives. The predictive value of a test is the test's accuracy in avoiding either false-positive or false-negative results. In terms of genetic monitoring, heterogeneity lowers the sensitivity, and the variable expression lowers the specificity.[7] Heterogeneity and variable expression also often show broad inter-individual variation. The predictive value of a test cannot be estimated unless one knows the frequency of the condition in the population to be tested – the prevalence. Some markers, despite high test sensitivity and specificity, will have little predictive value if they have a low prevalence in the study population.[8]

Table 17.2 shows the mathematical equations for the calculation of sensitivity, specificity and predictive value.[7] The mathematical definitions are as follows. Validity is the probability that the test will correctly classify true susceptible and true non-susceptible individuals. Sensitivity and specificity are the two characteristics presumed by validity. Sensitivity is the frequency with which the test will be positive when the genotype in question is present. Specificity is the frequency with which the test will be negative when the genotype in question is absent.[9]

Table 17.2   Sensitivity, specificity and predictive value of a test

		Disease		Total
		Present	Absent	
Test outcome	Positive	a (true positives)	B (false positives)	$a+b$
	Negative	c (false negatives)	d (true negatives)	$c+d$
	Total	$a+c$	$b+d$	

Sensitivity
$$= \frac{a}{a+c} = \frac{true\ positives}{true\ positives + false\ negatives}$$

Specificity
$$= \frac{d}{b+d} = \frac{true\ negatives}{false\ positives + true\ negatives}$$

Predictive value positive
$$= \frac{a}{a+b} = \frac{true\ positives}{true\ positives + false\ positives}$$

Predictive value negative
$$= \frac{d}{c+d} = \frac{true\ negatives}{false\ negatives + true\ negatives}$$

An example

Alpha-1 antitrypsin (AAT) deficiency can be mentioned as an example. Homozygous serum (AAT) deficiency is an important genetic factor in emphysema – a chronic lung disease characterised by the irreversible destruction of the walls of the smallest airways in the lungs (respiratory bronchioles) and of the terminal air sacs (alveoli). This is thought to be the result of excessive release of protein-digesting enzymes by macrophages and neutrophils. In heterozygotes AAT levels are 55–60% of their normal values. Epidemiological studies indicate that heterozygotic carriers of AAT deficiency (3% of the general population in the USA) display an enhanced risk of developing chronic obstructive pulmonary disease. The risk is exacerbated by smoking and occupational risk factors, such as grain dust[9] and asbestos.[10] A significant association between low serum AAT concentrations and byssinosis was found in a Danish cross-sectional study of respiratory disorders and atopy in 226 textile industry workers.[11] Data from this study have been applied in a calculation of predictive values of low serum concentration for respiratory symptoms, showing that approximately every fourth person can be relieved by excluding exposure, while – as shown in Table 17.3 – the number of false positives is very high (83%).

Table 17.3 Respiratory symptoms in textile workers exposed to dust, related to serum alpha-1 antitrypsin concentration

		Respiratory symptoms		Total
		Yes	No	
Serum alpha-1 antitrypsin	<35 μmol/L	5	13	18
concentration	>35 μmol/L	25	183	208
Total		30	196	226

Serum concentrations reflect genetic characteristics.

- Sensitivity: $5/(5+25)=5/30=17\%$
- Specificity: $183/(13+183)=183/196=93\%$
- Predictive value of low serum concentration vs. respiratory symptoms: $5/(5+13)=5/18=28\%$
- Predictive value of normal serum concentration versus no respiratory symptoms: $183/(183+25)=183/208=88\%$.

A Swedish study of 205 individuals who had never smoked who were suffering from alpha-1 antitrypsin deficiency (PiZZ) found an additive effect on decline in lung function from occupational exposures.[12] In a study of 2308 young Danish people living in rural areas, a gene or environment interaction was suggested between being in a farming occupation and the rare Pi alleles, leading to increased bronchial hyper-responsiveness in young farmers.[13]

Discussions of genetic testing for AAT deficiency as a way of screening all workers potentially exposed to dust, as opposed to post-symptomatic testing, are summarised in Table 17.4 and Table 17.5.

Table 17.4 Ethical implications of testing for AAT deficiency before employment

Stakeholder	Beneficence	Autonomy	Justice
Employee	Risk of false-positive result diminishing life quality. For true positive, benefit will consist of 28% avoiding disease due to non-exposure	The applicant has to undergo the test if job is seriously wanted, thus loss of autonomy	Since the predictive value is so low, this test is not justified as a genetic screening test
Family	Depends on whether the applicant was truly positive. If an increase in life quality can result from change of lifestyle, this will affect the family in a positive way	No autonomy, as above	
Employer	Since the predictive value is 28%, he will 'save' these, but will also erroneously deselect 72 potentially good workers	Some employers may choose the screening programme, others will decline	May take it as an alibi that the test is part of a programme approved by local authority, but this is a false justification
Colleagues	No effect	No effect	Not relevant
Society	As for employer	Scientifically unjustified pressure may be put on applicants	To be part of a legitimate programme the screening has to be justifiable
Occupational health practitioner	Marginally better knowledge of patient	Puts the practitioner in a dilemma if the test is part of duties	Sample has to be taken by a doctor
Testing laboratory	More tasks and data	Not relevant	Depends on legal situation

Table 17.5 Ethical implications of testing for AAT deficiency after respiratory symptoms

Stakeholder	Beneficence	Autonomy	Justice
Employee	Step in finding aetiology of disease	May be a voluntary offer	Proposed and used in several countries for diagnosing patients
Family	As above		
Employer	May identify general harmful exposures	May initiate action and diminish the exposures	
Colleagues	More knowledge about who will have the symptoms		
Society	Promotes prevention		
Occupational health practitioner	Greater knowledge about the patient		
Testing laboratory	More tasks and data		

The predictive value of a positive test is too low to justify screening, since this will be of minor beneficence to the study subjects (83% will test false positive), employer (the predictive value is too low, at only 28%) and the general public (the preventive potential is too low, there being too many diseased subjects, at 12%, showing a normal value). The autonomy of the study person can be secured by offering the test only upon request and with justification (based on family history, and symptoms indicating AAT deficiency).

Legislation

Workplace genetic testing is practised in a number of research projects, mostly covered by national ethical rules. The seriousness of the research and data protection are taken into account by a local ethical committee and data protection agencies. One of the outstanding questions relates to tissue banking and use of extra tissue, which often results from research projects. In the field of pharmacogenetics, the European Agency for the Evaluation of Medicinal Products has issued a position paper on terminology, which describes five different categories of samples. The codings, which are also relevant in the occupational health sciences, are: 'Identified'; 'Single coded'; 'Double coded'; 'Anonymised'; and 'Anonymous'.

For genetic testing as a part of pre-employment testing, Danish legislation contains a section requesting justification of the test (validity in relation to actual exposure). Also, informed consent is very important, and a 48-hour period is allowed for a job applicant to seek advice at alternative institutions before consenting to testing. The introduction of a genetic test must be scientifically justified, for example by documentation from specialists in genetics, stipulating the circumstances for testing and requiring the counselling of test persons with regard to risk.

In the preparation of Danish law, the special features of genetic testing, in relation to most other medical testing, were taken into account.

- Genetic test data are permanent and do not change during a person's lifetime.
- There may be a long latency period between analysis of a genetic test and manifestation of disease outcome.
- Genetic testing, either population-based genetic screening or individual-based genetic testing, also gives some information about the relatives of the person tested.

The various uses and potential applications of genetic testing give rise to a variety of ethical questions to be covered in future discussion of any workplace application.

- Ownership of data and samples. It has been proposed in Sweden that a third party, such as a governmental institution, should be set up to collect and store sensitive information. However, such centralised sensitive-data collectors are not practicable in countries like Germany and France for historical reasons.
- Use of genetic information as part of human integrity. This is probably inevitable, since individual job application is a matter of trust between employer and employee. Beneficial heritable characteristics may be one of several merits of a job applicant. For example, 'healthy family history' might be referred to as a qualification.
- Risk of discriminatory practices. This implies that the sifting out and rejecting of people with genetic characteristics are close at hand.
- Controversies between paternalism and autonomy of decision making. These are quite clear in cases where an employer requests information

on specific health characteristics when selecting workers on the basis of genetic testing results.

- Protection of confidentiality or anonymity. This may be secured by ensuring that an independent laboratory performs the test and counsels the applicant.
- Prevention of discrimination and stigmatisation. This is scarcely avoidable, since the primary aim of genetic testing is to select.
- Community considerations. Examples include safety aspects in relation to testing (such as colour blindness); they may become more dominant if safety aspects come to cover behaviours, and so on.
- Scientific quality requirements. These should be laid down by law and ensure the validity of any test.
- Commercialisation of genetic testing. This also poses specific ethical questions, which may be especially relevant to future possibilities of testing employees or insurance applicants. The applicant may be able to test his own genes, with poor counselling as a result.
- Need to consult specialists in genetics. This must be emphasised when considering ideas related to the planning and implementation of biogenetic monitoring and risk assessment.
- Previously, there was strong support for anonymity in genetic research as a privacy safeguard. Now, there is an increasingly popular school of thought opposed to anonymity – so as to preserve the individual's ability to withdraw and, if desired, obtain access to research results.[14]

Perspectives

Most genetic polymorphisms have no impact on health. However, some can be used as biomarkers of individual sensitivity to exposure and susceptibility to a specific disease. The Human Genome Project has brought about a quantum leap in the development of genetic markers of diseases and susceptibilities. The practical implications cannot presently be assessed with certainty.[15,16] It is therefore important to keep data protection optimal by ensuring the provision of information to all participants about the status of data and samples (respecting the right 'not to know').

Also, developments are not foreseeable in relation to workplace genetic testing. At present, no tests are sufficiently valid to justify selection of workers, but associations between unfavourable genotypes and increased risk of cancer or respiratory diseases have been reported. The possibility of the abuse of tests and use of test results for discriminatory practices should also be taken into account. Further, there is a temptation to replace preventive work by selection of staff. There is a risk that increasing public awareness and the commercialisation of genetic testing may force such testing into pre-employment testing programmes in an inappropriate manner. Suitable national and international regulation should be promoted to secure beneficence, autonomy and justice.

Considerations in situations involving genetic testing

Respecting the right to work, on the one hand, and the right to be protected against occupational hazards, on the other, speaks for the principle of 'first being employed and then tested' rather than that of 'first being tested and then employed' (the 'if test OK principle'). This, however, may conflict with the interest of the employer. A number of questions to be considered have been posed by Hermeren.[16]

* How is testing to be timed (before employment or after employment)?
* Who takes the initiative to test (employer or employee)?
* What is the purpose of the test (to diminish occupational disease or avoid employment of a person at increased risk)?
* What is going to be tested (a disease or risk indicators)?
* Who will be tested (all employees or only a selection of those at risk)?

Thorough information about the people who are to undergo testing is also a prerequisite. Danish law demands written informed consent with prior information about the purpose of the test, availability of any information derived from the test, correct data management and protection, and the right of the subject to know or not know the test result.

Employers considering genetic testing in employment programmes, and researchers including genetic testing in workplace studies should be encouraged to consult specialists in biogenetic monitoring and risk assessment.

European Initiative

In July 2003 the European Group of Ethics in Science and New Technologies (EGE) expressed its opinion to the European Commission concerning the ethical aspect of genetic testing in the workplace, making 19 points.[17] These points are very useful for a European frame, together with existing practice concerning good clinical practice and data protection.

References

1 McCunney RJ (2002) Genetic testing: ethical implications in the workplace. *Occupational Medicine.* **17**: 665–72.

2 Calabrese EJ (1996) Biochemical individuality. The next generation. *Regulatory Toxicology and Pharmacology.* **24**: 858–67.

3 Johnsen CR, Sørensen TB, Ingemann Larsen A *et al.* (1997) Allergy risk in an enzyme producing plant: a retrospective follow up study. *Occupational and Environmental Medicine.* **54**: 671–5.

4 Knudsen LE, Loft S and Autrup H (2001) Risk assessment. The importance of genetic polymorphisms in man. *Mutation Research.* **282**: 83–8.

5 Calabrese EJ (1991) Genetic predisposition to occupationally-related diseases: current status and future directions. In: P Grandjean (ed.) *Ecogenetics. Genetic predisposition to the toxic effects of chemicals.* WHO, Chapman & Hall, London.

6 Knudsen LE, Theilade MD, Gordon A, Mascaro J and Bruppacher R (2002) Will data privacy impact health research? *Drug Information Journal.* **36**: 465–80.

7 Ashford NA, Spadafor CJ, Hattis D and Caldart CC (1990) *Monitoring the Worker for Exposure and Disease. Scientific, legal and ethical considerations in the use of genetic biomarkers.* The Johns Hopkins University Press, Baltimore and London.

8 Schulte PA, Lomax GP, Ward EM and Colligan MJ (1999) Ethical issues in the use of genetic markers in occupational epidemiological research. *Journal of Occupational and Environmental Medicine.* **41**: 639–46.

9 Congress, Office of Technology Assessment (1990) *Genetic Monitoring and Screening in the Workplace.* OTA, Washington DC.

10 Sigsgaard T, Brandslund, I, Rasmussen JB *et al.* (1994) Low normal alpha-1-antitrypsin serum concentrations and MZ phenotype are associated with byssinosis and familial allergy in cotton mill workers. *Pharmacogenetics.* **4**: 135–41.

11 Piitulainen E, Tornling G and Eriksson S (1997) Effect of age and occupational expsoure to airway irritants on lung function in non-smoking individuals with alpha-1-antitrypsin deficiency (PiZZ). *Thorax.* **52**: 244–8.

12 Sigsgaard T, Brandslund, I, Omland Ø *et al.* (2000) A and Z alpha-1-antitrypsin alleles are risk factors for bronchial hyperresponsiveness in young farmers: an example of gene/environment interaction. *European Respiratory Journal.* **16**: 50–5.

13 Renegar G, Rieser P and Manasco P (2001) Family consent and the pursuit of better medicines through genetic research. *The Journal of Continuing Education in the Health Professions.* **21**: 265–70.

14 Hoffmann W, Latza U, Ahrens W *et al.* (2002) Biological markers in epidemiology: concepts, applications, perspectives. *Gesundheitswesen.* **64**: 145–52.

15 WHO Advisory Committee on Health Research (2002) *Genomics and the World Health.* WHO, Geneva.

16 Hermeren G (1995) Gentester i arbetslivet – risk, nytta, integritet (Genetic tests at work – risks, benefits, integrity). In: G Brunius *et al.* (eds) *Genetik, arbetsliv och etik. (Genetics, Working Life and Ethics)*. Fakta från Arbetslivsinstitutet. Stockholm, Sweden.

17 European Group on Ethics in Science and New Technologies to the European Commission (2003) *Opinion on the Ethical Aspects of Genetic Testing in the Workplace*. Opinion No. 18, 28 July. (www.etuc.org/tutb/fr/bts-info2.html#arret78) (French); (http://europa.eu.int/comm/european_group_ethics/docs/avis18compl-EN.pdf (English).

CHAPTER 18

Occupational health research

David Coggon

As with other areas of healthcare, good occupational health practice requires a sound basis in research. Many occupational health practitioners are involved at some stage in their careers in the collection or analysis of data for research purposes. And all have an ethical obligation to ensure that, in so far as it is practical, the advice that they give accords with the best available scientific evidence.

Ethical questions frequently arise in relation to the design and conduct of research, and health-related studies involving human subjects are routinely subject to review by independent research ethics committees. There is also an ethical imperative to ensure that the results of research are reported accurately, with honest acknowledgement of any limitations that impinge on their interpretation. Perhaps less obvious is the potential for ethical dilemmas to arise in the application of research findings.

To illustrate some of the difficulties that may be encountered, this chapter describes two cases relating to research on organophosphate insecticides.

Case 18.1: a postal survey to investigate risks to health

Concerns have been raised that organophosphate insecticides, in particular in sheep dip, may cause long-term neuropsychiatric illness. An extensive review in 1999 concluded that the balance of evidence did not indicate the occurrence of such effects, except after episodes of overt acute poisoning.[1] However, the possibility remained that chronic low-level exposure to organophosphates might cause disabling neuropsychiatric illness in a small minority of exposed people.

To address this question, a research team proposed to conduct a postal survey of 30 000 men randomly selected from the general population of rural areas in which organophosphates had been widely used, either in sheep or arable farming. The questionnaire would collect information about employment history (in particular, any work with pesticides in agriculture) and about various health outcomes that had been postulated to result from exposure to organophosphates. Conducting the study in the general population and not just in men currently employed as farmers would avoid a hazard being missed because the disability produced had caused those affected to give up work in agriculture.

To reduce the possibility of bias in the reporting of exposures and symptoms, the main purpose of the questionnaire would be disguised by asking also about non-agricultural occupational exposures and about other health variables that had not been linked to organophosphates. Analysis of this additional information would allow various secondary questions to be examined. The letter that accompanied the questionnaire would present the study simply as an investigation of health and work in rural populations.

Two possible methods were considered for identifying and approaching subjects. In the first (Option 1), general practitioners in the study areas would be invited to assist the study team by providing them with a computer file giving the names, addresses and dates of birth of men from their patient lists who were eligible for study, and a note of any who they felt should not be approached (e.g. because of recent bereavement). The researchers would then mail the questionnaires, including a covering letter from the subject's general practice as well as their own invitation to participate in the study.

With the second method (Option 2), the selection of subjects and mailing of questionnaires would be carried out on behalf of the study team by local health authorities, which hold details of all people registered with general practices in their area. Before the mailing, the general practitioners concerned would be told about the study, and given an opportunity to identify any of their patients who they believed should be excluded. However, the health authorities would not have the resources to chase general practitioners who failed to respond, and in the absence of a specific request for exclusion, the questionnaire would be sent.

Questions

The design of this study raised two ethical questions for the research team.

- How much information should participants be given about the exact purpose of the investigation?
- Which of the two proposed options would be the better method for identifying and approaching subjects?

Discussion

The main stakeholders in this scenario are: the members of the study population who would be invited to take part in the study; farmers and others who have used or might in the future use organophosphate insecticides; the general public, who through taxation contribute to the funding of medical research and also of healthcare for adverse effects of pesticide exposure; the general practitioners in the study areas; and the research team. Table 18.1 summarises the ethical implications for each of these parties under the headings of beneficence, autonomy and justice.

Table 18.1 Case 18.1: ethical implications for stakeholders

Stakeholder	Beneficence	Autonomy	Justice
Members of the study population	1 A longer, less focused questionnaire will require more of their time 2 A few may be distressed by receiving a questionnaire 3 Some may benefit from the research through the management of occupational health hazards	1 Incomplete information about the purpose of the study will reduce autonomy 2 Passing personal information to the research team without consent would be an infringement	
Farmers and others who use organophosphate insecticides	1 Lower response rates and biased participation in study would reduce potential benefit from improved control of organophosphate hazard		
General public	1 Lower response rates and biased participation in study would reduce its cost-effectiveness		1 If the study is less cost-effective this may divert resources from other deserving areas of medical research
General practitioners in the study areas	1 Option 1 for approaching subjects would entail a greater workload		
Research team	1 Lower response rates and biased participation in study could reduce the esteem in which the research is held and make it harder to obtain funding		1 Competing researchers in other countries may not face the same ethical constraints

Information for participants

The extent to which participants should be told the purpose of a study is a common problem in epidemiological research where such knowledge could adversely influence the findings of the investigation. It also arises sometimes in experimental psychology, where a subject's knowledge and expectations may be important study variables that the investigator wishes to control.

In the case described above, disguising the exact purpose of the study would infringe the autonomy of members of the study population in so far as they would not have full information on which to base their decision whether or not to participate. Moreover, the added demands on the time of those who took part, because of the greater length of the questionnaire, could be viewed as harmful to them, although only to a minor degree.

Against this, by restricting the explanation given to participants, the design proposed would be expected to give more reliable results. This could have benefits for users of organophosphates through better management of associated health hazards, for the general public in better value for money from the research, and for the research team in the higher value attached to their work by colleagues in the research community and potential funders of the investigation. Further, the elements added to the questionnaire to distract from its prime aim could lead to supplementary benefits for the general public (perhaps including some members of the study population) through improved control of other occupational hazards.

Importantly, the explanation of the study in the letter accompanying the questionnaire would not contain false information. A deliberate lie to potential participants would be a greater infringement of their autonomy, and harder to justify. If later publicised, a lie could also bring epidemiological research into disrepute, with harmful consequences for both the general public and the research community.

In deciding whether it would be acceptable to withhold information from participants as proposed, one test might be to ask how many subjects would alter their decision whether to take part if they were told more. It is possible that such information would encourage a few extra individuals with past exposure to organophosphates to complete the questionnaire. It seems less likely, however, that knowing the main purpose of the study would influence some men not to take part who otherwise would have done so (unless they mistakenly believed that this was the only object of the investigation).

For this reason, I believe that the design proposed was ethically acceptable. On this matter, the research ethics committee that reviewed the protocol agreed.

Method of selecting and approaching subjects

Choosing between the two proposed methods for selecting and approaching subjects is more complex.

The main disadvantage of Option 1 is that it would require general practices to pass information about members of the study population to researchers without their consent. It is unlikely that this would cause them any harm since the study team was based in a different part of the country and bound by a strict code of practice on confidentiality. Further, the information supplied on individuals would be only their name, address and date of birth, plus, in a few cases, an indication that the general practitioner did not wish the individual to be approached (no explanation would be required for such requests). There would be greater concerns if health data were included, especially if they related to sensitive topics such as sexual function. Nevertheless, passing on personal information without prior consent would infringe the autonomy of members of the study population. Option 2 would avoid this problem since names, addresses and dates of birth were already held by the health authority, and would not be given to the research team.

A second consideration is the harm that might be done to some members of the study population by writing to them. The topics covered in the questionnaire were not unusually sensitive, but for a few people, any sort of official letter might be a source of distress. In this respect, Option 1 offered the advantage that general practitioners would be more actively involved, and questionnaires would only be mailed after the general practitioners had excluded men whom they did not think should be contacted. There would of course be a cost, in the time that the doctors put into this exercise. Option 2 also gave an opportunity to general practitioners to identify men who should be excluded, but because they would be less closely involved in the study and could not be chased to respond, the task was unlikely to be carried out so thoroughly by all of the doctors concerned.

The third major issue is the impact of the method of approaching subjects on the quality of information obtained from the study. Experience from previous surveys suggested that response rates could be substantially higher when questionnaires were accompanied by a letter of introduction from the subject's own doctor. Also, if the mailing was carried out by health authorities then letters would have to be addressed impersonally ('Dear patient'), since the authorities did not have the secretarial and computing resource to address recipients by name. Again, this would be expected to reduce response rates. Where the response to a questionnaire is low, steps can be taken to assess the consequent potential for bias, for example by comparing the known characteristics of responders and non-responders, and by comparing information from those who respond early with that from subjects who only answer after a reminder. Nevertheless, there will still be more uncertainty in the interpretation of results than if the response rate is higher. In the case under discussion, greater uncertainty surrounding the results of the study would reduce its potential benefits for users of organophosphates, reduce the value for money that the public obtained from the investigation (possibly diverting resources from other deserving research topics), and place the research team at a disadvantage relative to other investigators who were able to obtain higher response rates.

In summary, the decision between the two possible study methods hinges on the balance that is drawn when a loss of autonomy and small risk of harm to members of the study population from Option 1 is weighed against an alternative risk of harm to members of the study population (again small), reduced benefits to organophosphate users, poorer value for money for the general public, and disadvantages to the researchers from Option 2. Over the past century, value judgements of this sort in Western countries have tended increasingly to favour the autonomy of the individual at the expense of benefits to the wider community. Nevertheless, my view is that Option 1 is ethically preferable. In this case, however, the ethics committee that reviewed the proposal took the opposite view.

Involvement of research ethics committees

A further issue raised by this case is the relation of the researcher to the ethics committee. In what circumstances is it appropriate for investigators to seek approval for a proposed study, and how much detail should they communicate to the committee about the study design?

Views on the need for independent ethical review have varied over time and between countries. For example, historically in the UK it was not considered essential to review studies that involved the analysis only of patient records and clinical material to which the researcher already had access. However, today this no longer applies, since the use of such information without prior consent could be viewed as an infringement of individual autonomy.

Interestingly, in this respect, a distinction is drawn between audit and research. Audit assesses the structure, function or outcome of a specific service against standards or benchmark comparators with the aim of optimising its performance. Research addresses questions of more general relevance, and application of its findings normally extends beyond the immediate setting in which it is carried out. For the purposes of audit, it is generally regarded as acceptable for occupational health departments to analyse data that they already hold on their own patients or clients without independent ethical review, although, of course, ethical principles apply in audit just as in any other aspect of practice. By contrast, prior ethical approval would normally be expected for research, even where the data analysed were obtained in the same way and were identical to those that might be used for audit.

If a research ethics committee is consulted, a good rule is that researchers should provide all information about the study that they consider would be relevant to the committee's deliberations. To help with this, committees often give guidance to researchers on the level of documentation that they wish to see, and on specific aspects of study design that they view as particularly important.

Case 18.2: use of research in the regulation of a pesticide

As in many other countries, the registration of pesticides for use in the UK is subject to periodic review. This entails the submission of scientific data by organisations (usually chemical manufacturers) that seek continued approval for products that incorporate the pesticide concerned. They are required to demonstrate the efficacy of the product, and to provide adequate reassurance that its use will not present unacceptable risks to human health, wildlife or the environment.

A major concern in the consideration of organophosphate insecticides is the possibility of acute toxicity in people exposed either during their use or through consumption of residues in foods derived from treated crops. In particular, organophosphates have the potential to cause illness through inhibition of the enzyme acetylcholinesterase in both the central and peripheral nervous system. Evidence on the risk of such toxicity and its relation to levels of exposure comes largely from experimental studies in laboratory animals. Results are then extrapolated to humans with the application of 'assessment factors' to allow for possible differences in susceptibility between species, and for the possibility that some individuals are more sensitive than others. In some cases, data may also be available from experiments in human volunteers, using doses that are not expected to produce symptoms or signs, but which may be sufficient to cause detectable inhibition of acetylcholinesterase in erythrocytes. The use of human data for risk assessment has the advantage of avoiding the uncertainties that are inherent in extrapolation between species.

In the case of one organophosphate insecticide, one of the studies submitted in support of continued registration had been carried out decades earlier in a group of prisoners. The participants were said to have volunteered for the research, but from the available documentation it was unclear whether their consent to take part had been properly informed and freely given.

Question

This raised a question for the registration authority of whether or not it was ethical to use data from the study of prisoners as part of its risk assessment.

Discussion

As well as the prisoners who took part in the study and the company seeking continued registration for the pesticide, the other major stakeholders in this decision are potential users of the product, the public more generally, participants in future experimental research, and other competing pesticide manufacturers. Table 18.2 summarises the potential impact of the registration authority's decision for each party concerned.

Among the stakeholders listed, the potential users of the product and the general public would both stand to benefit from use of the experimental data from prisoners for risk assessment. It might, for example, enable better control of a pest problem than could otherwise be permitted, with financial benefits for farmers and the production of cheaper and better quality food for public consumption. Alternatively, if the data indicated a higher risk than would otherwise have been anticipated, they could lead to controls on usage that protected the health of users and of consumers of food derived from treated crops.

For the company that produced the pesticide, the commercial benefits of enabling continued registration would probably be even greater than for users, but it would derive no benefit if use of the data on prisoners led to restrictions on usage, other than perhaps protection from later litigation.

Against the gains for these parties from using results of the study of prisoners must be weighed the potential adverse consequences for people who undergo experimental exposure to pesticides and other hazards to assist medical and scientific research. The risk of harm from experiments such as that carried out on the prisoners is small, but failure to obtain adequately informed and freely given consent detracts from the autonomy of participants. For the prisoners themselves, any damage of this sort will already have been done, and choosing to apply the results in risk management would not now add to their loss. Nevertheless, some would argue that

Table 18.2 Case 18.2: ethical implications for stakeholders

Stakeholder	Beneficence	Autonomy	Justice
Users of organophosphates	1 Information from the prisoner study might bring commercial benefits from continued use of the pesticide or prevent ill-health through restrictions on its use		
Prisoners who took part in the study	1 Participation entailed a small chance of injury from unexpected toxicity	1 Lack of information and pressure to participate would have reduced autonomy	
Participants in future experimental research	1 Acceptance of ethically flawed research from the past could lead to harm by encouraging unethical research in the future	1 Acceptance of ethically flawed research from the past could impair autonomy by encouraging unethical research in the future	
General public	1 Information from the prisoner study might bring benefits from continued use of the pesticide (through better or cheaper food) or through prevention of ill-health by restrictions on its use		
Company that produced the pesticide	1 Commercial benefit from sale and use of prisoners' data enabled continuing registration of the pesticide		
Other competing companies			1 Use of the prisoners' data to support continued registration might be unfair on competitors whose products are supported by more ethical research

it is wrong to apply the results of unethical research, even when doing so does not exacerbate the injury or loss of autonomy that has already been perpetrated. Moreover, it is possible that discounting damage that has already been done could encourage unethical research in the future because investigators conclude that their findings can have an impact even if derived by dubious means.

The concern for competing manufacturers is an issue of justice. It could be argued that, if it prevented restrictions on the pesticide, use of the prisoners' study for risk assessment would give the producer an unfair commercial advantage over competitors that did not rely on ethically dubious data to support their products.

In deciding whether to make use of the prisoners' data, one important consideration is the nature of the benefits that would be obtained. While continued use of a pesticide could be advantageous for several parties, the main benefit would be to the producer, and would be financial. Some people might place less value on commercial gains to a large company than on the prevention of illness that could result if a more extensive risk assessment led to use of the pesticide being restricted.

Another factor that may be relevant is the consensus of ethical opinion in the society and era in which the research on the prisoners was conducted. At the time the investigation was carried out, ethical review of studies was less stringent than nowadays, and less emphasis was placed on the level of information that had to be given to subjects before they consented to take part in research. It may well be that, at the time the research was conducted, most people would have considered it ethically acceptable. This is in contrast, for example, to human experiments carried out in Nazi concentration camps, which were clearly unacceptable by contemporary standards. Value judgements and views on what is ethically justifiable vary, not only between cultures but also within the same society over time. If we uncompromisingly apply current ethical standards to research from earlier epochs as a condition for using its results, we will forego benefits from the honest endeavours of our forefathers, and also run the risk that the full value of the research that we conduct today will not be realised.

My view is that if the effect of applying results from the study of prisoners was stricter regulatory control of the pesticide for the protection of users or the general public, the benefits in preventing illness or injury would outweigh any loss of autonomy suffered by those who volunteered for the research. Importantly, in this situation, the company that produced the pesticide would derive no commercial benefit from the use made of the research. Thus, the decision would not encourage the commissioning of unethical research by pesticide manufacturers in the future. Nor would it unjustly penalise competitors whose products were supported only by studies that were ethically robust.

However, I would only support application of the results of the study to enable continued use of the pesticide if it could be shown that the experiment on prisoners was ethically acceptable by the standards of the society and era in which it was carried out.

In coming to these views, I have taken account of the minimal risk of harm to the prisoners from taking part in the research. If the experiment had involved major risks to the health of participants, I would not support using its results unless there were overwhelming compensatory benefits to the health of others from doing so, and I was confident that the decision would not be an encouragement to seriously unethical research in the future.

Reference

1   Committee on Toxicity of Chemicals in Food (1999) *Consumer Products and the Environment: organophosphates.* DoH, London. (www.doh.gov.uk/cot.htm).

The ethics of health and safety services: a trade union perspective

Laurent Vogel

An atypical contribution

This is a very special contribution. I was asked to make it as a trade unionist as an input into the debate aimed at defining the ethical principles that govern the workings of health and safety activities. The trade union movement has no firm tradition of debate where ethical aspects of health and safety (or indeed many other) issues are concerned. Further, my own professional experience is not restricted to a specific country, and I can say with certainty that the way ethical issues are handled is subject to major cultural peculiarities. In these few pages, I shall undertake to outline a few criteria that the trade union movement deems vital in discussions of ethical principles underlying health and safety in the workplace. Whilst my thoughts are based on regular contacts with a large number of trade union officials responsible for such issues, they do not constitute an official viewpoint taken by the European trade unions. Personally, I doubt whether such a viewpoint could ever be drawn up.

In my opinion, when the actions in question do not belong to the strictly private sphere, and do not fall solely under a form of moral responsibility resting on individual values, ethics and politics are inseparable.[1] I do not think there is a common set of European values (or even a set that applies solely to the Protestant countries of northern Europe) that would suffice to define the rules governing the professional practice of occupational health professionals. Political views on their role can vary strongly, and such variation results in a hierarchy of priorities that has a crucial influence on the way ethical issues are treated. From a trade union viewpoint, the main role of occupational health professionals is to make a contribution to the struggle to reduce social inequalities related to health issues, which are partly determined by work conditions.[2,3] This means that occupational health services serve as an external factor contributing to society's and the public's control over companies. Obviously, there are other political concepts of occupational health preventive services (such as rendering a high level of productivity compatible with a high level of health protection, reconciling the employer's interests with a concern to safeguard the lives of workers and so on), and approaches utilising these concepts affect the debate. In any ethical dilemma, benefits and disadvantages are weighed against each other, so it is important to know what is being weighed up and on the basis of what values a judgement is made.

In some countries, ethical debates about health and safety at work have been closely linked to political debates about the roles played by the various actors involved in determining the nature of work conditions. This emerges particularly clearly in France, Italy and Spain. In France, the debate has focused on the missions of occupational health physicians, and resolution of the ethical dilemma concerning their determination of which workers are 'fit' or 'unfit'.[4] The context of these debates is extensively characterised by the implications of the asbestos scandal. Why did large numbers of workers continue to be exposed to this mortal danger when the potential consequences of such exposure had been known for at least 50 years? What lesson should we learn from this with respect to the activities of thousands of occupational health professionals and the system of health surveillance that covers all people working in France? In Italy, the link between ethics and politics becomes apparent in a more general framework. Changes affecting work organisation are discussed in relation to the more profound social changes in and major upheavals to the political system that was set up after 1945.[5]

From medical ethics to a broader view on multidisciplinary preventive services

An examination of the literature reveals the main characteristics of most documents on ethics in health and safety services.[6,7] Generally, they aim to apply rules established in the tradition of medical ethics to the specific area of health and safety at work, and – more specifically – to all activities where an individual decision about a worker is taken by a health and safety operator. What attitude should be adopted at a pre-employment examination? What kind of approach should be taken to drug testing? Under what conditions should a worker be considered unfit for work?

Medical ethics and occupational safety and health

This approach – which focuses on the noteworthy relationship between a specialist (usually a physician) and an individual who, to a certain extent, is comparable to a patient – can be explained largely by the following contradiction. For many years, occupational health physicians have had broad discretionary powers when it comes to choosing tests and other investigative methods. By contrast, strict rules have applied to decisions taken on the basis of the results of these tests. Generally speaking, the doctor has had to draw a conclusion (e.g. whether or not a worker is fit) without having an overview of the entire series of events involved. In most cases, deciding that a worker was unfit meant that the worker lost his or her job without the doctor being able to 'negotiate' the consequences of his or her decision. Interest in ethics was strongly encouraged by an awareness that a competent professional judgement can have negative consequences, and that perhaps such negative consequences should be taken into account when making the decision. Indeed, losing a job often has a negative impact on health. Consequently, a competent professional judgement made by an occupational health physician can incorporate this consideration into an overall assessment of the risks linked to a given job. Moreover, using ethical arguments is an important legitimising factor in relations with the other parties involved (employers, workers, other health and safety professionals, etc.).

This kind of approach is still valid, but it is no longer enough in the light of a number of new challenges.

- Health and safety services are tending to become multidisciplinary. References to ethics are less common among occupational health professionals who are not medical doctors or nurses. Safety engineers, hygienists and ergonomists do not generally use ethical arguments to legitimise their proposals or interventions. They tend to conceive their role mainly on the basis of technical expertise.
- The priority of health and safety activities is to transform collective work conditions. This considerably alters the usual framework for debate on medical ethics where the relationship between health practitioner and patient is central. Many factors in the context in which health and safety services operate are undergoing change. Just some examples are the growing trend by health and safety services to operate as companies on a competitive market, the growing standardisation of health and safety activities via certification systems or under pressure from insurance companies, and the growing integration of health and safety services into companies' overall management.

Workers' expertise

Consequently, the ethical debate on health and safety at work will not continue to focus so sharply on a system of ethics based on the relationship between doctors and their patients. As things currently stand, we can only note the difficulty of successfully building up collective multidisciplinary expertise between medical personnel and personnel who approach the issue of health and safety from a different perspective, for example ergonomics or industrial hygiene. And another factor must be taken into account in addition to intrinsic uncertainty. In a participatory strategy to improve work conditions, no scientific discipline can enable full validation of a given solution. The two reasons for this are that technical validation should usually be the result of interdisciplinarity, and should also be supported by the validation of workers themselves. In medical ethics, autonomy is traditionally conceived as respect for the subjective will of the individual (patient), who can enter into conflict with an objectively validated solution that might better contribute to his or her health. In the area of health and safety at work, this vision does not fully correspond to reality. Experience at work, and with both the pleasure and suffering linked to work, are contributions made by workers themselves. This is not a factor external to any definition of problems and solutions involving health at work. Workers' perceptions of what is acceptable and unacceptable, of pain, of their ability to cope with a given problem, of the support they find in relations with their co-workers and so on, are all part of the 'evidence' in evidence-based professional practices.[8] Of course, this does not mean that subjective perception is enough permanently to validate a given solution; a person can be exposed to carcinogens, and consider it perfectly normal and not really risky. Workers have their own form of expertise (individual and collective), and taking account of this expertise involves moving beyond the traditional view of a patient's autonomy. All this justifies a debate on the ethics of listening, in which each of the parties involved agrees to question his or her conceptions via the experience of other parties and, in particular, via the experience of subjects who are responsible for their own health under specified work conditions.[9] From this point of view, the autonomy granted to workers is not limited to taking account – as far as possible – of their freedom to make mistakes or cause harm. There is also the recognition that the will of workers is linked to specific knowledge that has a rational core, and which should enable a kind of synthesis between the viewpoint of health and safety experts and the viewpoint of workers.

The drug test: a story about the importance of setting limits

Let us start with a hypothetical scenario. I want to visualise a version of the story concerning Mrs A described in Case 11.1 in Chapter 11 (*see* p. 151). I will start with a hypothesis that is entirely compatible with the one you may already have read. Mrs A is an excellent worker, but her friends and family find her terribly boring. All she talks about is work. When she comes over to dinner, her mobile phone is always on and she is bound to have to interrupt the conversation to take calls from colleagues, who know that they can bother her at all hours. The other evening one of her sons decided to bake a very special cake. Partly as a practical joke, partly out of scientific curiosity, he put some cocaine in the flour. I wasn't there that evening. I don't know how Mrs A behaved during the meal. But the next day it was the same responsible, serious Mrs A who showed up at work. Naturally, she knew nothing about the ingredients of the cake. It was that day she was tested. You may know how the story ended, and I suppose that the 'happy ending' may well have something to do with the fact that Mrs A is a white woman, aged 41, with a career spanning 16 years. I am not sure whether a young Jamaican would have benefited from the same scrutiny.

Imagine a slightly different scenario. The test was conducted under ideal conditions. No error was possible. The urine clearly contained traces of cocaine and had come from Mrs A. I can see several major problems from an ethical point of view. There is nothing to prove that the standard procedure, which almost inevitably leads to dismissal, is justified from the viewpoint of safety. Other motives can play a role in this procedure – pressure from customers or a public authority for a tough policy on drugs, the desire to select staff on the basis of criteria associated with morality, and the ease of a procedure that is based solely on technology and keeps the role played by personal judgement to a minimum. There is probably no clear link between traces of a substance in someone's urine and a real danger from a safety point of view. It is possible that moderate consumption of a drug outside working hours has no influence whatsoever on the user's behaviour at work. Consequently, the established procedures may reflect a degree of moral and disciplinary control on the part of the employer that does not constitute a proportionate response to the potential safety problem caused by abusive consumption of certain substances. On the other hand, an occupational health professional should always take account of the inter-action between the person and their work environment. Isn't there also an ethical dilemma when co-operating with a procedure that precludes a specific assessment of this interaction? In the case in point, the presence of traces of cocaine in Mrs A's urine could have justified a discussion with her and with her colleagues. Perhaps it would have emerged that Mrs A had nothing to do with the safety problems. On the various occasions they had arisen, all she had displayed was professional calm and awareness. Her son's practical joke did not affect her competence or qualities.

The case involving Mrs A would lead to one of several possible decisions by the occupational health physician in the company's health and safety service. He could follow the standard procedure and indicate the positive result of the test, but also draw up a report to request that the procedure in question be quashed or significantly changed. In this case there is a major risk that Mrs A will be fired anyway. He could refuse to take part in the procedure, not divulge the results of the test and inform the employer of the reasons for the action. There is no guarantee that Mrs A will keep her job and that the doctor himself will not be dismissed. He could also lie and maintain that all the results were negative, whilst at the same time proposing that the verification procedure be abandoned. But lying like that itself raises ethical problems.

Setting limits to occupational health activities

The various contributions to this book raise the problem of setting limits to the activities of health and safety services – one among several important problems. Setting limits has become difficult due to the fact that health and safety policies have rapidly expanded to cover a much broader area. No longer limited to preventing industrial accidents and occupational disease, health and safety policies now impact on all aspects of work organisation.

My proposal with regard to limits has three components, all related to the 'mission' of occupational health services.

- The key mission of health and safety services is to improve work conditions in order to guarantee the health, safety and well-being of workers. This definition – with a slightly different wording – can also be found in documents issued by the International Labour Organization (ILO), such as Convention 161, and in the 1989 European Union framework directive. Health surveillance and inter-individual relations between occupational health professionals and workers form part of this mission. They are not ends in themselves, but focus on all work-related health problems.
- This mission of health and safety in the workplace fits into a broader setting in which health and safety services constitute just one

component of a public health system. The aim is to reduce social inequalities in the area of health by taking action in respect of work conditions. This implies that the responsibility of staff working in health and safety services is not limited to protecting the health of workers in the companies that they cover directly. The data gathered make it possible better to gear health and safety policies at other levels (e.g. at sectoral level, national level, European level, etc.).

- On the whole, health and safety services accomplish their mission by advising workers, employers, public authorities and other relevant parties, and by disseminating information and proposals on the basis of their autonomous professional skills and competence.

In the debate on ethics setting limits is often a key issue. There are constant pressures to have health and safety departments embrace priorities or constraints other than health and safety at work. I will give a few examples. Some may seem absurd or comical, others legitimate, but what they have in common is that they go beyond the area of preventive intervention and, in so doing, can lead to ethical dilemmas.

From reviewing the literature,[10–12] it appears that interventions led by occupational health services have been justified by:

- the 'company's well-being'
- reducing social security costs or workers' compensation costs
- an increase in the birth rate
- concerns regarding the morality of the workforce or some parts of the workforce (often women)
- protection of a specific ethnic group
- the need to ensure the recruitment of healthy 'soldiers' from the young generation
- the requirements of certification linked to quality assurance, etc.

The legitimacy of each of these objectives can be discussed. What is most important is to realise that they are extraneous to the mission of occupational health services. Historically, health and safety at work has often been organised within an ambiguous framework. Objectives such as consolidating employers' power, justifying dangerous work conditions, boosting productivity and recruiting labour characterised many practices that were presented as health and safety activities. There are plenty of examples – from the recruitment of foreign workers to go down the coal mines, where industrial health provisions were notoriously inadequate, through to the distribution of milk to workers exposed to lead.

Occupational health services play an important, albeit limited role. They help improve the health and safety of workers through their activities in the workplace. The direct beneficiaries of their activities are:

- individual workers
- workers in the company
- workers in the production process (e.g. when two companies co-operate, when a company subcontracts certain activities, etc.)
- workers and the general public in society at large.

Generally speaking, employers are indirect beneficiaries of occupational health activities. Obviously, they are concerned in so far as the services must provide them with an independent, competent opinion on the issues of health and safety at work. More rarely, they can be direct beneficiaries when their own lives and health are exposed to hazards in the workplace (which is usually only the case in small companies where the employer personally takes part in production). On the other hand, employers' economic interests do not, in my opinion, constitute a relevant criterion in ethical debates on the activities of health and safety services. In this respect, it should be observed that, as a rule, an occupational health service does not take decisions on the management of a company. It provides an opinion that will contribute to the decision-making process. It would be dangerous to try to include, in any such opinion, constraints that stem from the general management of the company – since this would limit the full professional independence of health and safety operators.

I have sought to draw attention to the ambiguity that I think can be found in most of the definitions of the word 'stakeholder' – or worse, 'customer' – in the debate on the activities of health and safety services. I believe we are under constant pressure, and that this is likely to skew the meaning of the terms used in discussions of the professional responsibilities and ethics of a health and safety service. This pressure is considerable when occupational health services are active on a competitive market, where employers decide to a large extent which missions will be assigned to which service. However, I would also like to emphasise the fact that there are many work-related health problems for which solutions cannot be found at company level alone. This paves the way for a debate on the ethics of responsibility. In many cases, occupational health professionals can see that problems are caused by political, economic and social decisions made outside the company. The evolution of the labour market, the setting of limit values, banning a hazardous substance, and stipulating the age from which a person can work, and also retirement age, are all examples of this. I think it is important for occupational health professionals to be supported in contributing, on the basis of their experience, to the debates on these issues. Given this perspective, making the issues of health and safety at work more broadly visible is not limited to 'whistleblowing'. It is more akin to building up a collective expertise that combines our professional experience and commitment as citizens.

References

1   Castoriadis C (1993) Le cache-misère de l'éthique (The concealing veil of ethics). *Lettre Internationale.* **37**: 2–8.

2   Borg V and Kristensen TS (2000) Social class and self-rated health: can the gradient be explained by differences in life style or work environment? *Social Sciences and Medicine.* **51**(7): 1019–30.

3   Conne-Perréard E, Glardon MJ, Parrat J and Usel M (2001) *Effets de conditions de travail défavorables sur la santé des travailleurs et leurs conséquences économiques* (Effects of adversial working conditions on workers' health and their economic consequences). Conférence Romande et Tessinoise des Offices Cantonuax de Protection des Travailleurs, Geneva.

4   Association Santé et Médecine du Travail (1998) *Des Médecins du Travail Prennent la Parole. Un métier en débat* (Occupational Physicians take to the floor. A profession under debate). Syros, Paris.

5   Polo G and Sabattini C (2000) *Restaurazione Italiana. FIAT, la Sconfitta Operaia dell'Autunno 1980 alle Origini della Controrivoluzione Liberista* (The Italian Restoration. FIAT, the setback for the workers in the autumn of 1980 at the beginning of the free-market counter-revolution). Manifestolibri, Rome.

6   International Labour Organization (1997) *Technical and Ethical Guidelines for Workers' Health Surveillance.* ILO, Geneva.

7   Ashford N, Spadafor C, Hattis D and Caldart C (1990) *Monitoring the Worker for Exposure and Disease: scientific, legal and ethical considerations in the use of biomarkers.* Johns Hopkins University Press, Baltimore, MD.

8   Lax M (2002) Occupational medicine: toward a worker/patient empowerment approach to occupational illness. *International Journal of Health Services.* **32**: 515–49.

9   Dodier N (1993) *L'expertise Médicale. Essai de sociologie sur l'exercice du jugement.* (Medical expertise. A sociologic essay on the exercise of judgement). Métailié, Paris.

10 Viet V and Ruffat M (1999) *Le Choix de la Prevention* (Making prevention the choice). Economica, Paris.

11 Weindling P (ed.) (1985) *The Social History of Occupational Health.* Croom Helm, London.

12 Grieco A and Bertazzi PA (eds) (1997) *Per una Storiografia Italiana della Prevenzione Occupazionale ed Ambientale* (For a historiography of occupational and environmental prevention). Franco Angeli, Milan.

CHAPTER 20

Employer attitudes to ethics in occupational health

Niki Ellis

Introduction

This chapter aims to improve understanding of employer attitudes to ethical issues in occupational health.

First, it argues that the growth of interest by employers in business ethics, and corporate social responsibility in particular, is a boost for health and safety. It is suggested that occupational health practitioners need to overcome any suspicions about employers' motivations for this, and focus more on using this current interest in business ethics and corporate social responsibility to maximise beneficial effects on the health of personnel, customers and neighbouring communities.

Second, against this positive background, the more problematic question of employer attitudes to some of the specific ethical dilemmas in occupational health is considered.

It is concluded that occupational health should renegotiate its position on the changed landscape of the modern workplace. It is proposed that corporate social responsibility, described in a recent report by CSR Europe as the need for the management decision-making process to 'take into account a wide range of criteria relating to the financial, environmental and social implications of business operations',[1] provides an opportunity to do this.

Business ethics, corporate social responsibility and occupational health

Obtaining true information about employer attitudes to 'motherhood' subjects – such as ethics, corporate social responsibility and occupational health – is very difficult. The reason for this is that employers who do not consider that responsibilities other than financial are of high priority to their business find it difficult to say so publicly. They tend to 'talk the talk' but not 'walk the walk'. Although individual chief executive officers and other senior managers are unlikely to express views that could be construed as unsupportive, organisations that represent them collectively may well do so. However, more penetrating attitudinal research aims to explore employers who do express support, why they do so, what are the benefits to their business, and also what they do, and can be quite revealing.

The following strategy was used to search for information on employer attitudes in these areas.

Searches on the websites of the following business organisations for information on safety, health and well-being.

- Leading business-oriented ethics organisations:
  - Business for Social Responsibility (BSR) – American based but international, considered to be the leading business-oriented organisation in the world in this area.
  - CSR Europe – leading European business-oriented organisation in Europe, also affiliated to BSR.
- Organisations representing business:
  - European Chamber of Commerce and Industry (ECCI).
  - Confederation of British Industry (CBI).

Search of the following business-press databases from January 2002 to February 2003 for information on corporate social responsibility:

- Business and Industry
- European Intelligence Wire.

How employers have positioned health in business ethics

Table 20.1 shows a breakdown of the topics of so-called 'White Papers' on the BSR website. Since most of the health-oriented ones are included under 'workplace', a further breakdown of papers on this subject is provided.

One of the introductory papers, entitled *Business Ethics*, describes how leading-edge employers consider there has been a shift in policy from corporate governance, in which employees were guided to follow compliance-based, legally driven codes, to the current situation where organisations develop 'values-based, globally consistent programs that give employees a level of ethical understanding that allows them to make

Table 20.1 Topics for policy papers and their frequency on the website of the leading international business-oriented organisation for corporate social responsibility*

Topic	Number of papers
Corporate social responsibility (introduction)	1
Business ethics	5
Community investment	16
Environment	14
Governance and accountability	6
Human rights	12
Market place	3
Mission, vision and values	1
Workplace	11
dependent care	
diversity	
domestic partner benefits	
downsizing: layoffs/closings	
flexible scheduling	
health and wellness	
HIV/AIDS in the workplace	
privacy (employee)	
religion in the workplace	
work life – balance	
workplace	
Total	69

* Source: www.bsr.org.

appropriate decisions'.[2] The benefits of investing in business ethics are listed as follows: strengthen financial performance; improve sales, brand image and reputation; strengthen employee loyalty and commitment; limit vulnerability to activists; avoid fines and other penalties; avoid loss of business; and greater access to capital. Although health *per se* is not mentioned in this paper, clearly strengthening employee loyalty and commitment is a key aim of ethical business practice. And, as will be demonstrated below, corporate social responsibility is one way of achieving this.

The BSR introductory paper on corporate social responsibility[3] – also listed in Table 20.1 – positions it as a value that might be adopted by an ethical business. Health is included in the expected benefits, as follows.

- Reduced costs – through improvements to operating environment and through reduced absenteeism.

- Increased productivity and quality – through health programmes.
- Reduced regulatory oversight, such as where US agencies reward companies who have demonstrated effective environment, health and safety programmes with fewer inspections or the fast-tracking of other procedures.

In the BSR White Paper *Sustainable Business Practices*[4] the link to health is even stronger. Here, health and safety strategies are regarded as an important way of achieving desired aims (as well as being included in discussion of expected benefits). For example, a set of principles of the 'Coalition for Environmentally Responsible Economies' is cited. These include:

- risk reduction – minimising environmental health and safety risks to employees and communities
- safe products and services
- environmental restoration – correcting conditions that endanger health, safety or the environment.

In general, the closer the subject of the paper comes to operations, the more likely it is to contain rationales for business ethics that relate to health. So, although a paper that provides a high-level strategic framework for business ethics might not mention health at all, it may well describe desired outcomes, including strengthening employee loyalty and commitment, which are relevant to health. This contrasts with subsequent papers that describe what businesses can do ethically to address health more directly in operations. A progressive workplace health and safety practitioner looking at the issues that make up the corporate social responsibility agenda, as illustrated in Table 20.1, would immediately see scope for a wide range of involvement. As well as the more obvious topics of health and wellness and environment, occupational health practitioners contribute to the management of diversity through their contributions to programmes to prevent racial harassment; to the management of downsizing, flexible scheduling and work–life balance (which brings in their expertise in human factors and occupational stress); to considering HIV or AIDS in the workplace; and to the protection of privacy (e.g. through the management of health information).

However, there is evidence that employers, even those who actively support corporate social responsibility, tend to define occupational health and safety within this agenda rather narrowly.

For example, the *Health and Wellness* paper on the BSR website[5] has a very limited, and rather reactive scope. The implementation steps described are to:

- promote health and wellness – establishing a positive health, safety and well-being culture

- provide health screening
- reward healthy lifestyles
- ban smoking in and around company premises
- encourage other cessation programmes – that is, not just smoking
- encourage healthy diets
- offer flexible health plans
- create an employee assistance programme
- promote healthy work habits (in a very low-key paragraph on safety and ergonomics)
- maintain high air quality
- encourage health club membership
- encourage healthy baby practice (pre-natal support)
- consider dependent care plans
- encourage conflict resolution
- assess and evaluate health and wellness programmes.

Another example – to illustrate the point that whilst progressive employers include health and safety dimensions in their broad strategic thinking they may still define the occupational health function very narrowly – is given by the BSR papers on downsizing,[6] flexible scheduling[7] and work–life balance.[8] Although modern occupational health practice sees issues of the nature of employment and work organisation or job design as probably the most important in terms of potential to influence health and well-being (*see* Chapter 1), employers – even those who are leaders in corporate social responsibility – appear not to see this connection to occupational health. The BSR papers on downsizing, flexible scheduling and work–life balance clearly show that the health dimension to work organisation has been understood. In all three papers, the expected benefits of having responsible restructuring, flexible scheduling and work–life balance programmes include improvement to health.

- Responsible restructuring – prevention of increase in disability claims, both work and non-work related, especially stress.
- Flexible scheduling – reduced absenteeism.
- Work–life balance – increased morale or job satisfaction (which is associated with longevity), reduced employee stress, reduced absenteeism and reduced healthcare costs.

Yet, the functions described in the BSR paper *Health and Wellness*[5] do not include or link in with work organisation at all.

So, it is certainly possible to conceptualise health and safety issues very broadly in business strategy. But, while corporate social responsibility strategies tend to do this, and occupational health practitioners may well be contributing to a diverse range of activities within an organisation, there is still a tendency for employers, and indeed many occupational health practitioners, to see the role of the occupational health function and its practitioners in very narrow terms.

It is interesting to note points of similarity and difference with the trade union perspective on occupational health and ethics provided in Chapter 19. Like this chapter, the former argues that to consider the ethics of occupational health service practice today adequately requires a broader view on occupational health to be taken. The chapter contains comments that the domain no longer just concerns the relationship between a worker or patient and a health provider, or even the prevention of work-related injuries and disease, but all aspects of work organisation. However, an important point of difference between the perspective of employers and trade unions arises from the fact that the corporate social responsibility movement is based on a 'win–win' philosophy – namely, that what is good for workers and community can also be good for business too. In Chapter 19 it is argued that the company's well-being is extraneous to the mission of a health and safety service.

Organisations representing leading-edge corporate social responsibility employers, and those that represent employers more generally, also differ in how they position safety, health and well-being in corporate social responsibility and business ethics. The Confederation of British Industry (CBI) provides a good example. The CBI is very active in occupational health, corporate social responsibility and business ethics. It positions occupational health and safety within corporate social responsibility on its website. However, it is seeking to limit the scope of occupational health services to the risk management of physical risk factors at work. For example, a statement in response to the *EU Commission Strategy on Occupational Health and Safety and Health for 2002–2006* is wary about the proposal to strengthen the links between occupational health and safety and corporate social responsibility, saying that the CBI is 'unhappy that the document does not convey a clearer sense of focus . . . The main objective stated, "to foster well-being at work", goes well beyond the sphere of the workplace'.[9] Another example that places the CBI in stark contrast with the corporate social responsibility employer organisations lies in the reluctance of the former to recognise the problem of occupational stress and tackle it through the reorganisation of work.[10] This illustrates the point made earlier on the need to dig a bit deeper in order to understand what employers mean when they show support for corporate social responsibility in order to improve their reputations as ethical businesses.

In conclusion, progressive employers who have responded early to demands for improved business ethics, including corporate social responsibility, clearly recognise the potential for improving health and well-being among their personnel, clients and neighbouring communities as an important means of achieving this outcome.

However, in terms of the potential contributions to be made by occupational health practitioners, it appears that employers more generally – and even employers with progressive attitudes to corporate social responsibility – are tending narrowly to define health in the workplace, particularly in excluding work organisation and occupational stress. Unless occupational health practitioners challenge this definition, the opportunity will be missed to contribute scientifically based public health knowledge to the development of the following:

- new technologies and new work processes
- new products and services
- new community initiatives.

Employer attitudes to corporate social responsibility as an indicator of perspectives on business ethics and occupational health

If coverage in the business press is any indication, no one can doubt the growth of interest by employers in business ethics and corporate social responsibility. In a European database of business and trade press (Business and Industry) citations for corporate social responsibility rose from zero in 1995 to 45 in 2002. This far outstripped citations for occupational health and safety, which were 21 in 1995 and 36 in 2002.

That employer interest in creating a broader social agenda, including health, is growing was confirmed by two surveys identified in the search of the business press databases described at the outset of this chapter. An article on 4 January 2002 on cause-related marketing in the journal *Marketing*[11] reported on the Corporate Survey III conducted by 'Business in the Community' (BitC). The article states that 400 business leaders were surveyed; 70% of CEOs considered corporate social responsibility to be essential to their business, and 89% of marketing directors said they believed that business should be involved in social issues (up from 81% in 1998). Two-thirds of all respondents expected cause-related marketing to increase over the following two or three years from when they were surveyed. The other survey identified was reported in the *Financial News* on 4 March 2003.[12] The Business Environment Survey of attitudes to the

Social Responsibility Index (SRI) – a tool used to compare businesses on this criterion – was employed. The survey aimed to assess attitudes of FTSE 100 and FTSE 250 companies. The article states that 'the BE results make it clear that, while making great strides, SRI has a long way to go, with several companies not disclosing data on their approach'.[12]

There is, however, a consistent dissenting voice to the view that corporate social responsibility, with its strong corporate health and safety platform, is an important part of business ethics. Once again, the CBI provides insight on the view of the whole population of employers, not just business leaders from multinationals. Its response[13] to the European Commission Green Paper on a European framework for corporate social responsibility[14] outlines its position in terms of the following.

- Support for business involvement in corporate social responsibility.
- A call for the development of corporate social responsibility to be voluntary – pressure will come for business to extend beyond profitability for shareholders to satisfy a wider range of stakeholders from the market (sustainable share value).
- The impossibility of corporate social responsibility being standardised (and therefore of it being regulated consistently).
- Limits to the role that business can play – business should not replace government in the social field.

But it is difficult to find such views expressed in the business press. A search of two European business press databases yielded 37 articles on employer attitudes to corporate social responsibility. Only six were classified as illustrating negative attitudes. The arguments for *not* further developing corporate social responsibility are consistent with those articulated by the CBI.

Reasons given for not embracing CSR

Corporate social responsibility is a cost for an activity which is peripheral to business

Clearly, the employers involved have not been persuaded by the arguments (and some research) that corporate social responsibility will bring benefits to the traditional 'bottom line'. For example, the citation below from an article in *Marketing Week* in November 2002 about the difficulty of staying on top in the market emphasises the cost and wide range of CSR activities:

> Market leaders are increasingly finding they must subscribe to an extraordinarily expensive and sophisticated CSR agenda, or suffer dire consequences to their

prestige. Whether it's child labour in the Far East, oil in the North Atlantic, obesity in North America, or perceived cultural and economic imperialism in France, is not a responsibility to be taken lightly.[15]

An article in *Investor Relations Business* on 4 November 2002 also reached the conclusion that many companies still see any matters other than financial as secondary to finances. The article was commenting on a survey of companies on the New York Stock Exchange and aimed to establish the extent to which they met proposed enhanced requirements for reporting on corporate governance, including corporate social responsibility. It states:

> The problem is that many companies still see corporate governance as a soft issue – an optional side to the financial meat and potatoes.[16]

Corporate social responsibility is an effort by government to transfer its social responsibilities to business

In an article in *The Guardian* on 26 September 2002, Andrew Wilson, Director of the Centre of Business and Society at Ashridge, was quoted as commenting on this attitude, saying:

> Business leaders are becoming concerned that government is trying to offload responsibility for tackling Britain's social problems on their shoulder. . . They are now keen to know exactly what limits are for corporate social responsibility compared to its own responsibility. Privately they are worried the government's view of CSR is infinitely elastic.[17]

There is cynicism about what is motivating business

Interestingly, there may be more cynicism within the population of employers and the business sector than outside. A Mori poll of consumers, reported in *The Guardian* on 25 October 2002,[18] found that 60% felt it was reasonable for business to benefit from its corporate social responsibility programme. However, the Which consumer organisation in the UK was concerned about the amount of money cause-led marketing programmes were making for business, compared with the amounts flowing to the charities – according to the article in *Marketing* on 4 January 2002.[12] Their comments were triggered by the findings of research that showed that the grocery chain Tesco's 'Computers for Schools' scheme led to significant increases in spending by consumers and was more effective than discounting as a marketing strategy.

Another citation illustrating this cynicism was found in an article on corporate social responsibility in *New Media Age* on 9 January 2003:

> In any discussion of CSR, cynicism can never be far away. Environmentalists have coined the term 'greenwashing' . . . . Small companies can be accused of green-washing in using CSR activities, like designing free sites for charities, as ways of drumming up business.[19]

Sensitivity towards this cynicism is illustrated by legal action to silence a report commissioned by the Institute of Public Policy Research on corporate social responsibility. *Marketing Week*, 31 October 2002,[20] reported that the Institute of Directors had a 'bellicose' reaction to findings that there may be a disparity between corporate social responsibility theory and practice.

There is resistance to regulation

Quoted in the *Birmingham Post*, 24 January 2003, the head of the CBI stated that the focus of business should be on the creation of jobs and wealth for 'returning mothers and criminals working to go straight'. He went on to call for business to be 'unfettered from regulation to do this'.[21]

Reasons given for embracing corporate social responsibility

Articles in the business press in 2002 and early 2003 were much more likely to be supportive of corporate social responsibility. Consistent with this is the finding in the Mori poll of consumers, mentioned earlier, that two out of three business journalists considered that not enough attention was being paid to corporate social responsibility. Statements that this was not just another management fad were common; this attitude is illustrated below by a citation from Jeff Lane, Partner, PricewaterhouseCoopers in *Brand Strategy* on 20 November 2002:

> If you'd asked me about the work we were doing four years ago, we'd have been evangelising about sustainability at board level, to get executives to realise that it is an issue. Now companies recognise sustainability and responsibility and realise that it isn't just a fad.[22]

Consumer demand for ethical products leads to increased sales, representing a success for cause-led marketing

According to the Co-operative Bank purchasing index, as reported in *Brand Strategy* on 5 December 2002, spending on ethical and environmentally friendly products increased by 19% in a year, whereas the UK economy grew by just 2.1%.[23]

Investors' demands for investment in ethical companies also drive the attitudes of fund managers

There was, for example, a report in *Private Equity Week* on March 11 2002[24] on a Californian pension fund, CalPERS, which was pulling out venture capital from Malaysia, the Philippines, Thailand and Indonesia because of pensioner sensitivity about how funds were being used. *The Express on Sunday* 9 June 2002 quoted the EU Commissioner for Social Affairs warning British bosses reluctant to adopt corporate social responsibility that they 'will be sanctioned by the market itself'.[25]

A good reputation will restore consumer and investor confidence

The following comments in an article on corporate governance in *Retail Banker International*, 4 December 2002, illustrate this argument:

> Good corporate governance cannot exist in isolation. Governance must be an expression of a company's corporate values and ethics. . . . Best practice banks pursue sustainable growth policies and corporate social responsibility.[26]

External relationships and access to new markets may be improved

The benefits of developing external relationships have been seen in terms of sales or partnerships. An extreme example is provided by an article in *The Herald* on 4 April 2002,[27] reporting on comments by the United Nations that the next untapped market for business was the world's poor, who are seeking to improve their standard of living. It was argued that only companies that are environmentally and socially responsible would be able to achieve this.

Improvement in processes through innovation leads to increases in productivity and quality

Another quote from the EU Commissioner for Social Affairs in *The Express on Sunday* illustrates this point: '[CSR will] fuel productivity and innovation which will have a positive impact . . . on employment'.[25]

There is an improvement to employee morale and also teamwork and skills

Corporate social responsibility strategies that target staff often aim to improve morale by improving work conditions. But advocates also argue that involvement in community-based projects improves morale as well. For example, the article on corporate social responsibility in the *New Media Age* (website), mentioned above, also states the following: 'It should be a natural fit as new media is full of trendy young liberals who do think about social responsibility'.[19]

There are gains to the bottom line

In a profile on Npower in *Brand Strategy* in August 2002, the journalist noted that Npower defended its corporate social responsibility programme in terms of contribution to the bottom line and quoted the representative as saying, '"The projects we run in our social responsibility mode such as Health through Warmth (a 10 million pound campaign to reduce fuel bills and increase energy and efficiency in 20 000 houses) or investing in youth cricket isn't just reputation management", he claims. "These can be very valuable business and relationship builders"'.[28]

Benefits to the community accrue

Some still think that helping the community should be sufficient. However, the corporate social responsibility agenda involves putting pressure on organisations to make their community work align better to business. Marks and Spencer, a UK retailing organisation with a strong tradition of philanthropy, has changed its approach to 'make its social behaviour relevant to its business'. 'M&S doesn't want to get involved in things that are not appropriate for the business or that stakeholders don't think are important for us', according to a profile in *Brand Strategy*, this time in May 2002.[29]

The above confirms the suspicions of some, including occupational health practitioners, that what is motivating employers to embrace business ethics in the form of corporate social responsibility has more to do with improving profits than providing benefits to staff and community. Despite some protagonists insisting that this is not just the latest management fad, we do not know how long corporate health and safety will have this 'moment in the sun' with senior management. Unless occupational health practitioners start to focus more on the positive effect on health and less on employers' motivation we may look back on this time as an opportunity lost.

Expectations of employers as a source of ethical dilemmas

This book has taken a practical approach to ethical issues in occupational health. Mostly, it is written from the perspective of occupational health practitioners. As the preceding chapters have shown, often the dilemmas are caused by the expectations of employers.

Four areas in which employer attitudes and behaviours do have a significant effect on ethical dilemmas are described below.

Risk assessment

In Chapter 4, Case 4.1 presents a situation where a worker is exposed to isocyanate, a chemical known to cause occupational asthma. In the first part of the story an occupational health physician responds to a worker's refusal to co-operate with risk control procedures by attempting to overrule the worker, thereby compromising the ethical principle of autonomy.

Failure of workers to take up risk control measures is a defence used commonly by employers found to be in breach of occupational health and safety standards. In some cases, such as the example given in Case 4.1, this is a reasonable defence. More often than not, however, the defence is unreasonable since it fails to take into account two fundamental principles of occupational health and safety, usually enshrined in law:

- that the employer, not his or her workers, has the overwhelming responsibility to create a safe and healthy work environment
- that the hierarchy-of-control principle means that in doing so employers must give priority to eradicating hazardous substances and processes, and to creating physical and administrative solutions that do not require the co-operation of the worker over solutions requiring the worker to observe safe work procedures or wear protective equipment.

In Case 4.1, the employer's perspective coincides with that of the occupational health physician. The principles of law and occupational health outweigh the worker's ethical right to autonomy.

Chapter 4 then moves on to a more complicated situation where controls are applied, presumably consistent with normal external standards (Case 4.2). Nevertheless, the worker is still at risk of occupational asthma, arguably due to some intrinsic characteristics. The ethical dilemma identified here is written more from the perspective of employers and workers than occupational health practitioners. It is one concerning distributive justice. Here, despite controls that meet external norms, that is, risk limits where most people would be protected from adverse health effects, a susceptible individual might experience occupational asthma from very small exposures. This case implies that there may be economic implications for the entire workforce if measures are taken to protect a few susceptible individuals.

Case 4.2 is an extreme example, made to illustrate the point. In practice, employer representatives involved in the social decision-making process of determining acceptable risk rely heavily on this argument to resist the lowering of threshold limit values, supported by an abundance of evidence about the relationships between employment and health, and unemployment and ill-health.

However, perhaps for the occupational health practitioners, the greatest difficulty that arises from employers' expectations is their desire for objectivity and certainty from this process. We in the profession know that risk assessment in practice is a combination of objective and subjective assessment but – when the complicating factor of risk perception is thrown in – it can become very personal indeed. Think of repetitive strain injury, electromagnetic radiation and man-made mineral fibres, to name just a few. As is mentioned in Chapter 4, people tolerate risks over which they have no direct control, for example those arising from their work, less well than those over which they have direct control, such as smoking. So, the balance of probability is often not enough to reassure workers under these circumstances. Interpreting scientific knowledge whilst keeping an eye on the employer's desire for certainty and the worker's right to know requires considerable pragmatic judgement and communication skills.

Health assessments and health surveillance

Chapters 6, 7, 8 and 9 all deal with the wide range of health assessments and surveillance undertaken in the course of employment. They include:

- new employment
- periodic health surveillance for health effects arising from work-related risk factors
- periodic health surveillance for health effects arising from non-work related risk factors
- work-disability assessments.

Ethical problems for occupational health practitioners identified in these chapters, to which employer attitudes and knowledge contribute, lie in the following principles.

- *Beneficence.* Protocols for the routine assessment of healthy workers in many circumstances cannot be justified in terms of contribution to health gain at a population level (i.e. they are not effective) nor often at an individual level. In some cases these interventions may lead to harm, for example cases of false positives and false negatives, yet they remain popular with employers and workers alike. This, combined with market pressure for commercialised occupational health units to sell services, means that employers often purchase unnecessary, inappropriate and ineffective health assessment and surveillance regimes.
- *Autonomy.* Periodic health surveillance for health effects arising from non-work related risk factors must be voluntary. Workers need to give informed consent, and there should not be explicit or implicit pressure from employers for them to participate. A problem sometimes faced by occupational health practitioners is that employers expect to have access to this health information and may want to use it in the context of decisions about employment. (*See* 'Confidentiality' below.)
- *Discrimination.* Some employers see it as a part of the employer's prerogative to deny employment, either to potential or existing employees, either permanently or temporarily, without adequate consideration of how disability relates to job demands and whether a reasonable adjustment to work would result in an ability–work match
- *Confidentiality.* Employers may have an expectation that information about health status, as opposed to fitness for a job or return to work, will be provided to them.

Often, these problems arise as employers have unrealistic expectations of the capacity of health assessments to predict future work ability, although worker enthusiasm for health assessments cannot be denied. Strategies available to occupational health practitioners lie in making employers better informed. Employers will be interested to know that whilst targeted health assessment programmes, designed in keeping with the principles of public health screening and equal employment opportunity, are both effective and cost-effective, more general, non-strategic health assessments are ineffective and costly.

Reduction of sickness absence

Chapter 10 analyses an intervention to reduce sick leave rates from the point of view of the company and the individuals within that company.

It is pointed out that a key dilemma was the difference in goals between the senior representatives of the owners, who wanted short-term profit, and the local business unit, who were looking for longer term, business sustainability. In doing so this case study comes to the nub of corporate social responsibility.

This is a common problem for occupational health practitioners working in the area of occupational stress and quality of working life.

When dealing with sickness absence, employers tend to prefer strategies within the domain of workers' rights and responsibilities, that is, attendance, whilst neglecting the other side of the equation, that is, the way work is organised and the way people are managed, which is within their sphere of control.

As a result, reviews of workplace interventions, such as the one led by Brian Oldenburg,[30] show that many workplaces have secondary prevention strategies (employee assistance programmes or team leader-led interventions to manage work absences very early), but few have primary prevention strategies (structured approaches to identifying high-impact, potentially remedial problems with the way work is organised and the way people are managed).

This is an issue of distributive justice. The contribution being requested of workers is greater than the contribution of employers to solving the problem. Yet, it is in the longer term interests of both parties for this problem to be solved.

For the occupational health practitioners the solution lies in encouraging employers to take a longer term view. These days most employers are interested in attracting and retaining staff, and this can be a useful driver on which to focus. Then a balanced strategy should be proposed, which tackles primary, secondary and tertiary prevention simultaneously. One argument for this is that if workers recognise that employers are prepared to improve the quality of the work environment from the point of view of health and well-being, they are more likely to be prepared to make a personal contribution, as was found in the WellWorks integrated health promotion and protection programme for cancer.[31] The comparable situation for reducing sickness absence is that if employers improve the way work is organised or the way people are managed, workers are more likely to review their own work attendance.

Compensation medicine

Chapters 15 and 16 address issues of compensation medicine. Chapter 16 presents an example that raises the dilemma of how an occupational health physician should advise a patient on compensation when a work-related condition is suspected (Case 16.1). Employers will be pleased to see this case. It is not uncommon for employers to be left with significant problems when workers have been given information that leads them to believe that they may have a work-related illness and be entitled to compensation, either *en masse* or individually. For example, a well-intentioned but poorly conceived health education programme in which workers are given information about hazards they may face at work and lists of symptoms they should look out for, without sufficient contextual information about risk and controls in place, or that they can and should use, may have disastrous consequences for employers and workers alike.

Chapter 15 addresses insurance medicine and has a focus on expertise and professionalism. As such, it opens a can of worms. With workers' compensation schemes around the world, including North America, the UK, Australia and New Zealand, facing economic pressure and in some cases collapse, long-held concerns of employers about the inadequacy of the medical role in adversarial systems are coming to the fore. Although employers' primary concerns are usually the cost of workers' compensation to them, they have also expressed dissatisfaction with:

- the 'hired gun' expert medical practitioners who tend to advise either the plaintiffs or the defendants and are not seen to be giving impartial advice
- the costly and excessive health assessments and investigations undertaken
- the time taken for medical evidence to be obtained
- outcomes of medical opinions on impairment, disability and handicap being subject to interpretation (they have an expectation of objective answers)
- the process itself encouraging illness behaviour.

Reforms being considered elsewhere in the world include:

- closer alignment of the principles of evidence in medicine and the principles of evidence at law

- establishment of processes in which medical evidence is collected independently for use by both parties (employer and worker)
- scientific validation of the tools for the assessment of impairment and disability
- better information to injured workers about the process and its likely outcomes in order to adjust unrealistic expectations
- scheme redesign to ensure that incentives are likely to lead to desired behaviours
- insurance company redesign to shift the role of claims officers from that of process administrator to injury or illness manager with a goal of appropriate return to work
- using networks of medical and health advisers known to have skills in workplace rehabilitation, rather than just expertise in the diagnosis and treatment of particular conditions.

For a description of concerns about traditional workers' compensation systems for employers and others, and also ideas for reform, see the report by the Australasian Faculty of Occupational Medicine on this subject published in 2001.[32] Future reforms of the structure of workers' compensation are likely to affect drastically the role of occupational health practitioners involved in medico-legal practice, and therefore the ethics associated with such practice.

In conclusion, employers' expectations of occupational health and safety can give rise to ethical dilemmas for its practitioners. Sometimes these expectations are unrealistic and can be addressed by, over time, giving honest and consistent accounts of what can and cannot be expected from the knowledge and methodologies available. An important part of creating more realistic expectations in employers will be saying 'No' to inappropriate requests. For example, there is the expectation that the occupational health department will sort out a performance problem simply because there is an ill-health dimension. However, perhaps the real ethical dilemmas for occupational health practitioners arise not so much from the unrealistic expectations of employers, but because the two clients that we serve – employers and workers – often have different needs, and we have not yet defined properly how we propose to relate to our clients in the changed world of the modern work environment.

With the decline of union power internationally and the growth of outsourced occupational health and safety services, occupational health practitioners are more in the control of employers than ever before.

The rise of corporate social responsibility – with its agenda of sustainable business and its central platform of health and well-being of staff, customers and neighbouring communities – can only support the renegotiation of the role of occupational health and safety practitioners with employers that this book has demonstrated to be necessary.

References

1 CSR Europe (Undated) *Exploring Business Dynamics*. Enterprise and Personnel, Ashridge.

2 Business for Social Responsibility (Undated) White papers: *Business Ethics*. (www.bsr.org).

3 Business for Social Responsibility (Undated) White papers: *Introduction to Corporate Social Responsibility*. (www.bsr.org).

4 Business for Social Responsibility (Undated) White papers: *Sustainable Business Practices*. (www.bsr.org).

5 Business for Social Responsibility (Undated) White papers: *Health and Wellness*. (www.bsr.org).

6 Business for Social Responsibility (Undated) White papers: *Downsizing: layoffs/ closing*. (www.bsr.org).

7 Business for Social Responsibility (Undated) White papers: *Flexible Scheduling*. (www.bsr.org).

8 Business for Social Responsibility (Undated) White papers: *Work–Life*. (www.bsr.org).

9 Confederation of British Industry (2002) *Issue Statement: EU Commission Strategy on Occupational Health and Safety & Health, 2002–2006*. 3 October 2002. (www.cbi.org.uk)

10 Confederation of British Industry (2002) *Issue Statement: work-related stress*. 28 October. (www.cbi.org.uk).

11 Good-causes deliver for brands: cause-related marketing. *Marketing*, 4 January 2002.

12 Fund managers snub BE survey on SRI attitudes. *Financial News*, 4 March 2003.

13 Confederation of British Industry (Undated) *Response to the European Commission Green Paper on Promoting a European Framework for Corporate Social Responsibility*. (www.cbi.org.uk).

14 Commission of the European Communities (2001) Green paper: *Promoting a European Framework for Corporate Social Responsibility*, July.

15 The top is only for the toughest. *Marketing Week*, 28 November 2002.

16 Most companies don't disclose governance policies online. *Investor Relations Business*, 4 November 2002.

17 Good-causes burden irks executives. *The Guardian*, 26 September 2002.

18 Mori poll company reputation. *The Guardian*, 25 October 2002.

19 Social benefit. *New Media Age*, 9 January 2003.

20 Reputations are difficult to mend. *Marketing Week*, 31 October 2002.

21 CBI chief asks for change to create change in society. *Birmingham Post*, 24 January 2003.

22 Sense and sensibility. *Brand Strategy*, 20 November 2002.

23 Co-operative bank purchasing index. *Brand Strategy*, 5 December 2002.

24 CalPERS pulls VC support from four nations. *Private Equity Week*, 11 March 2002.

25 EC for employment and social affairs announced a new social auditing plan. *The Express on Sunday*, 9 June 2002.

26 Corporate governance rises to the fore. *Retail Banker International*, 4 December 2002.

27 A better deal for the poor. *The Herald*, 4 April 2002.

28 Tightening the utility belt. *Brand Strategy*, August 2002.

29 M&S brand philanthropy. *Brand Strategy*, 20 May 2002.

30 Oldenburg B *et al.* (1994) Review of effectiveness of interventions for the management of stress at work. Unpublished research paper. Department of Public Health, University of Sydney, Australia.

31 Sorensen G *et al.* (1996) Worker participation in an integrated health promotion/health protection program: results from the WellWorks project. *Health Education Quarterly.* **23**: 191–203.

32 Australasian Faculty of Occupational Medicine (2001) *Compensible Injuries and Health Outcomes.* Royal Australasian College of Physicians, Sydney.

'Would you tell me, please, which way I ought to go from here?' asked Alice.
'That depends a good deal on where you want to get to,' said the Cat.
'I don't much care where – ' said Alice.
'Then it doesn't matter which way you go,' said the Cat.
' – so long as I get somewhere,' Alice added as an explanation.
'Oh, you're sure to do that,' said the Cat, 'if you only walk long enough.'

Alice's Adventures in Wonderland (Lewis Carroll, 1832–98)

CHAPTER 21

Whistleblowing

Tore Nilstun and Peter Westerholm

But it's no use now,' thought poor Alice, 'to pretend to be two people!
Why, there's hardly enough of me left to make one respectable person!'

Alice's Adventures in Wonderland (Lewis Carroll, 1832–98)

The term 'whistleblowing' refers to a warning issued by a member or former member of an organisation to the public about a serious wrongdoing or danger created or concealed within an organisation.[1] Anyone associated with an organisation, such as occupational health professionals, may find themselves in a situation where assuming the role of whistleblower is a possible line of action.

There are three essential elements to whistleblowing. The whistleblower: dissents from an action or practice within the organisation; breaches loyalties by taking the matter outside the organisation; and makes an accusation against an individual person or group of persons within the organisation.[2] Whistleblowing should be distinguished from internal dissent. In the former case, but not the latter, an external vehicle of warning is used (e.g. a newspaper), and there is a preparedness or even an intention to be named publicly.

The decision of an employee to inform on illegal or unethical practices in the workplace – to 'blow the whistle' – is difficult for several reasons.[2–4] Thus, questions can be asked about when whistleblowing might be prohibited, permissible, recommended, obligatory or supererogatory (i.e. to do more than what is required). Under what circumstances is the practice of 'going public' defensible – at least as a last resort after all internal reporting procedures have been exhausted? Employees asking such questions find that conflicting loyalties – personal, organisational and societal – can be agonising. Further, it is often difficult to determine the actual cause or causes of the situation that justifies whistleblowing.

Regardless of motive, accuracy of the charge or outcome, 'blowing the whistle' places whistleblowers in jeopardy. They usually lack power in the organisation, and may be exposed to extreme forms of retaliation – such as loss of employment, loss of promotion or demotion, reassignment, blacklisting, accusation of mental instability, harassment and shunning. Attempts have therefore been made to formulate guidelines, sometimes even laws, to protect whistleblowers.[5,6]

The position adopted in this chapter is that whistleblowing, as a general rule, indicates a failure at organisational level. The professional codes of ethics for occupational health professionals do not provide, in their present forms, any mechanism to overcome the need for whistleblowing.[7,8] In concluding, therefore, we address the needs to recommend fairly sophisticated approaches to organisational ethics, and to protect occupational health professionals who publicly speak out about illegal or unethical practices in the workplace.

A case of whistleblowing

There have been many cases of whistleblowing worldwide, but to our knowledge none that involves an occupational health professional blowing the whistle on people in a client company for which he or she has responsibility. Accordingly, we will use a case where a company employee did the whistleblowing. The case is real and has been publicly documented.[9]

The event took place at a sub-acute care unit in a New England hospital in the USA in 1996. A registered nurse, Barry Adams, blew the whistle on unsafe healthcare practices that he observed in his work setting. Nurse Adams became increasingly concerned about the inadequacies of the quality, safety and dignity of practices in patient care as the hospital implemented cuts in personnel resources. His observations were associated with what he regarded as increasingly inadequate staffing and a lack of proper supervision by inexperienced nurses. There was an increased incidence of patient falls, instances where patients were left to lie in their own excrement, treatment not being completed, and also serious medication errors. The frequency of such events was, in his view, immediately followed by a substantial increase in the number of patient assignments for each nurse.

For three months, Nurse Adams and his colleagues strictly followed the process outlined by the organisation to communicate concerns to hospital administrators. He soon realised that the administrators were not interested in using the information he provided to remedy the situation; indeed, he was harshly criticised even for collecting the information. He then decided to proceed on the basis of a variation of the traditional saying 'If it's not documented, it's not done'. He adopted the opposite approach: 'If it's not done, document it!'. Also, at one point, he refused to dispense a prescription for narcotic drugs issued by a technician acting on behalf of a physician – citing that this was against the Nurses Practice Act.

Adams was threatened with job dismissal, and – despite excellent previous performance reviews – he was eventually fired. He brought the case to court and won (his attorney was also a registered nurse). The hospital appealed and lost again. Five units in the hospital have since closed – 'for financial reasons'.

Psychology and ethics

Generally, whistleblowers present themselves as having the motive of protecting other individuals, or even society in general; their willingness to step forward publicly is evidence of such an honourable motive. Some whistleblowers, however, may be driven by a desire for revenge for real or perceived injustices that they attribute to the organisation – from personal grievances to ideology-based objections. The accuracy of the charges made by the whistleblower and the fairness of the accusations made against individuals are central ethical considerations. There is a fundamental ethical obligation on all who consider 'blowing the whistle' to have charges based on facts. But, and this is important, organisations can become so resistant to internal criticism that essential reform can only be accomplished via the pressure of external revelation, even to the point of public disclosure.

The possible harm caused by a public accusation can be significant and often irreparable – not only to the organisation involved, but also to whistleblowers and their families. Ethical guidelines in occupational health services require 'reasonable' action on the part of others in situations where value criteria are violated. From this, however, there does not follow a duty to extend action to the extreme of heroic self-sacrifice. In many cases, it is exceedingly difficult to calculate potential harms and benefits. Then, the decision on whether or not to blow the whistle must rely on reflection, individual conviction and practical wisdom.

In a discussion paper entitled *Whistleblowing to Combat Corruption,*[10] the Organization for Economic Co-operation and Development (OECD) issues a sobering general, introductory statement:

> Whistleblowing is relevant to all organisations and all people, not just those few who are corrupt or criminal. This is because every business and every public body faces the risk of things going wrong or of unknowingly harbouring a corrupt individual. Where such a risk arises, usually the first people to realise or suspect the wrongdoing will be those who work in or with the organisation. Yet these people, who are the best placed to sound the alarm or blow the whistle, also have most to lose if they do.

Unless culture, practice and the law indicate that it is safe and accepted for them to raise a genuine concern about corruption or illegality, workers will assume that they risk victimisation, losing their job or damaging their career. Firms and companies aware that a bribe has been solicited will fear not only that they will lose the contract if they do not pay, but that if they blow the whistle their future economic interests will be damaged and their people will be harassed.[10]

Ethical analysis

The basic question in analysis of this particular case is whether or not whistleblowing was justified under the circumstances. First, we identify the people involved or affected. Second, we apply the ethical principles formulated in Chapter 3 of this book as value premises in our analysis (Table 21.1).

Table 21.1 A matrix for the ethical analysis of whistleblowing: the case of Barry Adams

People involved or affected	Ethical principles		
	Beneficence	Autonomy	Justice
Barry Adams	A	E	I
Other employees	B	F	J
Patients	C	G	K
Employer	D	H	L

Beneficence

First, we will apply the principle of *beneficence* (Column 1, cells A–D in Table 21.1). The costs to Barry Adams for blowing the whistle were considerable. However, the costs and benefits for other employees are uncertain in the short term. Nevertheless, in the long run we are inclined to believe that the benefits will overweigh the costs. Patients will obviously benefit. The employer, who refused to take necessary remedial action and lost in court, had to carry his part of the costs.

Autonomy

The principle of *autonomy* (Column 2, cells E–H) requires that the preferences of those involved or affected should be taken into account when performing an ethical analysis. Barry Adams wanted a change and behaved accordingly. He acted simply as a straightforward autonomous agent. It is difficult to say what the other employees preferred, but the patients would obviously have wanted an improvement to the situation. They would probably have supported Barry Adams in his criticism of the healthcare institution (had they known about the case). The employer was reluctant to implement any change. Looking at the consequences of Nurse Adams' whistleblowing, his autonomy may have been either strengthened or restricted – depending on the future course of events. The same applied to the employer. In fact, the trial outcome entailed that a restriction was imposed on the employer's autonomy.

Justice

There are two basic requirements to the principle of *justice* (Column 3, cells I–L) – no discrimination, and solidarity. It might be argued that the way Barry Adams was treated, both before and after he blew the whistle, should be described as discrimination. He had to carry an unfair part of the costs required to improve the situation. Patients, both present and future, are primarily to be seen as a vulnerable segment of the population. Their situation, such as it was before the whistle was blown, represented an inequity, and thus a further burden with regard to their situation. Inequity in such a situation is a violation of the solidarity requirement, and also a cost to patients. The situation ought to be rectified. There seem to be no justice costs or justice benefits to other employees or to the employer.

Recommendations

Formulating a list of prerequisites for whistleblowing is both difficult and controversial. Any such list easily ends up requiring too much or too little. The one that follows, based on ethical analysis of a particular case, represents an outline for a pragmatic approach. It is defensible on grounds of health professional ethics.

- To minimise the need for whistleblowing, all organisations should create effective means for hearing complaints, protecting complainants, and acting expeditiously on valid complaints.

- Any indications of wrongdoing or danger must be documented accurately by the potential whistleblower.
- Potential whistleblowers should consult with trusted colleagues to confirm key facts before taking action.
- Potential whistleblowers should take reasonable steps to use methods of redress within the organisation before going outside them.
- The wrongdoing or danger that prompts whistleblowing must be substantial enough to outweigh the harms caused by a breach of loyalty.
- There must be good reasons to believe that public disclosure will end the wrongdoing or avoid the danger at stake.
- Potential whistleblowers should assess, beside their objectives, also their motives and the personal costs involved, including effects on their family and career.

But is whistleblowing an obligation? In countries where there is no official support for whistleblowers, we believe it is not an obligation, only a supererogatory duty. Blowing the whistle is desirable, but is it doing more than what *ought* to be done? We believe that all countries should have a public institution to help people who blow the whistle. Any such institution should provide essential security to the individual involved by having capacity to take immediate action. It must have power and economic resources. Only in this way can it prevent rumours and escalation of conflict. Representatives of the institution should act like referees in a football match.

Whistleblowing is about freedom of speech and democracy. If potential whistleblowers do not dare to use their freedom, the openness of society is under threat. Democracy is in danger! In our view, employees' freedom of speech has to be strengthened in most countries throughout the world. Given the existence of an appropriate institution that fulfils the requirements indicated above, we strongly recommend that occupational health professionals warn the general public about a serious wrongdoing or a danger created or concealed within an organisation.

It is an act of collegial solidarity to protect occupational health professionals from untoward effects and retaliations when they have opted to blow the whistle in a situation related to their professional practice. Professional occupational health organisations and societies should be prepared and willing to offer peer counselling, and provide for collegial discussions of events or developments where whistleblowing is considered by their members. They should also promote collective action in situations where members need to make their views publicly known on issues infringing their professional integrity or fundamental values concerned with professional ethics.

Concluding remarks

Ethical analysis of a specific act of whistleblowing involves consideration of breach of loyalty – not only to the organisation but also to the service rendered. Such analysis must take account of any wider and more significant loyalties that may be pertinent.

Organisational loyalty, taken to the point of a failure to recognise the implications of the wider and deeper personal commitments of staff members to the community or society, may lead to insensitivity or loss of social awareness within an organisation. This may be harmful to particular individuals, and even socially disruptive. Whistleblowing is not infrequent in organisations and enterprises, either in Europe or in other regions and countries of the world. It is worth noting that, in European universities and other public establishments and organisations, there are examples of principles for the handling of whistleblowing having been adopted for the guidance of management and personnel. One of the roles and responsibilities of professional organisations is to protect and support members who have, in their professional capacity, become involved in situations giving rise to dilemmas of loyalties and threats to their professional integrity.

References

1 Dougherty CD (1995) Whistleblowing in healthcare. In: WT Reich (ed.) *Encyclopedia of Bioethics*. Simon & Schuster Macmillan, New York, NY. 2552–3.

2 Bok S (1980) Whistleblowing and professional responsibility. *New York University Education Quarterly*. **11**: 2–7.

3 Bowin N (1982) *Business Ethics*. Prentice-Hall, Englewood Cliffs, NJ.

4 Duska R (1997) Whistleblowing and employee loyalty. In: TJ Beachhamp, N Bowie (eds) *Ethics Theory and Business*. Prentice-Hall, Upper Saddle River, NJ.

5 OECD (2000) *Whistleblowing to Combat Corruption*. OECD, Paris.

6 Public Concern at Work (1998) *Public Interest Disclosure Act 1998. An introduction to the legislation with authoritative notes on its provisions, section by section*. Sweet & Maxwell, London. (www.pcaw.demon.co.uk).

7 Faculty of Occupational Medicine of the Royal College of Physicians (1999) *Guidance on Ethics for Occupational Physicians* (5e). Royal College of Physicians, London.

8 International Commission on Occupational Health (1999) *International Code of Ethics for Occupational Health Professionals*. ICOH, Geneva.

9 Fletcher JJ, Sorrell JM and Cipriano Silva M (1998) Whistleblowing as a failure of organizational ethics. *Online Journal of Issues in Nursing* (www.nursingworld. org/ojin/topic8/topic8_3.htm).

10 Organisation for Economic Co-operation and Development (2000) *Whistle-blowing to Combat Corruption (OECD Labour/management programme)*. OECD, Paris.

CHAPTER 22

Education in ethics

Noks Nauta

Case 22.1: a serious problem

During the vocational training of occupational health physicians, one of the trainees tells a story. He has had a phone call from a Mr Taylor, an employer who asks him to visit Mr Smith, one of his employees. Mr Taylor has the idea that Mr Smith has a serious problem with alcohol, which is the reason for his frequent absence from work. Mr Taylor requests a report from the occupational health physician, and states, more or less explicitly, that he is going to fire Mr Smith if alcoholism is the problem. The trainee asks the group how to deal with the request from the employer.

What can occupational health professionals do when confronted by an issue of this kind? What educational advice might they be given? In this case, it is the occupational health physician who is directly subject to the problem. But other occupational health professionals also encounter situations where moral values collide. This applies to occupational health nurses, and also to social workers and occupational hygienists. In this book, many cases are presented in which several occupational health professionals are involved.

What methods are suitable for dealing with ethical problems, and how can we teach occupational health professionals to practise ethical deliberation in everyday practice? If we are going to start training courses, we have to know how much occupational health professionals actually know about ethics. In 1998, for example, Martimo et al.[1] performed a postal survey of Finnish occupational health physicians and nurses on their ethical values and problems. Both groups considered 'expertise' and 'confidentiality' as the most important core values of occupational health services. Only 41% of nurses and 36% of physicians had received some training in the ethics of occupational health service, and 76% of all respondents had never referred to available ethical guidelines.

The aims of this chapter are to give some background information on education in medical ethics and to give practical suggestions for training courses in ethics for occupational health professionals.

First, a short description is given of what is taught in medical curricula. What is known about the effects of teaching ethics for undergraduates? Is it effective?

Second, the question of what we might wish occupational health professionals to learn is addressed. What do we want to change in terms of knowledge, attitude and behaviour? (In fact, the authors of this book gave their opinions on this during a private conference in April 2003.)

Third, what is the best way to achieve the changes we want to take place? (For this purpose, both the experience of the author of this chapter and of other contributors to this book are employed.)

Fourth, there is a description of a Dutch method for moral deliberation by occupational health physicians that can also be used by all occupational health professionals. The method is described, accompanied by an account of why and how it was constructed. We give brief examples of cases and how the method can be used in such cases. The method is reported verbatim in the Appendix to this chapter. The method is used in audit groups and workshops. Experiences of employing the method are also described.

Education in ethics in medical and para-medical curricula

In medical curricula, ethics is a regular part of education. A literature review shows that there is consensus on the aims of education in medical ethics (at least for doctors). These aims are to:

- teach doctors to recognise the humanistic and ethical aspects of medical careers
- enable doctors to examine and affirm their personal and professional moral commitments
- equip doctors with a foundation in philosophical, social and legal knowledge
- enable doctors to employ such knowledge in clinical reasoning
- equip doctors with the interactional skills needed to apply insights, knowledge and reasoning to human clinical care.[2]

Ethics also forms part of the vocational training of other health professionals, such as nurses and social workers. We do not know if this is the case for hygienists, safety specialists and other (more technical) specialists. We assume, however, that – since they usually have no patient contacts – ethics will be only a minor part of their training.

Several curricular patterns are available for the teaching of ethics. All have their stronger and their weaker points. As known by educational specialists, teaching should be performed in such a way as to enable an easy transfer to practice. Case-centred teaching, especially during the clinical phase of education, is essential.[3] It seems doubtful, however, whether students can really learn to apply ethical principles if teachers do not provide the stimulation to ask questions.[4] Goldie[2] speaks of a 'hidden curriculum', by which he means that teachers and other educational staff have a role as positive role models outside regular teaching hours. In order to facilitate this way of learning, we need to be aware of the hidden curriculum.

What are the effects of teaching ethics? Goldie *et al.*[5] investigated the issue in Glasgow, Scotland, where ethics is taught during the first three years of the medical curriculum. The aims of the subject are to enable students to become familiar with the general theories of medical ethics, to apply these theories, and to ensure that students are aware of their ethical obligations in clinical reasoning. Evaluation of effects showed that the first year of training is particularly effective, and the authors suggest that subsequent years should focus more on small-group sessions.[5] Self and colleagues[6] had previously found that teaching medical ethics can increase students' moral reasoning skills, and that any such increase comes more from exposure to small-group case study discussion than from lecture-based courses.

In the medical curriculum in Rotterdam, the Netherlands, experiments using narrative forms – like stories, novels or films – are being employed. These are often more realistic or complex than written cases.

Perhaps it is also important to have ethical questions in the exams, because this might influence students' learning behaviours.[5] But how could such assessments be made? How can students prove that they have learnt enough and know how to use their acquired knowledge in practice? There are several options available, such as chart reviews, objective structured medical examinations, direct observations, videotaping, and simulated patients.[5] Questions in the forms of essay assignments seem more appropriate for the purpose. Multiple-choice exams are not suitable, since you will never know the underlying theme in any student's argumentation.

Although not much literature is available on education in ethics at postgraduate level, there seems to be agreement over the usefulness of small groups. *See*, for example, Nilstun and co-workers.[7] As with all postgraduate training, the link to personal practice is essential to the translation of what is learned into what is practised. Accordingly, application of cases from personal practice is essential.

What do occupational health professionals need to learn about ethics?

This book represents a start in making occupational health professionals aware of ethical values in their work. Many situations may never have been seen as having a moral aspect. One of the aims of (postgraduate) training is to show that moral values do operate in everyday situations. But people have to become aware of such values before they can even start thinking about them. Only then can they learn how to deal with them in daily practice. Health professional ethics in practice implies raising consciousness of choices and consequences.

'Everything has got a moral, if only you can find it.'

Alice's Adventures in Wonderland (Lewis Carroll, 1832–98)

Learning points

What should occupational health professionals learn about ethics? Learning points will differ beteen medical knowledge and medical capacity for treatment. They concern reflection on our own behaviours. The chapters of this book give more than enough examples of ethical dilemmas in the daily practice of occupational health professionals. What can we learn from them?

The authors gathered for a seminar in April 2003, and we discussed what we had learnt – from our experiences and each from writing our own chapters. Occupational health professionals might adopt the following points in training courses:

- taking an organisational approach to ethical issues
- identification of values, understanding of ethical values
- economy versus confidentiality
- systematic analysis, a systematic approach
- balancing ethics and law.

Other statements that suggested learning points were:

- occupational health is ethical when you co-operate as a team
- it is unethical to make a decision or to give advice without evidence-based practice.

From the list, we see that for occupational health professionals it is not only the professional–patient relationship that counts. There are different stakeholders, all of whom need to be taken into account. It is good to start all training programmes with the goal of making this clear. After that, moral values should be clarified; in some cases, it can be shown which values are present and which are conflicting. Business economics considerations are often important, but can go against confidentiality. The position of the occupational health professional in this game of forces needs to be worked upon. The game is quite different from that played in other healthcare arenas, where treatment of the patient is the first aim. Systematic analyses of the moral values of a case are important, as is the relationship between law and ethics.

Cases that can be used in vocational training courses

Examination of practical cases is a very good way of showing ethical dilemmas in educational courses.

The authors of this book were asked about which cases, in their opinion, were essential for vocational training courses. They mentioned the following topics or kinds of cases (in descending rank order, with most votes on top):

- business ethics
- periodic employee examination (assessment)
- confidentiality of clinical information records
- occupational disease recognition
- insurance medicine
- health surveillance
- work ability or disability assessment
- workplace risk assessment
- interventions
- blood-borne virus transmission.

We find that the tasks of an occupational health service are not fully the same across countries. On the other hand, the types of problems that occupational health professionals encounter are rather similar. All occupational health professionals work for firms that have their own ethics. Implementing ethical standards or practices that are not compatible with the ethics of the occupational health professional is a serious problem. Clearly, a case on business ethics seems a good one to use in training sessions.

Educational methods for teaching ethics in occupational health

Ethics should be an integral part of vocational training for occupational health professionals, and there should also be postgraduate training in ethics. Occupational health professionals should learn to reflect on ethical issues and do this on a regular basis. Table 22.1 shows the various phases and actions in education in ethics for occupational health professionals, and also the educational methods associated with each phase. It also indicates what is important to effect new ways of behaving among occupational health professionals, both in their own groups and in the context of employees and employers.

Table 22.1 Phases in education in ethics for occupational health professionals

Educational phase	Educational methods
Creating a positive attitude towards ethics in occupational health and towards the learning of ethics	Statements by associations of occupational health professionals: 'Ethics is important' Lecture by an experienced and well-accepted person from own group; showing advantages of using moral values for decision making Articles in professional journals
Knowledge on moral values that are present in occupational health	Lectures by professionals in ethics and in occupational health practice Articles and books
Competence 1: 'showing how to do it' (moral deliberation method possible)	Lecture with examples of moral dilemmas in occupational health and how to deal with them: • recognising • alternative actions or decisions • moral values, weighting • decision making

Continued

Table 22.1 Continued

Educational phase	Educational methods
Competence 2: 'doing it together' (moral deliberation method possible)	Small groups with experienced leader talk about cases: • recognising • alternative actions or decisions • moral values, weighting • decision making
Competence 3: 'doing it oneself' (moral deliberation method possible)	Small groups, no external leader, talk about cases: • recognising • alternatives of action or decision • moral values, weighting • decision making Retrospective plenary talk with experienced professional.
Reflecting, and stabilising new behaviour	Audit groups talk about cases Articles in professional journals: cases and ways to deal with them from a moral view Frequent statements by associations of occupational health professionals Explanations of ethical behaviours of occupational health professionals in brochures for employees or employers

Since ethics has to do with the recognising and weighting of moral values, the best way to learn is by using cases from daily practice. Learning ethics has little to do with resolving regular medical problems. Describing moral values should be antecedent to the first step (that of recognising the moral values). Some people do not see the difference between legal problems and moral problems. In fact, there is a small overlap, but it is still important to make the distinction clear.

Weighting values needs discussion, preferably in small groups. People have to feel safe. Audits are suitable for getting people to reflect on their own behaviours. They should know that there is not one single best way of acting when an ethical dilemma arises; it always involves a weighting process, and finally taking a decision based on the outcome of that process. Reflection (the ability to critically evaluate one's own performance) can be quite difficult for medical professionals. An occupational health unit is multidisciplinary by its very nature, and we think that educational courses should preferably also be multidisciplinary. At the authors' conference the following cases were found to be especially suitable for courses of this kind:

- workplace intervention
- business ethics
- employability, fitness for work and sickness absence
- drugs and alcohol
- workplace health promotion
- occupational health research.

The best cases come from participants' own practice. This enhances the transfer of what is learnt into use in daily practice. Case histories can be videotaped, and role play can be a powerful method for putting oneself in the position of another and seeing another perspective. Small discussion groups (four to six people) are to be preferred. After a case is worked through, values are defined and the dilemmas become clear. The group may offer several alternative ways of dealing with the problem. Each alternative has its own consequences, but what are the ethical implications?

We cannot tell how long the course should be. A series of shorter courses during the year might be more effective than one longer course. More experience is needed to evaluate this. It will obviously also depend on the characteristics of the target group, the objectives of training programmes and their settings, and other factors. Integration into other subjects addressed in course curricula is also important.

A method for stepwise moral deliberation

In the Netherlands, the Committee for Occupational Health Practice and Ethics (CBE) of the Dutch Association of Occupational Health Physicians (NVAB) developed a way to perform moral deliberation by occupational health physicians. The method presented here is an adaptation of the one used in Nijmegen Academic Hospital, which is similar to the ones used in other hospitals in the Netherlands. This method, used by clinicians, consists of a series of questions. We adapted it for the occupational health situation and tested it in an audit group of occupational health physicians with an evaluation afterwards. This led to some changes. The method can also be used in multidisciplinary groups of occupational health professionals.

Before we explain the method, two cases are presented. These cases will be used as examples of how to use the method. Cases like these can, of course, be used in educational settings.

Case 22.1: natural healing

An employee of an IT firm is on sick leave because of depression. A natural healer, a physician, treats him. The patient refuses to take antidepressive drugs because he 'wants to stay open to his emotions'. The occupational health physician advises him to seek psychotherapeutic help but the patient does not want this. He is happy with his talks with the natural healer. In these talks 'conflicts from his youth are being worked through'. He does not want to follow the advice of the occupational health physician to opt for what the latter regards as an 'adequate treatment' for depression. The employer, a small firm with financial problems, wants him back to work as soon as possible and wants to support his reintegration.

Would you, as an occupational health physician, tell the employer that the employee is not co-operating regarding his reintegration? It should be remembered that, in the Netherlands, payment during sick leave is regulated by law. Pursuant to statutory regulation, employees on sick leave should not hinder their own reintegration, and should not refuse a treatment that offers the only real possible way of getting better. Of course, there is a restriction on this when obvious medical or practical problems are involved.

Case 22.2: exposure to potential hazards

In a chemical firm the exposure to potential genotoxic chemicals is diminished as far as possible by taking hygienic precautions. In order to diminish the risk even more, the management asks the occupational health service to take blood from every new employee and test it for predisposition for genetic damage. What is the answer of the occupational health service?

The full text of the moral deliberation method is presented in an appendix to this chapter. In what follows, references are made to its distinct parts.

1 Problem

It is important to define the problem before you start. Sometimes, the problem is not the problem of the occupational health professional, for example because it is really legal by nature or not to do with medical ethics at all. Then you can refer the client elsewhere, and skip the problem. Sometimes, it is immediately clear that the occupational health professional is the person with the problem; sometimes, this takes some time to decide. Occasionally, time for information gathering and reflection will be necessary to become aware of possible special situations, although these will not often arise in occupational health practice.

2   Facts

During this step we have to obtain a careful diagnosis of the facts. We divide this step into several clusters. It is like the diagnosis of a problem of the kind to which we are accustomed in pure medical practice. We may not always do this any more because of the routines we have acquired, and the time it takes. In our experience this step does take a long time.

In Case 22.1 it is important to get an idea of the illness and the therapy. Also, there is a need to know the motives of the employee in not wanting to take antidepressive drugs. It is possible that he has certain prejudices or has heard alarming stories about such drugs. It is also important to know the facts about his work situation, both from himself and from his employer. You have to know these to get a good idea of the consequences of the advice you are going to give.

In Case 22.2 there are a number of pertinent facts. These include, for example: What chemical substances are used? What is known about the risk of genetic damage from these substances? What is the predictive value of a positive and a negative test? How many cases have been described in which an employee suffers genetic damage due to work? How effective are the hygienic measures? And what about the procedures: Who will have access to the results? How will the results be used – for the prevention of ill-health or for the selection of employees?

All these facts have to be collected in order to perform a thorough evaluation at the next step.

Sometimes, the problem changes during the collecting of the facts. For example, if during Step 2 in Case 22.2 an employee gives birth to a child with a genetic defect, the labour union might raise questions about the risk. Or a study might be published, indicating that the risk is higher than was stated in your report.

3   Valuing

This step is to check on the values involved in any possible decision or to try to anticipate the implications of alternative decisions and the moral values that might be violated. It is necessary to agree on the moral values that should be discussed. Do we use the same definitions?

If, in Case 22.1, an occupational health professional decides not to tell the employer, will that decision further the well-being of the employee? And if he or she does tell, will that infringe confidentiality and the autonomy of the employee? What would an occupational health professional do in other non-identical but similar cases? How autonomous is the employee in making his or her choice? Do you have to support autonomy? In this case, the occupational health professional has to deal with the following moral values: autonomy, justice, honesty, confidentiality and non-maleficence (doing no harm).

In Case 22.2 there are, again, several considerations. Could your decision harm potential employees? Will positively tested employees not get the jobs they want? Will employees become anxious that they are facing greater health risks? On the other hand, not testing may lead to higher risks with regard to genotoxic change. Are employees free to take the test or not? Will confidentiality be protected? Who will have access to the results of the tests? The moral values in this case are non-maleficence (doing no harm), autonomy and confidentiality.

All values that might be present in the case have to be weighed up against one another. It is important to remember that there is no single correct answer. Weighting is subjective but can be made more transparent by defining the values concerned.

4   Decision making

Now a decision has to be made. Of course, it may be possible to postpone it until the occupational health professional has more facts available. But that is also a decision in itself!

A decision can be made if values are defined and weighed up. For example, if doing good and not doing harm is the most important value in Case 22.1, you will try to find a solution in which the employee gets the therapy you feel is most suitable, and that will also have a good chance of a positive effect. But that does not necessarily mean that he has to take antidepressive drugs. On the other hand, if you think honesty and justice prevail, then you may want to tell the employer that the employee does not support his reintegration. In Case 22.2 non-maleficence (doing no harm) prevails; you will need to find good studies to know which decision leads to least harm.

We hope that when occupational health professionals take a decision after having followed this (or some other systematic) procedure, they will feel that they have thought about the issue thoroughly and can also present the arguments to the parties involved. At the very least, the decision will be more transparent.

The stepwise method can be used in several ways.

- When alone, you can follow the questions to reflect on a past decision or a decision you have to make.
- It provides a basis on which to talk with colleagues in your own occupational health service. Just as you ask for advice from your colleagues on medical questions, you can also ask them to think about moral problems. Of course, all occupational health professionals can use the method, and multidisciplinary use can be a very effective way of improving co-operation.
- It can be applied in audit groups of occupational health physicians.

The method can also be used in educational settings. In the vocational training of occupational health professionals, it can be employed in small groups for ethical reflection, where a tutor should be present to lead the discussion.

Our own experience with the method was in an audit group of about 6–10 occupational health physicians. One of the members of the group used a real case. We found that we needed at least 1.5–2 hours for thorough deliberation.

The *Facts* step, in particular, took a lot of time. Often, the doctors gave their opinions, and did not focus on the facts. We also found that many facts were missing. Participants realised they needed more information before they could make a good decision. In all the cases, physicians afterwards gave the opinion that they were much helped by the deliberation, which genuinely supported the decision or advice they would give.

With this method, and with moral deliberation in general, we want to achieve the following:

- support the practice of the individual occupational health professional
- improve the quality of care of the individual caregiver
- make policy consistent (and transparent)
- enhance the well-being of all parties.

Acknowledgement

The author wishes to thank Medard Hilhorst, Department of Medical Ethics, Erasmus Medical Centre, Rotterdam, for his useful comments on an earlier draft of this chapter.

References

1 Martimo K-P, Antti-Poika M, Leino T and Rossi K (1998) Ethical issues among Finnish occupational physicians and nurses. *Occupational Medicine.* **48**: 375–80.

2 Goldie J (2000) Review of ethics curricula in undergraduate medical education. *Medical Education.* **34**: 108–19.

3 Goldie J, Schwartz L and Morrison J (2000) A process evaluation of medical ethics in the first year of a new medical curriculum. *Medical Education.* **34**: 468–73.

4 Woodall A (2001) Closing the gap between professional teaching and practice. *British Medical Journal.* **323**: 47.

5 Goldie J, Schwartz L, McConnachie A and Morrison J (2002) The impact of three years' ethics teaching, in an integrated medical curriculum, on students' proposed behaviour on meeting ethical dilemmas. *Medical Education.* **36**: 489–97.

6 Self DJ, Wolinsky FD and Baldwin DC (1989) The effect of teaching medical ethics on medical students' moral reasoning. *Academic Medicine.* **64**: 755–9.

7 Nilstun T, Cuttni M and Saracci R (2001) Teaching medical ethics to experienced staff: participants, teachers and method. *Journal of Medical Ethics.* **27**: 409–12.

Appendix

Moral deliberation for occupational health physicians

Committee for Occupational Health Practice and Ethics (CBE) of the Dutch Society of Physicians in Occupational Health, May 2002. Based on the Nijmegen method for moral deliberation, Department of Ethics, Philosophy and History of Medicine, Nijmegen University (KUN).

Introduction

Occupational health physicians in the Netherlands find themselves experiencing a conflict of duties in the course of their work. There is a law on the agreement to medical treatment (WGBO) and there are labour laws. The physicians work in an occupational health service. In making a judgement about a particular problem these conflicting duties can lead to different actions. Besides there are other factors to be weighed up, such as: 'How do I know what is right? What should I do?'.

To help occupational health physicians be clear what to do in a conflict of duties and in ethical (moral) problems, we suggest working according to a method for moral deliberation.

The steps in this method are: name the facts, value the facts and then come to a deliberated decision.

The method can be used for reflection (with colleagues) or for inter-professional consultation.

This is the method step by step.

1   Problem
   - What makes the case a moral problem?
   - What is the task or role of the occupational health physician in this problem?
   - Who has the final responsibility?

   Special situations
   - Is there incompetence of will (inability to make decisions or take actions)?
   - Is the client able to judge reality?
   - Who determined possible incompetence of will or disturbed sense of reality?
   - Is this state temporary or permanent?
   - Who represents the interests of the client?

2   Facts
   Medical
   - What is the medical diagnosis and what (other factors apart) is the prognosis concerning complaints and capacity to be fit for work?
   - What is the medical diagnosis and what (other factors apart) is the prognosis concerning reintegration into his or her own work?

   Psychological
   - What is the psychological situation (symptoms, frame of mind)?
   - How does the client view his or her own complaints?
   - How does the client view work in general?
   - How does the client look at (in)capacity for work?
   - What is the client's outlook on life (religion)?
   - How can personal development be stimulated?

   Social private
   - What is the client's lifestyle? What are his/her social activities?
   - How does the client view own domestic tasks?
   - How is the (in)capacity for work seen by family, friends and other people in non-work relationships?

Information from the client about the working situation
- What are working relationships like? (with colleagues, with head of department)
- What is the content of the work in relation to the client's capacities?
- What are the conditions of work (financial)?
- What is the working environment like?
- What are the possibilities for reintegration in this company?

View of employer and/or head of department
- What are working relationships like? (with colleagues, with head of department)
- What is the content of the work in relation to capacities?
- What are the conditions of work (financial)?
- What is the working environment like?
- What are the possibilities for reintegration in this company?

Occupational health diagnosis
- What is the occupational health diagnosis?

Suggested plan
- Which occupational health plan is suggested?
- What is the expected effect (and the scope) of that plan on the prognosis for illness and the client's capacity for managing the work?
- What is the expected effect (and the scope) of that plan on the prognosis for reintegration?
- What is the prognosis if nothing is done?
- What is the likelihood that the suggested plan will succeed?
- Could the suggested plan damage the health of the client?
- What could be the consequences of the suggested plan on the client's psychological condition?
- What could be the consequences of the suggested plan on the client's social relationships?
- What could be the consequences of the suggested plan on the client's working situation?
- What is the likely balance of positive and negative effects?

3 Valuing
Well-being of the client
- What are the consequences of being (un)fit to work for the well-being of the client (joy of living, freedom of movement, physical and mental well-being, anxiety, etc.)?
- What could be the consequences of the occupational health plan for the well-being of the client?

Autonomy of the client
- Is the client well informed about the situation?
- Is the client adequately concerned with the procedure so far?

- What is the judgement of the client about the costs and benefits of the plan? Short term and long term?
- Which values and opinions of the client are relevant?

Well-being of the company
- Does the occupational physician have to take into account the interests of a third party in the company?
- What are the consequences of the occupational health plan for the well-being of the company?

Well-being of the social environment
- Does the occupational health physician have to take into account the interests of a third party in the social environment?
- What are the consequences of the occupational health policy for the social environment?

Responsibility of the occupational health physician (and perhaps other caregivers)
- Is there a difference in opinion between the occupational health physician and other caregivers (inside or outside the occupational health service)?
- Has there been enough consultation between the caregivers?
- Is the division of responsibilities clearly marked between the caregivers?
- How do the caregivers deal with confidential information? (Confidentiality)
- Has the client been adequately informed about the situation? (Openness)
- Can the suggested policy be justified in respect of other clients? (Justice)
- What are the relevant guidelines of the occupational group or the occupational health service?

4 Decision making
- What is the moral problem now?
- Are there any important facts that are unknown? Is it possible nevertheless to make a sound decision?
- Can the problem be conceptualised in terms of (conflicting) values?
- Is there a way out of this dilemma?
- Which alternative for action is most in agreement with the general medical ethical starting points (values)?
- What other arguments are important for the decision?
- Which action (based on the arguments) is preferred?
- What are the duties of all the persons concerned?
- Which questions are still unanswered?

CHAPTER 23

Ethical occupational health management and organisation

John Øvretveit

Introduction

Occupational health managers – people with direct responsibility for running an occupational health service – face unprecedented and conflicting demands. Ethics often appears as yet another demand and an unattainable counsel of perfection. Indeed, learning about ethics in management can make us feel more guilty and make the work even more stressful. This chapter, however, shows how ethics can help managers in their work. It builds on Chapter 2 in which the concept of 'ethical occupational health management' was developed. This is both a way of managing and a set of tools, which brings back meaning and integrity into the often lonely, difficult and thankless task of managing an occupational health service.

Chapter 2 proposed tools for developing more research-informed practice and quality improvement as part of the concept of 'ethical occupational health management'. These tools enable managers better to meet current demands and develop a more ethical service. This chapter adds two more tools to the concept – the idea of and methods for developing a health-enhancing 'social work architecture', and a simple ethical analysis method for managers. This complements the ethical analysis method for occupational health practitioners described in Chapter 3.

Occupational health managers face unprecedented demands. Their funders want lower costs. The different users of their service expect more. Company employees want higher quality services. There are ever more laws and initiatives to implement. Personnel working for occupational health services want better pay and work conditions, and also meaningful, fulfilling work. Competition is increasing for these personnel, including those from other kinds of occupational services. Occupational health services have to become more business-like, and there are increasing pressures to put income before the interests of clients. The services are becoming more multidisciplinary and the different occupational groups within them have different values and views about their work and service aims. The method described later in this chapter shows how to use ethics in everyday situations to help cope with competing demands in the operation of occupational health management.

Ethics and work organisation

Occupational health practitioners are experts in the many hazards to employees' health, and have a number of methods for diagnosing and intervening to protect health and promote well-being. The focus of occupational health services has been on physical and measurable features of the work environment. However, the profession has not sufficiently recognised that how work is organised and managed also affects employee health – for good and for bad. This is a feature of the work situation which is less tangible and more difficult to study, and where it is more difficult to relate outcome to cause. Where work organisation has been studied, there has been a tendency for research not to be used to develop practical ways of analysing work organisation or management in terms of their harmful or health-promoting features. The issue here is more than organisation and management as a 'stress factor', although this is one aspect of 'ethical organisation'.

Occupational health managers have a particular responsibility for addressing the health aspects of work organisation. As managers, work organisation is central to their own tasks and responsibilities; they are responsible for designing the work organisation of their own services, and also for giving advice to employers about health hazards.

Work organisation as a potential health hazard

In Chapter 2 it was proposed that one cause of quality problems is that individual patient care is not well organised as a system. Analysis often shows that a certain number of errors or mishaps are likely to happen regardless of the care and attention of the practitioner, simply because of how care is organised. This includes how different service providers do, or do not, relate with or communicate with each other.

A care organisation not designed for quality can harm patients. But employees' health is also affected by how their work is organised. Organisation affects occupational health workers and the employees they serve equally. We know that the amount and intensity of work, and the control that employees have over their own work are related to stress and affect health. We know that employees vary in their ability to cope with job demands; what for one is stressful is for another boring. We know that good employee and work matching is important to health and well-being. Health is affected by the way work is divided up and tasks are structured, and also the working relations necessary for performing the tasks. This is what we call the 'social work architecture'.

Work teams offer one example of 'social work architecture' and its effects. Like some marriages, a well-functioning team brings out the best in people and gives a satisfying and life-enhancing experience. The support and identity it provides are likely to promote health and to protect against harmful stressors. But a poorly functioning team with an unclear or inappropriate decision-making structure is the source of much distress and wasted energy. The experience, like that of a bad marriage, affects a person's entire well-being, and possibly his or her health if it is an unavoidable and large part of working life. Occupational health services are increasingly provided by multidisciplinary teams, and the way these are designed – or not designed – can cause stress, conflict and bad work conditions for occupational health employees. This, in turn, affects the services they provide to their clients.

The example of a good and bad team also illustrates that work organisation can be designed, diagnosed and subject to intervention. Teams are often formed without attention being paid to their organisation. A group with goodwill and good sense will evolve a 'social work architecture' that works on a functional and interpersonal level. With luck the group will perform well, enable its members to develop and continue to be satisfied. But many teams get caught up in power struggles, time-wasting and destructive behaviours, largely because basic features of organisation are neglected. The point is that teams and other aspects of work organisation can and should be designed – not just for efficiency but also for employee well-being.[1] The right 'social work architecture' enhances health and also helps to retain employees.

What is the primary cause of overwork or underwork and unfair work distribution? It is proposed in this chapter that the main cause is managerial inattention to work organisation. Some work and relations structuring is designed by managers (formal work organisation); some is not designed, but arises out of the nature of the tasks and situation; and some of the structure is created by employees themselves. Often there is a combination of all three. But sometime managers do not take any part in designing work organisation at all; they pay no attention to clarifying roles and working relations or to other features of work organisation that we know affect people's health and well-being. What is being proposed here is that occupational health services and managers of these services are in the best position to identify organisational aspects, report on the consequences of inattention or lack of awareness about work design to higher levels of client company management, and make interventions. There is a remarkable lack of 'organisational consciousness' in most organisations, and occupational health services can be one source for highlighting these issues.[2]

The effects of work organisation on health are less recognised than the effects of physical architecture and other tangible factors and hazards. If employees do not step in in order to organise the work appropriately, then the way work is organised will become a source of conflict, stress and damage to health. Further, inappropriate work organisation reduces confidence and trust, and also increases suspicion and negative 'political manoeuvring'.

The proposition here is not just that organisation can harm health or that managers have responsibility for a health-enhancing work organisation. The proposition is that an organisation is ethical in so far as it promotes trust, confidence and respect in others and brings out the best in people. Ethics is not just a matter of individual behaviour; it entails that work organisation can be judged as ethical or not according to whether it breeds mistrust, suspicion and conflict or enhances positive social behaviours and faith in others.

Ethical organisation is:

- a culture and a structure of work roles, tasks and working relations where people are matched to their roles, enabled to give their best and become the best that they can be, which builds trust and confidence
- designed to enable people to take responsibility, to recognise the results of others' efforts, and to develop abilities to meet others' needs in ways that increase trust and respect for others
- one that enables people to make decisions with an awareness of the consequences, and with consideration of the best way to minimise harm and maximise the benefits for and growth in others.

Poor management as a health risk

Sixty to 75% of employees in any organisation report that the most stressful aspect of their work is their manager.[3] This is irrespective of industry, sector, level or occupational group. Research shows that management practices can cause stress and other health-impairing conditions.[4] Poor management styles and behaviours can have a devastating effect on employee well-being, especially if a company does not have effective mechanisms for its employees to complain or take protective action.[5] A recent review of research found sickness absenteeism to be associated with 'poor management style'.[6] 'Bullying' by managers was reported to be widespread in a study of a UK NHS community trust, and associated with anxiety and depression.[7]

One question for occupational health practitioners and managers concerns their responsibility to report to client-company management issues that are likely to be harming health. One issue is whether occupational health services have methods for making reliable and valid assessments in this context. Another is whether the occupational health contract with the client includes a responsibility to make such assessments and to make reports. In other words, should the occupational health manager or practitioner 'blow the whistle' on managers whose style or actions are, in his or her judgement, affecting employee health if the company has no channels to deal with such issues?

The key question raised in this chapter is whether health-impairing management styles and behaviours are an ethical issue for occupational health services. Further, is it an issue that should be of particular concern to occupational health managers? There is no clear answer, not least because the research and assessment methods in this area are rudimentary. However, it is an important and increasingly relevant question to raise. The method for ethical analysis described later in the chapter provides one way of working through the issue in a particular situation.

The chapter has proposed, however, that there is clear evidence of a link between health and poor work organisation, and points out that it is managers who are responsible for such work organisation. Where managers do not meet their responsibility, employees often step in and work out how to organise the work. In some small work groups, especially those that have been trained in quality methods, the results may be good (i.e. the creation of an effective and satisfying work organisation). But this is a matter of chance; the resulting work organisation may or may not be health enhancing.

In other cases, a manager may take responsibility for designing work organisation seriously, but his or her objective is efficiency and not employee health. In the long term these two objectives might not be in conflict, but in the short term they often are. Few managers have knowledge about how work organisation affects health. It is the responsibility of occupational health practitioners and managers to advise other managers about the health impact of their work organisation. Further, action needs to be taken to help managers meet their responsibility for designing work organisation not just for efficiency but also for employee health. Occupational health managers are in a position to promote such recognition and to develop and use methods for analysing work organisation in this latter aspect. Arnetz[8] provides a useful research-based model for doing so. Managers should be made more aware of how this intangible aspect of working life affects health. It also needs to be pointed out that more industries are moving from the idea of management alone being responsible for work organisation to management sharing this responsibility with employees. This applies especially in industries using quality management methods. However, sometimes the move from management responsibility to joint responsibility results in a lack of clarity about and neglect of action to design work organisation. Multiprofessional work organisations, like occupational health services themselves, are particularly vulnerable in this respect.

In summary, it is increasingly recognised in law and good management practice that managers have a responsibility for employee health. What is less recognised is how work organisation and management behaviours can both harm health or enhance employee well-being. In particular, there is potential for such 'invisible' structuring to promote constructive and trustful behaviours rather than destructive, harmfully conflictual and paranoid ones.[9] 'Ethical organisation' enhances trust and well-being. The message of this section is that occupational health managers have a responsibility for making companies more aware of this, and for putting their own house in order; that is, for designing the right 'social work architecture' for their own service. Ethical management requires greater consciousness of the harmful and beneficial impacts of poor and good management respectively.

Practising ethical management

Ethical management supports evidence-based practice, and also improves quality and the 'social work architecture'. These are, in fact, specific ways of implementing the ethical principles presented in this book. However, ethical principles also help managers with the many everyday situations they face, such as confronting an employee's addiction habit, conflict with company management or difficult financial decisions.

Putting ethical principles into practice is difficult. The issue is not so much deciding how to apply a principle in an actual situation, but that following one principle often means violating another. The simple ethical analysis method described here shows how to use ethics in everyday management. Practice in using this method makes it easier to deal with many of the decisions and conflicts that managers currently face.

In the heat of the moment we often do not have time to pay much attention to ethical principles. A simple framework provides a way of working through ethical considerations to find the best action. The following assumes that, in many situations, the manager will consult with and work through the issues with his or her occupational health service colleagues before making a decision (if this is possible and time allows). In such cases a manager can prepare for discussions by carrying out the analysis beforehand to clarify the ethical issues.

Think of a real and difficult management situation that you face right now. Appreciating what follows depends on you having a real situation to think about. You might not be able to think of a current situation, in which case think back to a recent one, for example an employee constantly making mistakes, a patient complaining, a budget cut of 15%, a request from a colleague or friend for a favour or a higher-level policy which could have unethical consequences if you carried it out (such as one which requires your service to change its policy about giving certain information to an employer about patients).

Is more than one ethical principle relevant? There are few situations where only one principle applies, and even then this principle may not give clear guidance on how to act. Most difficult situations are difficult because they appear to, or actually do, involve conflicts between people or principles. More than one principle or interest is at stake, and any action will mean acting against at least one principle or against at least one person's interests. An ethical approach entails deciding which principle is the most important in the situation in question. The aim, however, is not to pick a solution, and then justify it *post hoc* by reference to an ethical principle, but that the solution should arise out of the relevant ethical principle.

What are the choices?

An ethical approach means living with the agony of deciding, rather than making a quick decision. It even means increasing the agony of deciding, since an ethical approach is not just to consider the alternative ways of acting that immediately present themselves. It means recognising and *creating* choices in a difficult situation, usually when everyone wants a quick decision, and is saying that good leadership requires fast decisive action. In fact, good leadership means resisting these pressures – so as to be able to seek an alternative that meets everyone's needs and interests (or at least harms the fewest). How much choice you have is as much to do with how you see the situation as with objective constraints. And how much choice we have is often a result of our psychology – how much we are able to bear the tensions of uncertainty and conflict in examining the options. Sometimes, time limits or budget constraints give us excuses to take the easy way out.

If we return to the difficult situation that you thought about, the first question above is whether an immediate decision was essential. There are few management situations where lives depend on a quick decision. Before deciding which principle is most important in the situation, check first that you have considered all the alternative actions and choices that might better meet people's needs. Take the example of changing your service's policy on giving information about whether an employee has asked for an HIV/AIDS test. The two obvious ones are to change the policy and give the information or to stick to the policy of not giving such information. But a third is to give the information under certain circumstances, e.g. if the employee agrees or if the employer can give a good reason for seeking the information. Are there other actions or alternatives that are conceivable? Acting ethically involves believing that there is always choice, and also creating choices. Listing the choices is the first step in the 'ethical analysis' summarised below. Presenting the alternatives in this way is important for thinking creatively about the options (even if some of them are unlikely ever to be adopted).

Which principles apply?

For each of these alternative choices, which principles are relevant? For example, there is the option of not changing the policy, and therefore not giving information about the seeking of HIV/AIDS testing to the employer. One relevant principle is respect for patient privacy. Another is the utilitarian principle of promoting the greatest good of the greatest number, provided that the employer can show that having the information would achieve this.

The next step is to consider which principle is the most important to uphold in the situation, and use this to choose which of the alternatives to pursue (*see below*). What then is the ethical justification for your behaviour or decision? What it consists in is that you have identified all the choices in the time you had available; you have decided which ethical principle was most important; and your choice was the one that upheld this principle. This is a more ethical way of acting than justifying the easiest option by means of a *post-hoc* ethical argument.

Steps in an ethical analysis

- Step 1: CHOICES
  List the choices or alternative actions.

- Step 2: ETHICS OF EACH OPTION
  List the ethical arguments for and against each option (referring to ethical principles).

	For	*Against*
Alternative 1		
Alternative 2, etc.		

- Step 3: IMPORTANCE
  Which ethical principle is most important in this situation? Why?

- Step 4: THE ETHICAL CHOICE
  Which alternative best upholds this principle? Why?

- Step 5: CONSEQUENCES
  What harm or hurt will come from implementing this alternative? Who will be disadvantaged?

- Step 6: SELF-INTEREST BIAS
  Does the alternative you chose also advance your personal interests?
  If it does, how do you know that this did not bias you? Does it matter?

- Step 7: JUSTIFICATION
  Is the alternative justified?

- Step 8: TIME
  Is it likely that spending more time to create other alternatives, or to get more information, might help you make a more ethical decision?

The above is described as an 'ethical analysis'. And if you have followed your example through, you will have just performed an ethical analysis of a management situation. You can use these simple steps in most management circumstances, which is often necessary where there is no code or any obvious over-riding ethical guidance on how to act. Although using this approach takes time and may be difficult at first, with practice managers report that they are able to use it quickly and informally in many situations. It helps to improve your decisions and your awareness of issues that you may not have considered.

As pressures and conflicts increase, there is a greater need than ever to consider ethical issues, but less time to do so. Occupational health management involves more than technical management skills; it involves personal consideration of the human consequences of managerial behaviours and decisions. By raising your awareness, ethics does not take away the pains and agonies of management decisions, but it does make it easier for you to live with yourself and your colleagues if you have worked through the ethical issues. It is also a technique that can be taught to and used by client managers to help them recognise the conflicts in their work and deal with the stresses.

Occupational health managers are sometimes overwhelmed by the responsibilities of their position, become hardened, and feel that they are going backwards professionally and personally. Developing an ethical approach to your work helps you to grow personally and professionally from the experience of being a manager. In a fragmented and difficult job, a sense of right and wrong, of what is important and why it is important is essential to being able to come back to work each day and to taking pride in your work. It is also important in creating the right organisational culture and for leading by example – by showing integrity in practising what you preach. Occupational health managers bear a heavy burden, and ethics sometimes seems a counsel of perfection. It is important to remember that the aim is not to be a saint, but to make better decisions than you would otherwise have made if you had not considered the ethical aspects.

Ethical occupational health management is *not*:

- being more *caring*
- using ethical arguments to obtain more resources
- using ethics to justify a decision *after* a decision is made without ethical consideration
- only for when *resources* are inadequate.

Ethical occupational health management: a summary

One message of this chapter is that ethical professional practice can be both greatly helped and greatly hindered by occupational health managers. Their leadership 'sets the tone' and culture of a service and signals whether ethics are to be practised or are only ineffectual and non-applied principles. Managers create the opportunities to practise ethically or unethically. Their awareness of ethics and their visibly carrying-through such awareness in different situations and in the work systems they create make a big difference to whether their personnel can or cannot practise ethically. Chapter 2 showed that developing research-informed practice and the use of quality improvement methods are tangible ways in which managers could both improve efficiency and enable more ethical practice. This chapter has presented a simple method for carrying out an ethical analysis, which is one tool that managers can use to develop their ethical leadership as well as to help with a specific issue they face.

A second message is that poor work organisation is a health risk, and that managers have a responsibility for creating a work organisation that enhances well-being rather than damages health. Work organisation here means both how an occupational health service is organised – referring to who does what and when, and working relationships – and also how clients organise work for their employees.

We know that certain physical and chemical environments are harmful, and that there is an ethical, if not a legal, duty for managers to protect employees from hazards. We know that some management practices increase stress. But we are also learning that the way work and working relationships are structured – the intangible 'social work architecture' of organisations – not only can bring out the best and worst in employees, but can also be either positively harmful or health promoting. Occupational health managers have a duty to apply this knowledge in the way they design the work organisation of their own service, and to utilise it in the industries they serve.

Even occupational health managers positively disposed to an ethical approach may feel uncomfortable with discussions of ethics. Ethical considerations burden them with yet more 'impossible' responsibilities. This is an understandable reaction. But the aim of this chapter, and of Chapter 2, is to shows that ethics can help managers to deal with the conflicting demands on them, and give coherence and meaning to a fragmented and over-busy work schedule. The ideas can be summarised in the concept of 'ethical occupational health management', which is about ensuring quality services, using ethics to aid decision making and designing work organisations that help people to give and to become their best. The concept can give a new focus to occupational health services. It is congruent with the research base that the services need to use, and also with the values of practitioners and managers in the services. It can also serve to unite practitioners and managers; successful changes to occupational health practices require that the two groups work together to plan and make changes to services so as to face the challenges ahead.

Conclusions

The chapter shows that 'ethical occupational health management' entails addressing organisational and management issues in the various organisations that occupational health managers are advising and serving. Occupational health managers need to be aware of how management and organisation affect the well-being of employees, and of how to intervene in their own and other organisations to prevent harm and promote the well-being that is influenced by as yet scarcely unrecognised management and organisational factors.

Managers of occupational health services want to be more effective in their work and to use modern management methods. However, many do not want to abandon the values that led them to enter the profession and the ethical principles that underpin their clinical work. This chapter and Chapter 2 show where ethics and managerial priorities come together in the concept of 'ethical occupational health management'. Such management encompasses research-informed practice, quality improvement, ethical work organisation and ethical analysis. These are all tools for occupational health managers to apply ethical principles in their work. They are effective ways that individual managers can use to respond to the demands and pressures on their service.

Managers' use of ethics in their leadership sets the tone and culture of their service. Ethical occupational health management involves creating a service that brings out the best in people, rather than harming their health. It provides a way for occupational health to adapt to current challenges, combining 'head and heart' and uniting practitioners and managers. It gives coherence and meaning, and also effective methods with which to face the challenging and sometimes thankless task of managing an occupational health service.

References

1   Carter A and West M (1999) Sharing the burden – teamwork in a healthcare setting. In: J Firth-Cozens and R Payne (eds) *Stress in Health Professionals: psychological and organisational causes and interventions.* John Wiley, Chichester.

2   Peck S (1993) *A World Waiting to be Born.* Bantam Books, New York.

3   Hogan R, Curphy J and Hogan J (1994) What we know about leadership. *American Pyschologist.* **49**(6): 493–503.

4   Firth-Cozens J (1999) The psychological problems of doctors. In: J Firth-Cozens, R Payne (eds) *Stress in Health Professionals: psychological and organisational causes and interventions.* John Wiley, Chichester.

5   West M (2002) Quality and human resource practices. *Health Management.* **August**: 13–14.

6   Michie S and Williams S (2002) Reducing work related psychological ill health and sickness absence: a systematic literature review. *Occupational and Environmental Medicine.* **60**: 3–9.

7   Quine L (1999) Workplace bullying in an NHS community trust, staff questionnaire study. *British Medical Journal.* **318**: 228–32.

8   Arnetz B (1999) Stress and physicians' work. *Social Science and Medicine.* **52**: 203–13.

9   Jaques E (1989) *Requisite Organization.* Casson Hall, Arlington, VA.

CHAPTER 24

Professional codes of ethics

Kit Harling, Peter Westerholm and Tore Nilstun

In this chapter we will briefly present and comment on a few selected codes and guidance documents on professional ethics for health personnel, with a particular view to occupational health. The relationship between ethical theory and codes of practice is complex. The former deals with many abstract concepts while the latter tries to convey rules of behaviour. As legislators will readily agree, writing explicit rules is difficult, as small changes in circumstances often change the outcome dramatically.

Three ethical principles or shared moral beliefs have been applied in this book to common dilemmas for occupational health professionals. These principles have been developed over centuries, more particularly over the last 200 years.

The process is not complete. There are new developments in ethical theory – both in a general sense and more particularly in the field of biomedical ethics. Changes in medical practice cause us to re-evaluate past ethical analyses and, through the virtuous circle of development, lead to new insights. A hundred years ago, the principle of distributive justice would not have featured as prominently as it has in these chapters.

For most of us, the demands of a busy job do not permit the luxury of developing from first principles the ethical response to a given set of circumstances. It is helpful to have codified rules from which we can learn and from which we can derive standards of normal behaviour in our day-to-day work. Hence, we have seen the development of codes of ethics, which help us by describing standards of behaviour in common situations. The codes form a reference document. Most occupational health professionals will not need to refer to the codes on a regular basis; their content will be familiar to them. They form, however, a point of departure or a source of principles, which helps when facing an unfamiliar ethical scenario.

Guidance on Ethics for Occupational Physicians – issued by the Faculty of Occupational Medicine, London

The Faculty of Occupational Medicine of the Royal College of Physicians was established in 1978 with the objective of ensuring the highest standards of professional competence in occupational health physicians for the public benefit. As soon as the Faculty was created, the importance of clear ethical guidelines was recognised and the first edition of *Guidance on Ethics* was published two years later as the first professional statement of the fledgling organisation.[1]

The Faculty set up an ethics committee, composed mainly of senior occupational health physicians but also including representatives (including the President) from the parent Royal College of Physicians. Another key feature was the inclusion of one or more non-medical or lay members, who it was thought would have a key role in ensuring the general applicability of the guidance.

The other important context for the creation of *Guidance on Ethics* was *Ethical Guidance* published by the General Medical Council (GMC) in London, which was intended to regulate the behaviour of all doctors. Often wrongly characterised at the time as being only concerned with 'the three As' – alcohol, advertising and adultery – the rules give general guidance about the way doctors are expected to behave.

It was soon recognised that to command respect from major stakeholders it was necessary to recruit other members. The Trades Union Congress (TUC), representing most trade unions, is the authoritative voice for workers' representatives in the UK. A high-level representative from the TUC has for many years provided this particular insight. The organisation has been less successful in recruiting an employer's representative.

The relationship between ethical codes and the law is complex. In a representative democracy, compliance with the law is generally a civic duty, and sometimes there is a conflict between the requirements of the *Guidance on Ethics* and the law. For example, it has been held that an occupational health physician conducting a pre-employment health assessment does not owe a legal duty of care to the applicant. It remains the view of the Faculty (and the GMC) that the doctor owes a professional duty of care to the prospective employee. It is certainly the case that the professional code of ethics places a higher moral duty on a doctor in specific circumstances than is required more generally in society. The Ethics Committee has had a strong legal input – so as better to identify the conflicts, real or imagined, between the different requirements.

Over the last 25 years, change in medical practice has been huge. The founders of the Faculty and the first members of the Ethics Committee noted in the first edition of *Guidance on Ethics* that 'the statements made in this document may have to be revised from time to time as attitudes in society continue to change'. This is not the place to rehearse all the changes over that period but suffice it to say that the Faculty will shortly publish the sixth edition.

The aim of the *Guidance* has been to insert the ethical rules that apply to all doctors into the context of occupational health practice. It is argued that whatever role you have in an organisation, if you carry the title of 'doctor', those who may consult you are entitled to expect the same standard of moral behaviour as they would from any other medical practitioner. Thus, where the context allows, the guidance of the GMC should be followed. This principle is set out in the first section of *Guidance on Ethics*, entitled General Principles. The *Guidance* is not in itself a declaration of the roles, relationships and responsibilities of occupational health practice; rather, it is guidance on regulating these factors in a broader context. The factors themselves are set out in other Faculty publications, such as its academic syllabuses.

Given that many occupational health encounters involve not only the individual but also – to a greater or lesser degree – the employer, specific advice on the application of confidentiality to occupational health records forms the second and largest section of the guidance document.

Most medical practice in the UK has, for more than 50 years, taken place within the National Health Service (NHS), where issues such as confidentiality and the safe-keeping of records have become institutionalised. But the bulk of occupational health practice in the UK lies outside the NHS, where such traditions and arrangements do hold sway; to this day, questions about the storage, ownership and access to records are the largest group of queries submitted to the Faculty.

The *Guidance* establishes explicitly that occupational health records are just like other clinical records in the guardianship of the clinician; the employer and other third parties have no more access to the records than is permitted by law. Employers' legal advisers, in particular, often find this restriction burdensome. In light of the central importance of the subject of these records in regulating access, transfer of records when the worker changes employer or the employer changes occupational health provider, the principle of consent is considered paramount.

Also, the tripartite relationship – doctor/employee/employer – and the fact that many employees are asked to visit occupational health services by their employer rather than deciding themselves that they need advice have led to the development of sections on the provision of opinions on fitness for work, on health surveillance, and on special tests. The principles of consent, transparency and informed consent are emphasised again. Employees must know what is going to happen to them, why, according to what standards, and with what consequences.

Health surveillance at work, particularly that involving invasive procedures, must not be introduced without widespread discussion amongst all stakeholders ensuring that any proposed scheme complies with the general criteria for screening processes.

Changes in the style of occupational health practice over the last 25 years have been rapid. From a position where most occupational health physicians worked in large medical services in nationalised industries, such as coal mining and steel making, small private practices and larger occupational health companies are now the norm. There has also been an increase in occupational health services in the public and service sectors. A new section of the *Guidance* was introduced as an amendment to the fourth edition to cover business ethics, relationships between organisations, advertising, and the transfer of services (particularly as applied to occupational health businesses).

From the beginning, the *Guidance on Ethics* emphasised the importance of ethical relationships with other healthcare professionals. Over the years, the Faculty's *Guidance* has been unofficially adopted by other groups of occupational health professionals. This led the Faculty to invite occupational health nurses to join the committee as full members in their own right. Their contribution has been so valuable that this membership is currently being strengthened.

The Committee and its guidance will continue to evolve. Its roots will remain in the general ethics of healthcare provision in the UK, but with a focus on the particularities of occupational health practice

ICOH's *International Code of Ethics for Occupational Health Professionals*

The International Commission on Occupational Health (ICOH) is an international non-governmental organisation for occupational health professionals, founded in 1906, whose membership comprises both researchers and practitioners in the occupational health sciences and fields of practice. In 1992 ICOH adopted an *International Code of Ethics* for the many categories of professionals active in research institutions or carrying out tasks in enterprises and organisations concerning safety, health, hygiene and the environment in relation to work. This *Code*, henceforth referred to as the ICOH *Code*, has been updated since then, and a revised version was adopted by the ICOH Board in March 2002.[2] The updating process has included consultation with the scientific committees of the ICOH.

The target group, occupational health professionals, for the ICOH *Code* is referred to as a broad category of persons whose common vocation is professional commitment in pursuing an occupational health agenda. The ICOH *Code* applies to such professionals regardless of whether they operate in a free-market context or within public-sector organisations.

The ICOH *Code* represents an attempt to translate into terms of professional conduct the fundamental values and principles of occupational health on an international level. Its aim is to set a reference level of professional practice with regard to ethics by which evaluation can be carried out and to provide guidance in elaboration of national codes or codes for use in sectors or branches of labour markets and in enterprises. The following abstract from the ICOH *Code* will be restricted to indication of its key features.

The introductory part of the ICOH *Code* consists of 12 paragraphs describing the purpose and the context of the document in the perspective of the tasks of occupational health professionals in a changing world. On this follow three paragraphs referred to as Basic Principles.

- The purpose of occupational health is to serve the health and social well-being of the workers individually and collectively. Occupational health practice must be performed according to the highest professional standards and ethical principles. Occupational health professionals must contribute to environmental and community health.
- The duties of occupational health professionals include protecting the life and the health of the worker, respecting human dignity and promoting the highest ethical principles in occupational health policies and programmes. Integrity in professional conduct, impartiality and the protection of the confidentiality of health data and of the privacy of workers are part of these duties.
- Occupational health professionals are experts who must enjoy full professional independence in the execution of their functions. They must acquire and maintain the competence necessary for their duties and require conditions which allow them to carry out their tasks according to good practice and professional ethics.

Following this, the body of the ICOH *Code* text is presented under two headings: Duties and obligations of occupational health professionals (articles 1–15) and Conditions of execution of the functions of occupational health professionals (articles 16–26). Articles 1–15 deal with subject matter under the following headings: Aims and Advisory Role; Knowledge and Expertise; Development of a Policy and a Programme; Emphasis on Prevention and on a Prompt Action; Follow-up of Remedial Action; Safety and Health Information; Commercial Secrets; Information to the Worker; Information to the Employer; Danger to a Third Party; Biological Monitoring and Investigations; Health Promotion; Protection of Community and Environment; Contribution to Scientific Knowledge.

Articles 16–26, under the heading 'Conditions of execution of the functions of occupational health professionals', deal with the subject matter of ethics under the 13 headings of: Competence, Integrity and Impartiality; Professional Independence; Equity; Non-Discrimination and Communication; Clause on Ethics in Contracts of Employment; Records; Medical Confidentiality; Collective Health Data; Relationships with Health Professionals; Combating Abuses (of occupational health data or of confidential information); Relationships with Social Partners; Promoting Ethics; and Professional Audit.

These headings of the articles of the ICOH *Code* well reflect their contents. They are largely self-explanatory. The reader is, however, referred to the *Code* text for detailed study. The clause on Ethics (para 19) deals in particular with aspects related to professional independence and measures to be taken for its protection.

In adopting the *Code*, the ICOH Board has emphasised that the instrument needs to be regularly updated or revised. Account should be taken of changes in work conditions, and political and social developments globally and in different regions and countries of the world. The importance of such continuous quality improvement of the ICOH *Code* was also recognised by the ICOH Board in its update of 2002. The *Code* text reflects a clear awareness and recognition of the implications, real or potential, of the ongoing changes in the world at work on professional ethics and professional conduct of occupational health professionals at work.

The International Code of Conduct (Ethics) for Occupational Safety and Health Professionals[3]

This code of ethics, conceived and written by a group of 40 international occupational health experts – most of whom are US based – has been published with the explicit objective to 'overcome inadequacies of extant codes'. The Code text is supplemented with 'A Declaration of Conflicts of Interest', with a view to be used by health and safety professionals.

The code text is structured into eight sections.

1 Purposes and goals.
2 Definitions.

3 Responsibilities.
4 Right to know.
5 Reports and declaration of conflict of interest.
6 Compliance programs.
7 Transparency policy.
8 Enforcement provisions.

The Code text is supplemented by a form containing a 'Declaration of Conflict of Interest' to be signed and used by the professionals concerned. In an appendix to the Code, instructions are given for the use of this 'Declaration of Conflict of Interest' by World Health Organization experts. In the published article presenting the Code[3] the American Industrial Hygiene Association *Code of Ethics for the Practice of Industrial Hygiene* is appended as Appendix II and the American College of Occupational and Environmental Medicine (ACOEM) *Code of Ethics* as Appendix III. The ICOH *International Code of Ethics* from 1997 is appended as Appendix IV.

The Code has a particular focus on conflicts of interest and requirements for transparency in seeking to identify loyalties leading to such conflicts. It encourages above-board dealings and disclosure of loyalties with the objective of making it possible to discuss openly potential or real biases inherent in such relationships. The Code thus requires a transparency policy for the organisations to which the occupational health service and safety professional belongs and also that a 'Declaration of Interests' be signed and reviewed on a regular basis. The enforcement provisions of the Code include a requirement for organisations adopting the Code to limit membership in their organisation to professionals who agree to abide by the provisions of the Code.

This Code bears a name with close resemblance to the *International Code of Ethics for Occupational Health Professionals* issued by the ICOH described earlier in this chapter. There is, in consequence, a possibility that they are mistakenly believed to be one and the same document. They are, however, separate documents, produced by two different organisations and resulting from differing processes.

General comments

A fundamental argument underlying the conception of this book lies in the view that all the moral obligations a responsible agent in occupational health care should recognise in a given situation are difficult to articulate in a formal set of rules. This applies both for rules issued by the state in forms of legislation and for codes of practice elaborated by non-governmental organisations, such as professional bodies or enterprises. Such instruments are of a general nature and there are, in consequence, limits to what they can achieve, taking into account all relevant considerations in a situation at hand. It is preferable to see such codes as simply guidance. If challenged, it must be open to occupational health professionals to argue their behaviour has had a morally defensible outcome even if the precise wording of any particular code has been breached.

One implication of this, speaking in principle, is that the codes may – in unquestioning implementation – rule out most reasonable practical solutions and also permit unfair or immoral practices. Rules with the nature of legislation in many countries usually have the strength endowed by the instrument of coercion or sanction controlled by the state. This sanction instrument is commonly kept in reserve for non-compliers. The limits of what can be achieved by enforcement of law and fiscal regulations are well known and need not be elaborated here. So, codes cannot replace the individual responsibility of occupational health professionals to decide on each case in the light of moral obligations, expectations of stakeholders and their own sets of professional values. Nevertheless, codes, and in particular professional codes, have their place. First, they are commonly more determinate and specific, in the sense of addressing situations at hand, than rules of legislation. Second, they are communicable in public and by means of professional networks. Third, they are open to public criticism and collective action within professional bodies; they can undergo changes or even radical revision if needed. See, for example, the work of Griffiths and Lucas from 1996.[4]

The bottom line is, however, that professional codes, including codes of ethics, represent the crystallised conceptions of what is to be seen as good professional practice at a particular point in time. Professional codes provide strong incentives for compliance, in particular when they have been internalised by members in an active communication process or where the punishment for non-compliance is severe. In this perspective they can contribute to defining what considerations need to be brought into play in situations marked by complexity and ethical dilemmas. On this basis, codes may be helpful and even sometimes necessary as a moral compass – providing guidance and important reminders. In orienting health professionals in necessary choices in situations where sometimes fundamental convictions and values – which may reside in the subconscious mind – have to be brought to the surface, it therefore seems important to recognise that a set of principles, such as those provided by the National Commission for the Protection of Human Subjects,[5] the Appleton Consensus document,[6] and professional codes do not represent an articulation of one single ethical theory. They can, however, come close to this in presenting something that lies at the heart of a vast number of beliefs and policies.

References

1 Faculty of Occupational Medicine of the Royal Society of Medicine (1999) *Guidance on Ethics for Occupational Physicians* (5e). Royal Society of Medicine, London.

2 International Commission on Occupational Health (2002) *International Code of Ethics for Occupational Health Professionals 1992.* (Updated version of Code (2002) available (English and French languages) on ICOH website www.icoh.org.sg)

3 Ladou J, Tennenhouse DJ and Feitshans IL (2002) Codes of ethics (conduct) in occupational medicine. *State of the Art Reviews.* **17**: 559–85.

4 Griffiths JR and Lucas JR (1996) *Ethical Economics.* Macmillan Press Ltd, London.

5 National Commission for the Protection of Human Subjects of Biomedical and Behavioral Research (1978) *Belmont Report: ethical principles and guidelines for research involving human subjects.* US Government Printing Office, Washington.

6 The Appleton International Conference (1992) Developing guidelines for decisions to forgo life-prolonging medical treatment. *Journal of Medical Ethics.* **18**: Supplement (Guest editor: John M. Stanley).

CHAPTER 25

Concluding remarks

In essence, this book is based on descriptions of practical cases occurring in occupational health services practice. The cases presented represent model situations that constantly recur, in various contexts and forms, in occupational healthcare. They confront occupational health professionals with the challenges of making choices and acting in accordance with their fundamental professional values. The cases selected for this book do not, for obvious reasons, represent the full range of situations or difficulties that present themselves to occupational health services or the occupational health professionals in such services. The field of occupational health practice is broad in scope, and there are innumerable variants on complex tasks to perform and issues to resolve. Further, it should be remembered that the multidisciplinary activities of occupational health services involve health professionals of differing educational backgrounds (vocational or academic) and with varying professional experiences in the field.

The cases selected include coverage of the prevention of disease or injury caused by or related to work conditions, workplace health surveillance, risk assessments of workplace exposures, infectious diseases, workplace health intervention, rehabilitation, workplace management of alcohol abuse, drug testing in the workplace, genetic bio-monitoring, work capacity assessment, sickness absence surveillance and recognition of occupational disease as an issue in insurance medicine. Some selected issues in occupational health research – including those related to informed consent – are addressed in the book. One chapter introduces an employer or management perspective on professional ethics in occupational health, another a trade union view. Separate chapters deal with matters of education and training of occupational health professionals in ethics and the issues related to whistle-blowing and codes of ethics. We have chosen not to deal with professional ethics in relation to curative treatment in primary healthcare, often – in practice – provided by occupational health professionals.

When we first discussed the outline of this book, our inclination was to go for a set of case descriptions that would provide a framework within which many analogous cases might be discussed. By implication, this would provide an entry point for reflection over possible actions and application of the ethical values by which they might be underpinned. By means of analyses of cases, our principal aims were to improve insights into occupational health professional value systems, and show how these are mobilised as problems arise in day-to-day work.

Basic values

In analysis and the taking of a professional stance when ethical challenges arise at work, the two essential points of departure in arriving at a decision are to:

- assess the facts of the case
- consider the values involved.

Here, the facts refer to a range of information on the health of the people involved, their work conditions and other relevant contextual knowledge. They include available information on risk- or health-determining factors that are known well or reasonably well, and also knowledge that is not scientifically validated but still judged to be pertinent.

With regard to values, we have – for the purpose of structuring the case discussions – reduced them to the following set:

- beneficence (including non-maleficence)
- autonomy (i.e. the right to self-determination)
- justice (including equity).

First, we shall recall the basic ethical principles as stated in the Belmont Report (1978). In this report the three principles of respect for person, beneficence and justice are presented. With the birth of the Appleton Consensus Guidelines these principles were internationally accepted. In this document the ethical value criteria of beneficence, non-maleficence, autonomy and justice are used as value premises. They were included as fundamental elements in this consensus document, which was later to assume significant importance as a reference basis, both in academic discussions and in practical development of medical ethics. This document, first published in 1989, was originally a product of representatives of 10 countries, convened to draft a model set of guidelines aimed at implementation in medical ethics committees internationally. The document was designed specifically to address the issues of foregoing medical treatment, including life-prolonging treatment, precipitated by autonomous requests by patients or their surrogates and issues of foregoing medical treatment as a result of pressures caused by resource scarcity. It is thus noteworthy that the original intention of the consensus meeting in 1988 was aimed at quite specific issues, which were remotely, and only by implication, related to the practices of occupational health.

In the preamble to the international document entitled *Ethical Background*, the following consensus statement was agreed:

> In caring for patients, doctors and other healthcare professionals, as individuals and representatives of their professions, shall act with respect for human life and with integrity in providing medical treatment within certain norms of care and concern.

In the preamble of the Appleton Consensus Guidelines it was emphasised that these four principles do not comprise a single ethical theory. Indeed, they often conflict and require interpretation and balancing. The four principles are given different weights in different cultures, and some cultures would wish to add additional principles or values to be taken into account. There are also likely to be substantive disagreements within cultures on the weights of these four principles. It was also acknowledged that analyses of specific circumstances in individual cases might enhance the understanding of both ethical and cross-cultural perspectives, which are not directly derived from these four ethical principles. The Appleton Consensus document has been of significant importance in having had a notable impact on development of ethical thinking in biomedical sciences and practices in health professions.

We, the three editors, agreed at the outset to use the set of three principles in the examination of each of our cases and to reflect on their practical usability. Thus, all authors were presented with the task of confronting these three principles and offering an ethical analysis of a case (or cases) on the basis of them. For us all, this requirement was an obvious challenge. To condense a complex and multifaceted real-life situation in all its ethical aspects into a framework comprising these three value criteria is certainly no easy task. Thorough reflection was called for. But this proved not to be enough. In addition, a scrutiny of our own values and professional self-image became necessary. Our eventual conclusion, having examined all the cases presented to us, is that this triple value set remains a valid and useful tool in practical analyses of occupational healthcare situations.

Some of the authors in this book have used the three principles as a point of departure in their ethical analyses, others have not. Thus, different approaches have been adopted. We believe that such diversity of methods of ethical analysis will be of benefit to readers. The various methods well reflect what actually goes on in practical implementation of the principles of medical ethics. No single ethical theory is universally accepted for the practice of occupational health prevention and health promotion.

Universality

One issue to be reflected upon is the universality, or otherwise, of applications of the set of three value criteria mentioned above. Universality, in the present context, refers to principles or values that are not restricted to cultural, national or religious boundaries, but which in some sense are intercultural or international. A fundamental requirement of universality is the existence of a set of shared values or even agreements on moral norms that reflect a commonality of values. Both basic human needs and many social conditions, including work characteristics and work conditions, are globally shared, thus providing a basis for shared values in important regards. It is worthy of reminder that the World Commission for Culture and Development of the UNESCO, in a report entitled *Our Cultural Diversity* and edited for the UNESCO conference in Stockholm 1998, drew attention to many important perspectives that would underpin a new global ethics. This cross-cultural commission dismissed the claim that the United Nations Conventions on Human Rights are, in their conception, too Western, too liberal and too individualised. Instead, the Commission emphasised that moral convictions, such as to protect individual autonomy and to respect individual vulnerability, are generally applicable principles and an integral part of all major value systems. For the very idea and practice of the United Nations and the UNESCO, an ethical foundation in universality was seen as one of the core issues in this age of diversity.

Our contribution to this debate is, clearly, modest. It carries the limitations inherent in a small body of cases and in a group of authors recruited exclusively from affluent northern European countries. In terms of shared understanding, however, we found ourselves converging, with ease, in using the set of three ethical value criteria for examination of dilemmas drawn from the sphere of occupational health practice. Human rights are, obviously, a central source of inspiration in framing the ethical requirements. Pursuant to these rights every person, regardless of age, race or sex, must be treated with dignity – as an end and not only as a means. We recognise this as one solid foundation for professional ethics in the occupational health field. Important globally shared principles spring from this, such as human dignity, justice and beneficence as core values in professional health practice.

The role of occupational health professionals

The role of an occupational health professional – as a counsellor to primarily the employer or manager of an enterprise or other organisation, and also to other stakeholders and interested parties – has ethical implications. It should be recognised that the professional is an important agent in this capacity. The principal task of an employing organisation is to manage activities in such a way that the organisation survives even under conditions of sharp market competition, while securing healthy and safe work conditions for the people it employs. Any occupational health professional, in the same organisation, has the related and legitimate task – through use of professional experience and competence – of sustaining and improving the health of the labour force. This is aimed, as well as promoting health in its own right, at improvement of the productivity of companies in a broad sense. This double agenda may, however, lead to ethical dilemmas in that the occupational health professional is commonly expected to provide consulting services not only to the employer and the collective body of employed staff and their trade union representatives, but also to individual employees. For occupational health physicians, there is the added responsibility imposed by the fiduciary nature of the relationship between the physician and personnel as individual persons when curative primary care services are provided. And further, the tasks of occupational health physicians also include providing counselling services to outside bodies and organisations, such as social security agencies and insurance companies. For all occupational health professionals concerned with health and safety matters within an enterprise, the scope of their considerations may extend beyond company boundaries in situations where health hazards involving third party interests arise. Such parties include the general public, a specific community and society at large.

A multitude of stakeholders and the role of serving clients whose interests and aims are very different and sometimes incompatible set the stage for the operations of occupational health services and work of occupational health professionals. Balancing and resolving divergent interests and underlying values, while safeguarding professional integrity and independence, will remain one of the most difficult problems in applying professional ethics in occupational health service. There is no generally accepted theory for adjudicating between various interests when it comes to matters of occupational health practice. The hallmark of occupational health professionals lies in their ability to arrive at well-reflected, ethically founded solutions and decisions, which are then perceived as both fair and equitable.

Another critical issue is how far the occupational health professionals are to go towards meeting the increasingly dominating criterion of efficiency in organisations. At what point does compliance become incompatible with principles of professional medical ethics? Efficiency is a recognised determinant of competitiveness in a market situation, and is also increasingly promoted in public service organisations by many governments worldwide. For example, occupational health professionals may have to confront difficult ethical dilemmas arising from conflicts between stakeholder expectations during the downsizing and reshuffling of organisations.

The occupational health professional in a market setting

One feature of developments in the field of occupational health, and within the expert bodies referred to as occupational health services, is the establishment of private organisations providing similar services on market terms. This entails that occupational health services are subject to competition with other service providers. This trend is in line with that of private financing initiatives in public sector organisations, where the National Health Service (NHS) in the UK provides an obvious example. Adapting to an increasingly free-market economy implies that professional staff and the organisation itself have to make their living from salaries and service fees, respectively, that are set by the market. A market-based existence may give rise to ethical problems for occupational health professionals. Assuming that the first principle for ranking priorities is to allocate services according to the health needs of the populations they serve, occupational health professionals may have to confront situations where client demand is a more powerful determinant of allocation than client need. This gives rise to a dilemma in situations where demand does not correspond with an important health need of a client or in a client system. Providing services that are not based on the needs of a target population may amount to questionable practice as seen from the perspective of professional ethics.

Comprehensive responsibility of the occupational health professional

The ultimate role and proper conduct of occupational health professionals are clearly presented in professional codes of conduct, such as the *International Code of Ethics of Occupational Health Professionals* adopted by the International Commission on Occupational Health (ICOH). Such codes are commonly conceived and published by professional bodies. They aim at establishing a basic set of ethical norms of conduct for their members, and – in the case of occupational health specialists – also provide specific knowledge to clients and client enterprises. The core message of the codes lies in the explicit and clear reminder they give of the particular responsibilities of health professions in their service of humanity, in particular with regard to the protection of the health and dignity of the human labour force. In fact, the task of the health professional actually extends beyond this, so as to include – at the level of principle – involvement in matters related to the lives of citizens in society. Life at work in the modern world is hard to separate from, and is in many ways interconnected with, life outside work. The tasks of occupational health professionals go beyond making companies healthy and profitable. They include the aim of improving the 'world at work'.

In concluding, we see – both globally and in Europe in particular – growing indications of increasing attention being paid to ethical issues of life at work, with special regard to aspects of health and safety. It is a noteworthy observation that this has occurred in an era when the limits to human conduct set by traditional moral norms are perceived by many to have become increasingly ambiguous.

In our developed societies, where individualism is cultivated and an attitude of relativism to the ethical values of beneficence, autonomy and justice is adopted by many, the risk arises of ethical decisions in the occupational health arena being taken on the basis of proven scientific facts alone.

We are some of the many researchers and practitioners involved who find that the scientific, technical and social development of life at work leads us every day into situations that confront us with issues of considerable complexity from both a practical and an ethical perspective.

Accepting this as a point of departure implies a need to meet the challenge of opening up and organising meeting points for human beings to reflect on the implications of the way the world is developing, in particular with regard to conditions in the workplace.

For us an integral part of expert occupational health professional work is actively to participate in discourse, and to contribute to improving our ability to make well-reflected and well-judged decisions. In this regard, those representing occupational health science and those representing practical professional expertise in the field have a common value base in rationality. Professional ethical conduct in an occupational health and safety setting is, to a large extent, a matter of reasoned and reflected examination of the facts at hand and the ethical principles involved. Reflection and rationality of approach are to be seen as cornerstones of the ethos of occupational health professionals. Without this, many of us risk losing our identity and sense of direction. And this we need in a world at work subject to constant changes, innovations and new approaches. To this we may add the countless ramifications of globalisation affecting our lives at work.

It is difficult to finish a book like this. There is much more to say. There are aspects we have not even touched on. In the midst of this ongoing process of change, we are, however, obliged to leave you here.

So now goodbye. We have much work undone. We still have much to learn and, when we meet again, we will have much to discuss.

Peter Westerholm, Tore Nilstun and John Øvretveit
February 2004

Index